PROTEIN NUTRITIONAL QUALITY OF FOODS AND FEEDS

NUTRITION AND CLINICAL NUTRITION

A Series of Textbooks and Monographs

EDITOR

Robert E. Olson, M.D.

School of Medicine
Saint Louis University
Saint Louis, Missouri

Volume 1: PROTEIN NUTRITIONAL QUALITY OF FOODS AND FEEDS
(in two parts):

Part 1: Assay Methods—Biological, Biochemical, and Chemical

Part 2: Quality Factors—Plant Breeding, Composition, Processing, and Antinutrients

Edited by Mendel Friedman

Additional Volumes in Preparation

PROTEIN NUTRITIONAL QUALITY OF FOODS AND FEEDS

PART 2
Quality Factors—Plant Breeding, Composition, Processing, and Antinutrients

Edited by

MENDEL FRIEDMAN

Western Regional Research Laboratory
Agricultural Research Service
U.S. Department of Agriculture
Berkeley, California

MARCEL DEKKER, INC.   New York

PROTEIN NUTRITIONAL QUALITY OF FOODS AND FEEDS
Part 2: Quality Factors--Plant Breeding,
Composition, Processing, and Antinutrients

Proceedings of the American Chemical Society Symposium
on Chemical and Biological Methods for Protein Quality Evaluation
held in Atlantic City, New Jersey, September 9-11, 1974,
with supplemental invited contributions.

MARCEL DEKKER, INC.

270 Madison Avenue, New York, New York 10016

LIBRARY OF CONGRESS CATALOG CARD NUMBER: 74-33549
ISBN: 0-8247-6282-7

Current printing (last digit):
10 9 8 7 6 5 4 3 2 1

PRINTED IN THE UNITED STATES OF AMERICA

CONTRIBUTORS TO PART 2

MARVIN R. ALVAREZ, Department of Pathology, College of Medicine, University of Florida, Gainesville, Florida

MARY E. AMBROSE, Southeast Utilization Research Center, National Marine Fisheries Service, NOAA, U.S. Department of Commerce, College Park, Maryland

D. BALLESTER, Departmento de Nutricion y Tecnologia de los Alimentos, Universidad de Chile, Santiago, Chile

G. H. BEATON, Department of Nutrition and Food Science, Faculty of Medicine, University of Toronto, Toronto, Canada

ROBERT BECKER, Western Regional Research Laboratory, Agricultural Research Service, U.S. Department of Agriculture, Berkeley, California

J. G. BERGAN, Departments of Food and Nutritional Science and Food and Resource Chemistry, University of Rhode Island, Kingston, Rhode Island

E. M. BICKOFF, Western Regional Research Laboratory, Agricultural Research Service, U.S. Department of Agriculture, Berkeley, California

A. N. BOOTH, Western Regional Research Laboratory, Agricultural Research Service, U.S. Department of Agriculture, Berkeley, California

H. G. BOTTING, Foods and Nutrition Division, Health Protection Branch, Health and Welfare Canada, Ottawa, Ontario, Canada

G. A. BRODERICK, Department of Animal Science, Texas A&M University, Texas Agricultural Experimental Station, College Station, Texas

iii

HORACE K. BURR, Western Regional Research Laboratory, Agricultural Research Service, U.S. Department of Agriculture, Berkeley, California

C. O. CHICHESTER, Department of Food and Resource Chemistry, University of Rhode Island, Kingston, Rhode Island

JIMMY H. CLARK, Department of Dairy Science, University of Illinois, Urbana, Illinois

D. DE FREMERY, Western Regional Research Laboratory, Agricultural Research Service, U.S. Department of Agriculture, Berkeley, California

R. H. EDWARDS, Western Regional Research Laboratory, Agricultural Research Service, U.S. Department of Agriculture, Berkeley, California

R. E. FERREL, Western Regional Research Laboratory, Agricultural Research Service, U.S. Department of Agriculture, Berkeley, California

ELISABETH FORSUM, Institute of Nutrition, University of Uppsala, Uppsala, Sweden

MICHAEL R. GUMBMANN, Western Regional Research Laboratory, Agricultural Research Service, U.S. Department of Agriculture, Berkeley, California

L. P. HANSEN, Western Regional Research Laboratory, Agricultural Research Service, U.S. Department of Agriculture, Berkeley, California

MURIEL L. HAPPICH, Eastern Regional Research Center, Agricultural Research Service, U.S. Department of Agriculture, Philadelphia, Pennsylvania

DANIEL T. HOPKINS, Ralston Purina Company, St. Louis, Missouri

P. H. JOHNSTON, Western Regional Research Laboratory, Agricultural Research Service, U.S. Department of Agriculture, Berkeley, California

CONTRIBUTORS TO PART 2

DONALD D. KASARDA, Western Regional Research Laboratory, Agricultural Research Service, U.S. Department of Agriculture, Berkeley, California

B. M. KENNEDY, Department of Nutritional Sciences, University of California, Berkeley, California

J. E. KNIPFEL, Research Station, Research Branch, Agriculture Canada, Swift Current, Saskatchewan, Canada

B. E. KNUCKLES, Western Regional Research Laboratory, Agricultural Research Service, U.S. Department of Agriculture, Berkeley, California

G. O. KOHLER, Western Regional Research Laboratory, Agricultural Research Service, U.S. Department of Agriculture, Berkeley, California

RALPH H. KURTZMAN, Western Regional Research Laboratory, Agricultural Research Service, U.S. Department of Agriculture, Berkeley, California

TUNG-CHING LEE, Department of Food and Resource Chemistry, University of Rhode Island, Kingston, Rhode Island

IRVIN E. LIENER, Department of Biochemistry, College of Biological Sciences, University of Minnesota, St. Paul, Minnesota

B. S. LUH, Department of Food Science and Technology and Department of Nutrition, University of California, Davis, California

J. M. McLAUGHLAN, Foods and Nutrition Division, Health Protection Branch, Health and Welfare Canada, Ottawa, Ontario, Canada

SAIPIN MANEEPUN, Department of Food Science and Technology and Department of Nutrition, University of California, Davis, California

P. MARKAKIS, Department of Food Science and Human Nutrition, Michigan State University, East Lansing, Michigan

WILDA H. MARTINEZ, Southern Regional Research Center, Agricultural Research Service, U.S. Department of Agriculture, New Orleans, Louisiana

EDWIN T. MERTZ, Department of Biochemistry, Purdue University, West Lafayette, Indiana

JACKSON C. MIERS, Western Regional Research Laboratory, Agricultural Research Service, U.S. Department of Agriculture, Berkeley, California

R. E. MILLER, Western Regional Research Laboratory, Agricultural Research Service, U.S. Department of Agriculture, Berkeley, California

F. MONCKEBERG, Departmento de Nutricion y Tecnologia de los Alimentos, Universidad de Chile, Santiago, Chile

ALFRED C. OLSON, Western Regional Research Laboratory, Agricultural Research Service, U.S. Department of Agriculture, Berkeley, California

S. J. PINTAURO, Departments of Food and Nutritional Science and Food and Resource Chemistry, University of Rhode Island, Kingston, Rhode Island

N. W. PIRIE, Rothamsted Experimental Station, Harpenden, Hertfordshire, England

Y. POMERANZ, U.S. Grain Marketing Research Center, Agricultural Research Service, U.S. Department of Agriculture, Manhattan, Kansas

JON REYNIERS, Department of Pathology, College of Medicine, University of Florida, Gainesville, Florida

R. B. RUCKER, Department of Food Science and Technology and Department of Nutrition, University of California, Davis, California

R. M. SAUNDERS, Western Regional Research Laboratory, Agricultural Research Service, U.S. Department of Agriculture, Berkeley, California

S. SCHWIMMER, Western Regional Research Laboratory, Agricultural Research Service, U.S. Department of Agriculture, Berkeley, California

DENNIS D. SHORT, Department of Pathology, College of Medicine, University of Florida, Gainesville, Florida

VIRGINIA D. SIDWELL, Southeast Utilization Research Center, National Marine Fisheries Service, NOAA, U.S. Department of Commerce, College Park, Maryland

S. O. S. THOMKE, Department of Animal Husbandry, Agricultural University, Uppsala, Sweden

JOSEPH R. WAGNER, Western Regional Research Laboratory, Agricultural Research Service, U.S. Department of Agriculture, Berkeley, California

BIRGIT WIDSTRÖMER, Department of Animal Husbandry, Agricultural University, Uppsala, Sweden

J. CARROLL WOODARD, Department of Pathology, College of Medicine, University of Florida, Gainesville, Florida

E. YANEZ, Departmento de Nutricion y Tecnologia de los Alimentos, Universidad de Chile, Santiago, Chile

K-T. YUANN, Departments of Food and Nutritional Science and Food and Resource Chemistry, University of Rhode Island, Kingston, Rhode Island

PREFACE

The nutritive value, food value, or protein quality of a food
protein depends not only on its content of amino acids but also on
their physiological availability. Protein is a dietary essential.
We think we know the general requirements--different for different
animals--namely, adequate amounts of certain essential amino acids
with a reasonable balance among all. However, availability varies
with the protein source, processing treatments (especially heating),
and interaction with other diet components. Availability also
depends on the condition of the animal. Limitations of protein
supplies make the hunt for new protein sources and their quality
evaluation urgent. The need for reliable protein quality determination is further emphasized by new Food and Drug Administration
requirements for nutritional labeling. For all these reasons, it
is imperative that chemical analyses be critically compared with
animal and human feeding studies.

Scientists from many disciplines--physicians, biochemists,
physiologists, pharmacologists, pharmacists, nutritionists (both
general and clinical), animal scientists including veterinarians,
and food scientists including food technologists, dieticians, and
home economists--in fact, anyone seriously interested in nutrition--
all need reliable measures of protein quality. Because the subject
matter is so broad and encompasses so many disciplines, when I
organized this Symposium on Chemical and Biological Methods for Protein Quality Determination, I sought participants with the broadest
possible range of interests. Thirty-five, including six from abroad,
accepted this invitation. To supplement the verbal presentation, the
Proceedings include several closely related, invited contributions.
The papers are being published in two parts under the general title

PREFACE

PROTEIN NUTRITIONAL QUALITY OF FOODS AND FEEDS with the following subtitles: Part 1--Assay Methods--Biological, Biochemical, Chemical; Part 2--Quality Factors--Plant Breeding, Composition, Processing, and Antinutrients. The two parts are intended to be complementary as much as possible but their interests necessarily overlap.

The first part encompasses chemical and physical assay methods for amino acids, especially for essential amino acids, e.g., available and unavailable lysine, tryptophan, and methionine; biological tests, including human, animal, microbiological, and biochemical assays; feeding tests and test methods for protein quality; and methods for estimating the available energy of amino acids and proteins.

Nutritive evaluation of specific proteins, protein-containing foods and feeds, effects of processing on protein quality, "anti-nutritional factors," the nutritional quality of protected amino acids and proteins for ruminants, the use of enzymes to improve protein-containing foods, and the utility of protein:energy ratios as guidelines for assessing protein nutritional quality are the main subjects of the second part.

I want to record some considerations supporting the diversity of subject matter and of the contributors' backgrounds and interests represented in these volumes. I believe that the widest possible interaction of viewpoints and expertise is needed to transcend present limitations as expeditiously as possible. Scientists from related disciplines need one another's results and improved methods; results with different animals, including human beings, need to be compared; people responsible for practical application need to share experiences and problems with researchers. These volumes bring together elements needed for such interactions. The range of material includes a great variety of specific and general interests. This should interest at least a similar range of readers, but we challenge them to look also at the articles beyond their primary interest. We hope and expect everyone to profit by a broader overview.

I am particularly grateful to Wilda Martinez, Chairman of the Protein Subdivision of the Division of Agricultural and Food Chemistry of the American Chemical Society, who invited me to organize

PREFACE

this Symposium, to all contributors and participants for a well realized meeting of minds, to Carol J. Snow and Margaret M. Goss for typing the final draft of the manuscript and for editorial assistance, and to Dr. Wilfred H. Ward for valuable contributions to the preparation of these books. I also take great pleasure in thanking my son, Alan D. Friedman, for his help in alphabetizing thousands of index cards for the author and subject indices.

I am very hopeful that PROTEIN NUTRITIONAL QUALITY OF FOODS AND FEEDS will be a valuable record and resource for further progress to better human condition. If it is, the effort will be most worthwhile.

The ideas expressed are those of various authors, and are not necessarily approved or rejected by any agency of the United States Government. No official recommendation concerning the subject matter or products discussed is implied in this book.

Mendel Friedman

The eyes of all look to you expectantly, and you give them their food when it is due. You give it openhandedly, feeding every creature to its heart's content.

Psalm 145:15-16

CONTENTS OF PART 2

CONTENTS OF PART 2

CONTENTS OF PART 2

CONTENTS OF PART 1

CONTENTS OF PART 1

CONTENTS OF PART 1

CONTENTS OF PART 1

BREEDING FOR IMPROVED NUTRITIONAL VALUE IN CEREALS

Edwin T. Mertz

Department of Biochemistry
Purdue University
West Lafayette, Indiana

Cereal proteins are inferior nutritionally to the proteins in milk, meat, and eggs because of inadequate levels of the amino acid lysine. With the discovery ten years ago by Mertz et al. (1964) that the maize mutant *opaque-2* had nearly twice as much lysine as ordinary maize, scientists realized that cereal grain proteins could be improved in quality by genetic manipulation. The recent discovery of high lysine mutants of barley and sorghum raises the hope that all cereals can be improved in protein quality. If we assume that the FAO (1973) pattern of 5.2% lysine is the ideal level of lysine for the infant, high lysine maize and barley approach or equal this ideal, oats has approximately 73%, rice 71%, high lysine sorghum 63%, normal maize, barley, and wheat 50%, and normal sorghum and millet 35% of this level. Triticale, an artificial genus synthesized by combining the genomes of wheat and rye, has a substantially higher level of lysine per unit of protein than wheat. Other high lysine wide crosses between cereals are possible in the future. As the plant breeder selects for better cereal grains, it is necessary that the chemist carefully monitor the seeds used in the breeding program to insure that the level and quality of protein is maintained.

INTRODUCTION

All agricultural scientists agree that more efficient use of the earth's land resources is required if world food production is to keep pace with world population. One way to use the land more efficiently is to replace present cereal grains with grains of higher protein quality. The use of a high-quality protein cereal such as *opaque-2* maize (Mertz et al., 1964) in the diet of humans provides protein previously available only from a good mixture of normal cereals and legumes, or from meat, milk, and eggs. The latter three require much larger areas of land per calorie of food, and legumes are usually lower yielding than the cereal grains.

If we assume that the FAO (1973) pattern of 5.2% lysine is the ideal level of lysine for the infant, it is possible to compare the lysine content of common cereals and selected high lysine mutants. This comparison is shown in Table 1, based on data that we obtained in our laboratory. In Table 1, the protein levels of the various cereals are shown in column 3, and the percent of the ideal FAO level is shown in column 4. On the basis of these data, the best of the cereal grains, oats, has about 73% of the ideal level, and the poorest of the grains, sorghum and millet, 36% of the ideal level. The sample of high lysine barley that we analyzed contained 5.6% lysine, which is an excellent level. Normal maize contains 52%, whereas *opaque-2* maize, as currently produced in Mexico, contains 87-90% of the ideal level. Sorghum contains only 35% of the ideal level, but high lysine sorghum contains nearly double this amount (63% of the ideal level). The data in Table 1 indicate that wheat contains about 57% and current varieties of rice 71% of the ideal level of lysine.

It is obvious from the data in Table 1 that the plant breeder, by appropriate manipulation of the gene pools, can increase the lysine content of several cereals to a level which approaches that found in meat, milk, and eggs.

CEREAL BREEDING FOR IMPROVED NUTRITION

TABLE 1

Lysine Content of Cereals
and Selected High Lysine Mutants

Cereal grain	Protein %	Lysine g/100 g protein	% of ideal level
Maize 4858[a]	10.5	2.7	52
Maize 4855, high lysine[a]	10.9	4.5	87
Maize 4856, high lysine[a]	10.1	4.7	90
Sorghum, normal[b]	13.1	1.8	35
Sorghum, high lysine[b]	18.5	3.3	63
Barley, normal[c]	19.8	3.3	63
Barley, high lysine[c]	19.4	5.6	108
Rice BB, normal[d]	6.9	3.7	71
Rice BP1761, high protein[d]	15.4	3.4	65
Wheat, Genesee, normal[e]	12.1	3.0	58
Wheat, Purdue 4930, high protein[e]	17.3	2.9	56
Oats, Noble, normal[f]	18.9	3.8	73
Millet[g]	14.5	1.9	36

[a]4858: CIMMYT normal yellow flint synthetic. 4855: CIMMYT yellow hard endosperm *opaque-2* synthetic. 4856: CIMMYT yellow soft endosperm *opaque-2* synthetic. From CIMMYT, Mexico City.

[b]Normal sorghum kernels. High lysine sorghum: high lysine (hl hl hl) kernels from F_2 segregating heads derived from crosses between "normal" (low lysine) plants and the high lysine sorghum line IS 11758.

[c]Normal barley: Bomi barley variety. High lysine mutant: mutant 1508 from Risø, Denmark.

[d]Normal rice: Blue Bonnet variety. High protein rice: BP1 761 from IRRI.

[e]Normal wheat: Genesee, variety of New York soft wheat. High protein wheat: Purdue 4930-A6-28-2-1.

[f]Normal oats: Noble, a Wisconsin variety.

[g]Millet: Finger millet, variety from Uganda supplied by Dr. S. A. Eberhart, Iowa State University, Ames, Iowa.

EXPERIMENTAL PROCEDURE

The cereal chemist is especially interested in knowing more about the chemical changes which occur in the proteins to bring about these increases in lysine. In order to learn more about the nature of these changes, we fractionated the endosperm proteins in the various cereal samples by the Landry-Moureaux method (1970). This method is outlined in Table 2.

TABLE 2

Landry-Moureaux Fractionation Sequence D

Fraction	Solvent[a]	Time of agitation min	Protein fractions
I	NaCl 0.5 M (4°C)	60	Albumins
		30	Globulins
		30	
		15	
	Water	15	
II	Isopropanol 70% (v/v) (20°C)	30	
		30	Zein
		30	
III	[Isopropanol 70% (v/v)	30	
	+ 2-ME 0.6% (v/v)] (20°C)	30	Zein-like
IV	[Borate buffer pH 10	60	
	+ 2-ME 0.6% (v/v)] (20°C)	30	Glutelin-like
V	[Borate buffer pH 10	60	
	+ 2-ME 0.6% (v/v)	30	Glutelin
	+ SDS 0.5% (w/v)]	15	Residue

[a]2-ME: 2-mercaptoethanol. Borate buffer: borate, NaOH, NaCl μ 0.5. SDS: sodium dodecylsulphate.

CEREAL BREEDING FOR IMPROVED NUTRITION

RESULTS

Table 3 shows the results of fractionating the endosperm proteins in the isogenic mutants *opaque-2*, *floury-2*, the double mutant of *opaque-2* and *floury-2*, *brittle-2*, and the double mutant of *opaque-2* and *brittle-2* in the Ohio 43 background (Misra et al., 1975). Results are also shown for the fractionation of the high lysine mutant *opaque-7* and the double mutant of *opaque-2* and *opaque-7* in the W22 background (Misra et al., 1975). These data show that the introduction of the *opaque-2*, *floury-2*, *brittle-2*, or *opaque-7* genes into a normal background increases the level of saline-soluble proteins, decreases the level of zein, and increases the level of glutelin (Fraction V). Since the saline fraction (Fraction I) and Fraction V contain about 6 grams of lysine per 100 grams of protein, and Fraction II, zein, contains about 0.1% lysine, it is obvious that these changes will increase the lysine content of the mutant endosperms. It can also be noted that the double mutants, *floury-2/opaque-2* and *opaque-7/opaque-2*, show changes which resemble the changes observed with *opaque-2* without giving an effect on lysine higher than that observed with *opaque-2* alone. In contrast, the double mutant *brittle-2/opaque-2* shows substantially higher increases in saline-soluble and glutelin levels and an almost complete disappearance of the zein fraction. Here one observes an additive effect of the *opaque-2* and *brittle-2* genes to give a product with substantially higher levels of lysine than are found in either *opaque-2* or *brittle-2* alone.

We have extended these studies to include *sugary-1*, *shrunken-1*, *shrunken-2*, *shrunken-4*, and *brittle-1*, and the double mutants of these single mutants with *opaque-2*. These data are shown in Tables 4 and 5. The changes in fractions I, II, and V are similar to those observed with *brittle-2* (see Table 4). However, the levels of lysine in the double mutants (Table 5) are much higher than those observed in the single mutants and resemble the levels found in the double mutant of *opaque-2* and *brittle-2*.

TABLE 3

Nitrogen Distribution in Maize Endosperm[a]

Fraction	Inbred:	Ohio 43						W22		
	Genotype:	+	o-2	fl-2	fl-2/o-2	bt-2	bt-2/o-2	+	o-7	o-7/o-2
I (saline)		5.8	13.6	9.2	17.0	12.1	22.3	6.9	16.6	17.6
II (zein)		59.0	26.9	49.1	25.0	26.1	2.9	40.6	20.3	8.7
III (zein-like)		5.8	8.4	9.0	15.2	15.4	5.5	15.3	12.0	15.1
IV (glutelin-like)		12.7	14.0	7.6	9.9	8.7	12.2	12.8	18.8	21.3
V (glutelin)		13.8	29.2	22.0	24.8	27.9	48.0	21.0	29.5	33.3
Total N extracted		97.1	92.1	96.7	91.9	90.2	90.9	96.6	97.2	96.0
Lysine (g/100 g protein)		1.6	3.5	2.7	2.7	3.3	5.3	2.3	3.8	3.5

[a]Percent of total nitrogen.

TABLE 4

Nitrogen Distribution in *Opaque-2* and Several Non-Floury Endosperm Mutants[a]

Fraction	Endosperm genotype:	+	o-2	su-1	sh-1	sh-2	sh-4	bt-1	bt-2
I		5.8	13.6	11.9	8.2	12.3	25.7	8.8	12.1
II		59.0	26.9	27.1	43.7	29.4	30.8	36.0	26.1
III		5.8	8.4	21.9	12.3	9.4	7.7	16.4	15.4
IV		12.7	14.0	9.1	14.4	15.0	8.3	8.3	8.7
V		13.8	29.2	22.8	16.3	23.6	23.6	27.4	27.9
Total N extracted		97.1	92.1	92.8	94.9	89.8	96.1	96.9	90.2
Lysine (% of total protein)		1.6	3.5	1.8	1.9	2.7	3.0	2.3	3.3
Tryptophan (% of total protein)		0.3	0.8	0.3	0.6	0.7	0.8	0.5	0.7

[a]Percent of total nitrogen in endosperm.

TABLE 5

Nitrogen Distribution in Endosperm of Double Combination Mutants of Maize[a]

Fraction	Endosperm genotype:	su-1 /o-2	sh-1 /o-2	sh-2 /o-2	sh-4 /o-2	bt-1 /o-2	bt-2 /o-2
I		22.7	39.9	25.3	43.3	23.3	22.3
II		3.0	1.8	1.2	6.5	2.7	2.9
III		9.0	1.6	1.1	3.9	2.5	5.5
IV		14.2	16.4	26.1	8.7	13.1	12.2
V		45.3	32.2	35.4	26.8	50.2	48.0
Total N extracted		94.2	91.9	89.1	89.2	91.8	90.9
Lysine (% of total protein)		3.9	4.8	4.2	4.0	4.8	5.3
Tryptophan (% of total protein)		0.8	1.2	1.2	1.2	1.4	1.3

[a]Percent of total nitrogen.

8

CEREAL BREEDING FOR IMPROVED NUTRITION

Studies with the developing endosperms of the double mutant *opaque-2/brittle-2* indicate that at no time during development, from 14 days post-pollination on, is there any evidence that zein is being produced (P.S. Misra, E.T. Mertz, and D.V. Glover, in press). This has been confirmed with acrylamide gel electrophoresis which shows the complete lack of the two normal components of the zein fraction, one with a molecular weight of approximately 24,000 and the other with a molecular weight of approximately 22,000 (P.S. Misra, E.T. Mertz, and D.V. Glover, unpublished data).

Table 6 shows the results of fractionating normal and high lysine sorghum (Singh and Axtell, 1973). Here again, one observes in the high lysine sorghum an increase in Fraction I, a decrease in Fraction II, and an increase in Fraction V.

The Landry-Moureaux fractionation of high lysine mutant barley number 1508 (Ingversen et al., 1973) also shows an increase in the saline-soluble fraction, a decrease in the prolamine, hordein, and an increase in the glutelin fraction (Table 7).

It is obvious from these data that the maize, sorghum, and barley high lysine selections all have shown similar changes in the protein patterns, and it is the change in the protein pattern rather than the development of any new proteins that is primarily responsible for the increase of the lysine content of the grain.

TABLE 6

Protein Distribution in High Lysine Sorghum[a]

Sorghum	Fraction I	Fraction II	Fraction III	Fraction IV	Fraction V
Normal	15.3	26.4	26.5	4.3	22.5
High lysine	22.4	13.7	20.2	4.3	33.5

[a]High lysine values average of assays from 5 segregating heads using high lysine (hl hl hl) kernels from F_2 heads derived from crosses between normal plants and high lysine sorghum line IS 11758. Lysine content of normal sorghum: 1.8 g/100 g protein; lysine content of high lysine sorghum: 3.3 g/100 g protein.

TABLE 7

Protein Distribution in High Lysine Barley[a]

Samples	Albumin/Globulin		Prolamine		Glutelin		Lysine	
	Mutant	Normal	Mutant	Normal	Mutant	Normal	Mutant	Normal
Ingversen	46	27	9	39	39	39	7.0	4.7
Mertz	46	27	3	33	32	28	5.7	3.3

[a]Percent of the total nitrogen in fractions. Purdue values based on Landry-Moureaux fractions: albumin/globulin = Fraction I, prolamine = Fractions II + III, and glutelin = Fractions IV + V. Bomi barley (normal) and mutant 1508 kindly supplied by H.W. Ohm, Purdue University. The former contained 18.5% protein, the latter 19.8%. Ingversen's samples contained 10.2 and 10.1%, respectively.

One exception to these findings has been observed; the high lysine mutant barley, Hiproly, must be produced by a different set of genetic events. In this case, there is no drop in the level of prolamine, but there are marked increases in several high lysine-containing proteins in the saline-soluble fraction (Munck, 1972).

In those high lysine types where there is a marked reduction in prolamine, it has been observed that there is also a floury or soft type of endosperm. It is possible, however, by selective breeding to select for hard endosperm at the same time that one is selecting for high lysine. A successful opaque-2 hard synthetic type has been developed by the International Maize and Wheat Improvement Center, Mexico City (CIMMYT). It is theoretically possible that one could also breed for hard endosperm types of high lysine sorghum and high lysine barley.

With the advent of hard endosperm types of high lysine cereals, the cereal is difficult to distinguish by physical means from its normal counterpart. We recently developed a rapid test for high lysine mutants based on the unusually high levels of free amino acids found in high lysine mutants. The test reagent is ninhydrin (Mertz et al., 1974) which gives a much stronger reaction with high lysine maize, sorghum, and barley samples than with the normal counterparts. The ninhydrin screening test should be useful in the marketplace to identify high lysine types of cereals and in the research laboratory as a screening tool to search for other high lysine types based on a reduction in prolamines in the endosperm.

It is my opinion that breeding for improved nutritional value in cereals has a bright future. A search should be made for the *opaque-2* type of mutant in all economically important cereal grains. There is a good possibility that such types exist in millets and that they could also exist in wheat. Another promising approach is the use of wide crosses between cereal grains to add the genes of the high lysine maize, barley, and sorghum types to cereal grains in which high lysine types have not been found to date. For example, a wide cross between high lysine barley and wheat would certainly improve the lysine content and raise it to a level intermediate between that of wheat (3%) and high lysine barley (5%). It has been reported that such a wide cross has been achieved recently (Bates et al., 1974). A successful wide cross immediately available for exploitation is triticale, an artificial genus synthesized by combining the genomes of wheat (genus *triticum*) and rye (genus *secale*). The lysine level per unit of protein in this wide cross is higher than that in wheat (Hulse and Laing, 1974).

The major factor which is slowing down acceptance of high lysine cereals for human diets is the yield reduction of 10-15% encountered with these mutants when compared with their normal counterparts. Plant breeders are working to eliminate these yield differences. In the meantime, however, government agencies in the developing countries should encourage farmers to cultivate these cereals as a specialty crop for babies, preadolescent children, and pregnant mothers, by absorbing the 10-15% extra cost of production. The cost of supplying the high quality protein of these cereal mutants to children and pregnant mothers would be far less than supplying an equivalent amount of protein from meat, milk, or eggs, all of which are in extremely short supply in the developing countries.

ACKNOWLEDGMENT

This work was supported by the Agency for International Development under contract "Inheritance and Improvement of Protein Quality and Content in Maize."

REFERENCES

Bates, L.S., A.V. Campos, R. Rodriguiz and R.G. Anderson. 1974. Progress towards novel cereal grains. Cereal Sci. Today 19:1283.

FAO Nutritional Meetings Report Series No. 52. WHO Technical Report Series No. 522. 1973. Energy and protein requirements. Rome, Italy.

Hulse, J.H. and E.M. Laing. 1974. Nutritive value of triticale protein. IDRC Publication 021E, International Development Research Center, Ottawa, Canada.

Ingversen, J., B. Koie and H. Doll. 1973. Induced seed protein mutant of barley. Experimentia 29:1151.

Landry, J. and T. Moureaux. 1970. Hétérogénéité des glutélines du grain de mais: extraction sélective et composition en acides aminés des trois fractions isolées. Bull. Soc. Chim. Biol. 52:1021.

Mertz, E.T., L.S. Bates and O.E. Nelson. 1964. Mutant gene that changes protein composition and increases lysine content of maize endosperm. Science 145:279.

Mertz, E.T., P.S. Misra and R. Jambunathan. 1974. Rapid ninhydrin color test for screening high lysine mutants of maize, sorghum barley and other cereal grains. Cereal Chem. 51:304.

Misra, P.S., E.T. Mertz and D.V. Glover. 1975. Studies on corn proteins. VI. Endosperm protein changes in single and double endosperm mutants of maize. Cereal Chem. 52:161.

Misra, P.S., E.T. Mertz and D.V. Glover. Studies on corn proteins. VII. Developmental changes in endosperm proteins of high lysine mutants. Cereal Chem. (In press).

Munck, L. 1972. Improvement of nutritional value in cereals. Hereditas 72:1.

Singh, R. and J.D. Axtell. 1973. High lysine mutant gene (hl) that improves protein quality and biological value of grain sorghum. Crop Sci. 13:535.

PROTEINS AND AMINO ACIDS OF BARLEY, OATS, AND BUCKWHEAT

Y. Pomeranz

U.S. Grain Marketing Research Center
Agricultural Research Service
U.S. Department of Agriculture
Manhattan, Kansas

INTRODUCTION

Most discussions on the nutritive value of cereal proteins center around the major crops: wheat, corn, and rice. This is justly so, since these crops comprise more than 75% of the world production of cereal grains (Pomeranz and MacMasters, 1970). However, there is also justification for learning about the proteins of the minor cereal crops. They are well adapted to, and grown in, many areas of the world; they are rich in proteins (oats), or the amino acid composition is better balanced (oats and buckwheat) than in the major cereals, or they are uniquely suited (isogenic lines of barleys) for studies of factors and mechanisms which govern the biosynthesis, contents, composition, and nutritive value of cereal proteins.

This chapter updates a brief review on proteins in barley, oats, and buckwheat published recently (Pomeranz, 1973). The studies which are reviewed concerned cultivars and selections (including promising lines rich in both protein and lysine), distribution of proteins and amino acids in grain tissues, and changes that occur during maturation and malting. Results of surveys on amino acids in barleys, oats, and buckwheat were used to compare the amino acid balance in cereal grains, buckwheat, and peas.

GENERAL

Quantitatively starch is by far the most important food reserve material in cereal grains. Consequently, it has been argued (Carpenter, 1970) that cereal grains should be regarded primarily as sources of metabolizable energy rather than as sources of protein. However, as pointed out by Thielebein (1969), cereals provide 80 million tons of protein--about one half of the annual human requirement. The cereal proteins have a relatively low biological value. Consequently, even a small increase in the amount of protein or improvement in the biological value of that protein could make an important contribution to solving the worldwide problem of protein malnutrition.

According to Miller (1958), the average protein content of corn is only 10.4%; barley and oats average over 13% (Table 1). These data, for barley and oats, are much higher than the data given in Table 2 for protein in grain grown in England (Whitehouse, 1973).

TABLE 1

Protein Percentages in Commercial Lots of Cereal Grains[a]

Cereal	Protein percentage (air-dry basis)		No. of samples
	Mean	Range	
Barley	13.1	8.5-21.2	1,400
Corn	10.4	7.5-16.9	1,873
Oats	13.3	7.4-23.2	1,850
Rye	13.4	9.0-18.2	112
Sorghum	12.5	8.7-16.8	1,160
Wheat	12.0	8.1-18.5	309

[a]From Miller (1958).

TABLE 2

World Production of Cereal Grain and Cereal Protein (kg x 10^9)[a]

Item	Wheat	Barley	Oats	Rye	Maize	Sorghum and millet	Paddy rice	All grain crops
Grain[b]	333	131	54	33	251	85	284	1180
Protein (% of fresh weight)[c]	12	10	10.5	12.5	10	11	8	10.2
Protein	40	13	6	4	25	9	23	120

[a]From Whitehouse (1973).

[b]Food and Agriculture Organization, United Nations (1969).

[c]Adapted from Kent (1966).

No reliable statistical data are available on world production and average protein content of buckwheat.

The protein efficiency ratios (PER) for cereal proteins vary with the crop (Table 3). Buckwheat proteins have a very high PER value; the PER of oat proteins is higher than the PER of all regular cereal grains; the PER of barley is somewhat higher than the PER of regular corn, wheat, and sorghum (Frey, 1973). The PERs of the

TABLE 3

PER of Cereal Proteins in Diets of Rats[a]

Protein source	Protein percentage in ration			
	7.5	9.5	9.0-10.0	8.0-10.0
Barley	1.7	--	1.6	2.0
Corn	1.6	--	1.4	--
Oats	2.1	2.5	1.8	2.2
Rye	2.2	1.8	1.3	--
Sorghum	--	--	0.7	--
Wheat	1.4	1.7	0.9	1.7

[a]From Frey (1973).

proteins from different cereals seem to be related to the proportion of the alcohol-soluble prolamine fraction which is very low in lysine, the first limiting amino acid in practically all cereal grains (see also discussion under Scoring Procedures). Percentages of prolamine fractions in proteins of various cereal grains are shown in Table 4 (Mosse, 1966).

Up to 80% of the protein in the cereal grain is stored in the endosperm. The embryo proteins are rich in albumins and globulins and have a relatively balanced amino acid composition. The endosperm proteins are rich in prolamines and glutelins. The glutelins contain slightly more lysine than the prolamines. Increasing the protein content of cereals by cultural practices increases primarily the prolamine fraction and thus lowers biological value.

Proportions of amino acids, required by fast-growing chicks, in proteins of six grain crops are given in Table 5 (from Whitehouse, 1973). The data in Table 5 on net protein utilization by rats indicate that oats and barley are comparable and that both are lower than rice. Table 6 summarizes data, from several sources, on the proportions of albumins, globulins, glutelins, and prolamines in cereal grains and the lysine contents of those fractions.

TABLE 4

Percentages of Prolamine Fractions
in Grain Proteins of Various Cereals[a]

Crop	Prolamine	
	Name	Percent of protein
Barley	Hordein	40
Corn	Zein	50
Oats	Avenin	12
Rye	Secalin	40
Sorghum	Kafarin	60
Wheat	Gliadin	45

[a]From Mosse (1966).

Amino Acid Composition[a] of Grain Proteins[b]

Amino acids essential in some diets	Ideal composition for chicks	Rice[c,f]		Oats[c,d]		Barley[c,d]		Wheat[c,d]		Maize[c,d]		Sorghum[c,e]	
Lysine	5.0	3.5	3.7	4.0	3.7	3.7	3.4	2.6	2.7	2.7	3.0	1.8	2.0
Methionine + cystine	3.5	3.4	3.5	4.8	3.2	4.1	3.5	3.6	3.7	4.6	4.2	3.0	2.3
Threonine	3.5	3.3	4.1	3.6	3.4	3.6	3.7	3.0	2.9	4.0	4.2	3.6	3.0
Isoleucine	4.0	4.5	3.9	4.0	4.6	3.7	3.8	3.4	3.8	3.8	4.0	4.5	3.8
Leucine	7.0	8.0	8.0	7.1	7.0	7.1	6.9	6.8	6.4	10.6	12.0	11.6	13.1
Valine	4.3	5.4	5.7	5.1	5.4	5.3	5.0	4.6	4.3	5.0	5.6	5.4	4.9
Phenylalanine + tyrosine	7.0	10.3	8.5	8.4	8.8	8.6	8.5	7.6	7.8	8.7	8.8	5.2	6.4
Tryptophan	1.0	0.6	1.4	0.9	1.3	1.3	1.4	1.1	1.3	0.7	0.8	0.8	0.7
Histidine	2.0	2.2	2.3	2.2	1.9	2.2	1.9	2.3	2.1	2.6	2.4	2.0	2.1
Arginine	6.0	7.8	7.7	6.1	6.6	5.4	5.0	4.7	4.3	4.3	5.0	3.4	2.7
Net protein utilization by rat (%)		66		59		59		53		51		48	

[a] Grams per 16 g N.

[b] From Whitehouse (1973).

[c] Data in first column for each crop from Eggum (1969).

[d] Data in second column for oats, barley, wheat, and maize from Hughes (1960).

[e] Data in second column for sorghum (except for tryptophan) from Lykes (1970).

[f] Data in second column for brown rice (except for tryptophan) from Juliano et al. (1964).

TABLE 6

Protein Fractions and Their Lysine Content in Some Cereal Grains[a]

Cereal Grain	Protein fraction: Albumin		Globulin		Glutelin		Prolamine	
	Soluble in: Water		Salt		Alkali		Alcohol	
	(b)	(c)	(b)	(c)	(b)	(c)	(b)	(c)
Rice	5	4.9	10	2.6	80	3.5	5	0.5
Oats	1	--	78	--	5	--	16	--
Barley (normal)	13	7.9	12	6.3	23	4.8	52	0.8
Barley (Hiproly)	18	8.2	14	6.1	22	4.6	46	0.5
Wheat	5	--	10	--	16	1.9	69	0.6
Maize (normal)	4	3.8	2	6.1	39	3.4	55	0.2
Maize (opaque-2)	15	4.1	5	5.2	55	4.7	25	0.1
Sorghum (normal)	8	4.5	8	4.6	32	2.7	52	0.5
Sorghum (160-Cernum)	6	--	10	--	38	--	46	--

[a]From Whitehouse (1973).

[b]Protein fraction as % of total protein.

[c]Lysine as % of protein fraction.

YIELD, PROTEIN CONTENT, AND AMINO ACID COMPOSITION

The plant breeder who wishes to improve nutritional value of cereal grains must consider both the quantity and quality of the protein (Johnson et al., 1968). Increasing the quantity of protein is of limited value if that increase results in an impaired amino acid balance. The reverse is also true. The benefit from an improved amino acid balance is reduced if protein content of the grain is decreased. Finally, agrotechnical considerations must be considered. The yield is of utmost importance because: a) the amount of available protein depends largely on the quantity of grain which is produced, and b) the nutritionally improved crop must reap an adequate economic return to the farmer.

Whitehouse (1970) emphasized that in a free society economic forces largely determine which species and varieties are grown. If grain of special chemical composition or nutritive value does not receive price support there is much likelihood that the new varieties will be neglected by the farmer. The reason is that adding new selection criteria (i.e., chemical composition) limits the choice of plant breeding material and may result in selections which fall behind in yield. Total yield of grain per unit area of land is the most obvious measure of success or failure of any cereal crop.

According to Frey (1973), a review of literature shows that, almost universally, grain yields and protein contents in the grains are negatively correlated. However, White and Black (1954) suggested that the seemingly negative correlation between grain yields and grain protein percentages was the result of inadequate availability of soil nitrogen in most experiments. The implication is that the reported negative correlations are phenotypically real, but not genotypic in origin. According to Frey (1973), the numerous reports of negative correlations between grain yields and protein percentages for cereal grains are artifacts of experimental conditions. In wheat, some new cultivars combine, under U.S.A. conditions, high yield and high protein levels. Experiments conducted by Frey (1973) on oats indicated increased nitrogen fertilization requirements if the genetic potentials for high yields and high protein percentages in new cultivars are to be exploited.

Whitehouse (1970) stated that the high protein, high yielding wheats developed and tested in the U.S.A. may be inferior to accepted cultivars which yield 5-6 tons per hectare (ha) under conditions of Great Britain.

This assessment was reiterated more recently. According to Whitehouse (1973), in all cereal crops there is negative correlation between grain yield and protein content of the grain. Conditions which raise the yield of grain increase the amount of carbohydrates more than they increase the amount of protein. A common cause of high protein content may be an environmental restriction of growth. In some cases, the high protein content is genotypic in origin (i.e., poor endosperm development in *Avena sterilis*, in Hiproly, and in early triticale selections).

Protein yields are normally higher when total yields are higher. Correlations between grain yield and protein yield are usually positive. Whitehouse (1973) showed that this positive correlation was much stronger for genetic than for environmental differences. On the other hand, the negative correlations between grain yield and protein content were stronger for environmental comparisons. These results suggest that a change from a poor to a good environment results in a bigger increase in carbohydrate production than in protein production; a change from a poor to a good variety increases both components. Thus, protein yields can be increased more effectively through breeding than through cultural means.

As protein levels increase, the percentage of lysine in the protein falls (see data on Barley Cultivars in this chapter) although the total amount of lysine in the grain is still higher than in a low-protein sample of the same variety (Whitehouse, 1970). Only limited data are available on the percentage of lysine in the protein of high-lysine corn and barley cultivars grown under different conditions and as affected by cultural practices.

BARLEY

Changes in Developing Grain

Knowledge of changes that occur during development of cereal grains is essential to any sound plant breeding program. In addition, fractionation and characterization of components in developing grain can help in better identifying the components present in mature grain and help in devising methods of biological "agroengineering" of cereals with desirable composition and overall quality (i.e., by using proper quantity, type, and timing of fertilizers, or by other cultural practices).

Changes in amino acid composition of maturing barley have been the subject of several investigations. Danilova and Pleskov (1968)

determined 17 amino acids in proteins of maturing barley grown on
different soils. Soil type did not affect amino acid composition.
During ripening, glutamic acid, proline, and glycine increased and
lysine, histidine, arginine, and valine decreased. Somewhat
different results were found in investigations conducted by Pomeranz
and Robbins (1972b) on changes in amino acids of three barley cultivars grown for two years. Moisture contents at the time of harvest,
kernel weights of freeze-dried kernels, and protein contents of
samples from 11 stages of development in one crop year are given in
Figure 1. Protein content, on a moisture-free basis, decreased during the first two weeks after heading, increased during the third
week, and remained constant after 23 days. Full kernel weight was
attained after about three weeks.

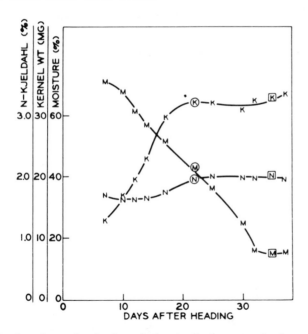

FIG. 1. Some physical and chemical characteristics of barleys
harvested at various stages of development in 1969. Averages for
three varieties; M, moisture (%); K, wt in mg of kernels dried to a
moisture of about 12%; N, Kjeldahl N (%) on a moisture-free basis.
Circled figures denote samples at physiological maturity; squared
figures, combine-ripe samples. From Pomeranz and Robbins (1972b).

Changes in average (for three cultivars) concentrations of
seven amino acids and of ammonia are given in Figures 2 and 3.
Practically in all cases, illustrated in Figures 2 and 3, changes
which took place in amino acid composition were completed within the
first three weeks after heading; this coincided with the time at
which full dry-kernel weight was attained. The largest average increases during maturation were in glutamic acid (from 16.1 to 24.0%),
proline (4.9 to 11.6%), and cystine (0.5 to 1.5%); the largest decreases were in alanine (not shown here, from 8.3 to 4.3%), lysine
(6.9 to 3.9%), and aspartic acid (9.8 to 6.9%). Concentration of
threonine decreased from 5.1 to 3.5%, phenylalanine increased from
4.3 to 5.1%, and ammonia increased from 2.7 to 2.9%. Additional
decreases in concentrations in the proteins were in serine (5.6 to
4.0%), glycine (5.4 to 4.2%), valine (6.2 to 5.3%), isoleucine (4.3
to 3.7%), and leucine (7.7 to 6.7%). Concentrations of other amino
acids remained fairly uniform or varied in an irregular manner:

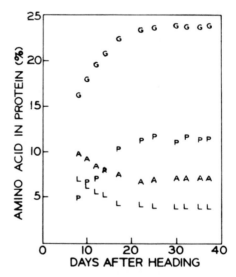

FIG. 2. Aspartic acid (A), glutamic acid (G), lysine (L),
and proline (P) concentrations in proteins of maturing barley
(averages for three varieties from the 1969 crop). From Pomeranz
and Robbins (1972b).

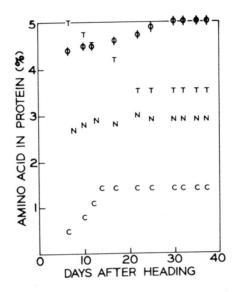

FIG. 3. Ammonia (N), cystine (C), phenylalanine (ϕ), and threonine (T) concentrations in proteins of maturing barley (averages for three varieties from the 1969 crop). From Pomeranz and Robbins (1972b).

histidine, 2.2 to 2.5%; arginine, 5.1 to 5.9%; methionine, 2.1 to 2.5%; and tyrosine, 2.3 to 3.0%.

Decrease in aspartic acid was smaller than increase in glutamic acid; consequently, increase during maturation in the sum of glutamic and aspartic acids was from 25.9 to 30.9%. Assuming that most of the ammonia was from glutamine and asparagine, about 89.0, 83.0, and 79.3% of the two dicarboxylic acids were in the form of amides 7, 14, and 37 days after heading, respectively. However, those values might have been affected significantly by the formation during hydrolysis of high levels of ammonia in samples from early stages of maturity.

Ivanko (1971), who reported similar changes, has shown that these changes occurred mainly as a result of increases in concentration of barley prolamines (hordein) which are characterized by high concentrations of glutamic acid and proline and low concentrations of aspartic acid, alanine, and lysine.

23

Barley Cultivars

The two limiting amino acids in barley protein are lysine and threonine (Howe et al., 1965). The low lysine in barley protein is primarily due to the virtual absence of lysine in hordein, the alcohol-soluble protein fraction (Folkes and Yemm, 1956).

Bishop reported as early as 1928 that hordein increases as the total protein content of barley increases. More recently, Munck et al. (1969) found correlations of -0.89** and -0.50* between protein content in the grain and lysine percentage in the protein for 16 commercial cultivars and 18 experimental lines, respectively. Viuf (1969) tested 650 barley cultivars and found that cultivars with 9.5-10.9 percent protein had 4.2 percent lysine in the protein, whereas those with 17.8-18.1 percent protein had only 2.7-3.1 percent lysine.

The two main types of malting barleys (depending on the arrangement of the grains in the ear) are 2-rowed and 6-rowed. In the U.S.A., approximately 90% of malt is made from the midwestern 6-rowed Manchurian type barley or varieties developed from it. These barleys are relatively small-kernelled, medium high in protein, and produce high enzymatic activities during malting (Kneen and Dickson, 1967). The western 2-rowed barleys have a medium-sized, uniform, plump kernel with a thin hull. The best samples are relatively low in protein and high in starch. Protein content is an important specification in malting barley; high protein levels impair modification of malt, decrease malt extract, and affect beer quality. According to recommendations of the Malting Barley Improvement Association (1971), preferred upper protein limit (dry basis) for midwestern 6-rowed types is 12.5% and for western 2-rowed types is only 12.0%.

Day and Dickson (1957) studied linkage associations between nitrogen percentages and several visible morphological characteristics of known inheritance. They found that nitrogen percentage was associated with the 2-rowed versus 6-rowed character. In a series of Alpha X O.A.C. 21 crosses, the 6-rowed segregates had a mean

PROTEINS AND AMINO ACIDS OF BARLEY, OATS, AND BUCKWHEAT

barley nitrogen percentage significantly lower than that of the 2-rowed segregates. In a survey of 1110 samples of barleys grown in 1969, evaluated by the National Barley and Malt Laboratory, the average grain protein was 11.9 and 12.6% in 6-rowed and 2-rowed barleys, respectively (Standridge et al., 1970).

Pomeranz et al. (1973a) determined kernel weight, protein content, and amino acid composition in isogenic pairs of 2-rowed and 6-rowed barleys, in 2-rowed and 6-rowed barleys, and in 2-rowed and 6-rowed backcrosses to a 2-rowed barley cultivar (Bonneville). The 2-rowed selections were higher both in kernel weight and in protein content than the 6-rowed selections. In addition, the proteins in 2-rowed selections contained more glutamic acid and proline (and less of most of the other amino acids) than the proteins of the 6-rowed selections. Amino acids were determined in proteins of 15 2-rowed and 21 6-rowed cultivars (grown for two years), each from two locations which consistently produced barleys varying widely in protein content. The results showed that the amino acid composition in the two types of barleys (2-rowed and 6-rowed) depended on their protein contents. It was concluded that amino acid composition in proteins of 2-rowed and 6-rowed barleys was governed by the total protein content rather than type of barley. There was a highly significant, positive correlation between the lysine and aspartic acid contents of proteins in all types and groups of barleys that were studied (Table 7).

Kernel weight, protein content, and amino acid composition were determined (Pomeranz et al., in press) for 113 barley cultivars from the USDA World Collection. Two-rowed covered spring, 6-rowed covered winter, 6-rowed hull-less spring, and 6-rowed covered spring types were represented within the 113 cultivars. Two-rowed barleys were higher than 6-rowed barleys in kernel weight and produced more protein and lysine per 1,000 kernels. Winter barleys were inferior to spring barleys for protein and lysine metameters. In comparison with covered barleys, hull-less cultivars were lower in kernel weight but higher in protein content and yielded more lysine per

TABLE 7

Simple Correlation Coefficients[a] Between
Lysine and Four Amino Acids in Proteins of Barleys[b]

Groups of barleys	Lysine vs			
	Aspartic acid	Glycine	Alanine	Glutamic acid
Isogenics				
2-rowed	0.912	0.893	0.672	-0.814
6-rowed	0.869	0.784	0.807	-0.568
Backcrosses				
2-rowed	0.931	0.972	0.925	-0.852
6-rowed	0.930	0.982	0.886	-0.971
Uniform nurseries				
2-rowed Delta, Colorado	0.686	0.575	0.701	-0.809
2-rowed Corvallis, Oregon	0.592	0.526	0.709	-0.588
6-rowed Morris, Minnesota	0.701	0.596	0.653	-0.780
6-rowed Carrington, N. Dak.	0.755	0.678	0.538	-0.822

[a]All correlations were significant at the 1% level.
[b]From Pomeranz et al. (1973a).

gram of barley sample. A close relationship between lysine and
glycine was found over different barley types. Decrease in lysine
concentration accompanying increase in protein content indicated a
curvilinear relation (Figure 4). A similar curvilinear relationship
between protein content of wheat endosperm and lysine content of the
protein was reported by Kent (1969). Large differences in kernel
weight, lysine, and protein within and between types of barleys indicated that the cultivars tested would provide a rich source of
germplasm for plant breeders.

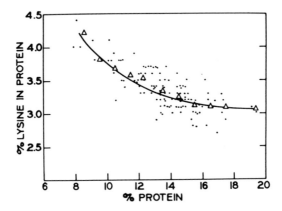

FIG. 4. Plot of relation between percent protein and percent lysine in protein of 113 barleys from the USDA World Collection. Dots represent individual samples; triangles are averages of percent lysine in protein for 1% intervals in protein content.

High-Protein, High-Lysine Barleys

Investigations of Munck et al. (1970) have led to the discovery of a high-protein, high-lysine barley line (Hiproly) with improved nutritional value. The Hiproly barley, C.I. 3947, is of Ethiopian origin; it is an erectoid type with naked, slightly shriveled seeds, and requires a long photoperiod. A sister line to Hiproly, C.I. 4362, has a similar growth habit, but has smoother, heavier seeds. Both lines are high in protein, but C.I. 3947 has substantially more lysine in the protein and a higher nutritional value than C.I. 4362. Kernel weight, protein content, and amino acid composition of C.I. 4362, Hiproly, and average of 113 samples from the Barley World Collection are compared in Table 8.

The high-lysine--high-protein trait markedly reduces the hordein content of barley but the reduction is not as large as the reduction in zein caused by the *opaque-2* trait in corn. According to Munck (1971), the Hiproly trait increases lysine, aspartic acid, and methionine and decreases glutamic acid, cystine, and proline. Feeding experiments with rats and mice confirmed the improved nutritional quality of Hiproly lines.

TABLE 8

Kernel Weight, Protein Content,

and Amino Acid Composition[a] of Barleys

Parameter	C.I. 4362[b]	Hiproly[b]	World Collection[c]
Kernel weight (mg)	46.7	35.0	43.2
Protein (N x 6.25) (%)	19.3	20.1	13.6
Lysine	3.0	4.3	3.4
Histidine	2.0	2.2	2.1
Ammonia	3.2	2.9	3.3
Arginine	4.0	4.8	4.4
Aspartic acid	5.4	7.4	6.3
Threonine	2.7	3.2	3.1
Serine	3.4	3.7	3.5
Glutamic acid	29.5	25.5	27.4
Proline	15.3	11.9	12.3
Cystine/2	1.1	0.8	1.2
Glycine	3.3	3.8	3.8
Alanine	3.5	4.7	4.1
Valine	4.3	5.1	5.0
Methionine	1.9	2.1	2.6
Isoleucine	3.3	3.6	3.6
Leucine	6.2	6.5	6.5
Tyrosine	2.3	2.3	2.5
Phenylalanine	5.7	5.4	5.2

[a]Grams amino acid per 100 g amino acids recovered.

[b]From Pomeranz et al. (1972).

[c]From Pomeranz et al. (in press); average of 113 samples from the Barley World Collection.

Protein content and amino acid composition were determined at five stages of development in seven barley populations including the high-lysine/low-lysine pair, Hiproly, and C.I. 4362 (Pomeranz et al., 1974). During seed development, concentrations (in the protein) of lysine, aspartic acid, alanine, and valine decreased more rapidly and concentration of glutamic acid increased to higher levels in C.I. 4362 than in Hiproly. However, amounts of some of the amino acids (i.e., lysine and aspartic acid) per kernel were identical in mature kernels of the pair. The results indicate that differences in concentrations of certain amino acids of the barleys may have resulted from differences in kernel development and protein deposition in the whole kernel or in specific kernel tissues.

The poor agronomical characteristics of Hiproly preclude, at present, its commercial cultivation. Plant breeders are highly interested in developing acceptable crosses between Hiproly and commercially grown cultivars. Hopefully, such crosses would combine the excellent amino acid balance of Hiproly with overall acceptable agronomic characteristics in cultivars useful for food, feed, and malting purposes. However, even if that objective is met, the content of the second limiting amino acid, threonine, would not be improved.

Erectoides mutants are more commonly induced than any other type of viable morphological mutants in barley. Mikaelsen (1972) produced a number of erectoides mutants by ionizing radiations (gamma and fast neutrons) and chemical mutagens (EMS and DES) in the barley variety Union. One of these mutants, H-14, showed a pleiotropic effect of the mutation. In addition to a dense spike, the mutant has a shorter and stiffer culm with superior lodging resistance compared with the mother variety. The mutant was tested in yield trials at two localities over three years. The mutant has retained the yielding capacity of the mother variety and the 1,000-kernel weight was only slightly lower. In all trials, seed protein content of the mutant was significantly higher (8%) than that of the mother variety.

The Riso mutant 1508 was found in 1970 by screening the Danish 2-rowed spring barley variety Bomi treated with ethyleneimine (Ingversen et al., 1973). The mutant was about 10% inferior to the parent in yield; the kernels were somewhat smaller. The lysine content of the protein (6.25 x N) ranged from 5.18 to 5.42% in the mutant compared with 3.64 to 3.82% in Bomi. The genetically stable increase of about 40% in lysine was accompanied by about 35% increase in the second limiting amino acid, threonine. Fractionation of proteins indicated that the albumin plus globulin contents were 46% in the mutant and only 27% in Bomi, the prolamine content decreased from 29% in Bomi to 9% in the mutant, and the glutelin content was 39% in both. While the amino acid composition of the albumin plus globulin in the mutant and Bomi was similar, there were great differences in the composition of the glutelins and especially prolamines. The lysine content of the prolamines and of the glutelins in the mutant was 192 and 36%, respectively, above the values for the parent variety.

Effects of Fertilizers

Numerous investigations have demonstrated that if nitrogen fertilizers are applied in the seed-bed the yield, but not the protein content, of the grain is increased (Foote and Batchelder, 1953). If, on the other hand, the fertilizer is applied during growth the effect is on the nitrogen content of the barley (McBeath and Toogood, 1960).

Doubling the quantity of nitrogen applied as top dressing increased seed nitrogen by 10-17% and yield by up to 13.5%. There were small differences in varietal responses and environmental conditions were of greater significance than nitrogen application (Woodham, 1973). Generally, an increase in protein was accompanied by a decrease in lysine (and possibly histidine and arginine) in the protein. The inverse relationship between protein and lysine was pronounced between the 8 and 11% protein levels but did not hold for very high protein barleys.

Barley Tissues and Fractions

Protein contents and amino acid composition of whole (hulled) barleys and barley fractions are given in Table 9. The results are

TABLE 9

Yield, Protein Content,[a] and Amino Acid Composition[b]
of Whole (Covered) Barley and Barley Fractions

Assay	Whole kernel[c]	Lemma[d]	Palea[d]	Germ[c]	Dehulled-degermed[c]
Yield (%)	100.0	7.3	3.1	3.7	85.9
Protein	12.4	1.7	2.0	35.0	12.3
Lysine	3.9	6.0	6.1	7.2	3.6
Histidine	2.2	1.5	1.8	3.1	2.2
Ammonia	3.0	3.2	3.4	2.3	3.1
Arginine	4.4	4.9	5.0	9.5	4.4
Aspartic acid	6.8	11.6	11.7	10.6	6.3
Threonine	3.4	5.5	5.5	4.5	3.5
Serine	3.7	5.9	6.1	4.4	3.7
Glutamic acid	26.1	12.8	13.1	14.6	27.0
Proline	11.4	4.9	3.8	3.9	11.8
Cystine/2	1.0	0.1	0.2	0.7	1.1
Glycine	4.2	7.4	7.5	6.7	4.0
Alanine	4.4	7.7	7.9	7.0	4.1
Valine	5.3	7.1	7.1	6.0	5.2
Methionine	2.6	2.0	1.8	2.3	2.6
Isoleucine	3.8	4.5	4.4	3.7	3.8
Leucine	7.1	8.3	8.1	6.9	7.1
Tyrosine	1.9	2.5	2.3	3.0	2.2
Phenylalanine	5.4	4.7	4.5	4.3	5.4

[a] $N \times 6.25$, %.

[b] Grams amino acid per 100 g amino acid recovered.

[c] Average of 2 samples.

[d] Average of 4 samples.   From Robbins and Pomeranz (1972).

averages of analyzing 2-4 barley cultivars. No consistent varietal
differences could be established. The hull layers, lemma and palea,
which comprised slightly over 10% of the kernel, were low in protein; the palea was slightly, but consistently higher in protein

than the lemma. The germ had, as expected, the highest protein content.

There were only small differences in amino acid composition between the lemma and the palea; the largest difference was in proline. The hull fractions resembled the germ fraction in their high lysine and aspartic acid and low glutamic and proline contents. Both hull fractions and the germ differed substantially from the whole kernel in amino acid composition. The major differences were in the concentrations of the main amino acids (glutamic acid, proline, and aspartic acid). Shifts in the major components were accompanied by significant changes in most of the other amino acids.

Conventional roller-milling of hulled barley yielded four major fractions, varying widely in protein content (Table 10). A 65%-extraction flour and tailings contained more protein than the whole kernel. The relatively high protein content of the 65%-extraction flour resulted from incomplete separation of the starchy endosperm from the rest of the kernel and from the fact that some tailings' flour was added to prepare the 65%-extraction flour. The bran was particularly low in protein, indicating high hull and pericarp contents. Proteins in the shorts and in the bran contained more lysine, aspartic acid, threonine, serine, glycine, alanine, and valine; and less glutamic acid than the proteins of the whole kernel, the 65%-extraction flour, or the tailings' flour. The bran proteins were particularly deficient in histidine and cystine, amino acids present in lowest concentrations in hull proteins.

Significant shifts in protein content and amino acid composition resulted from air classification of the 65%-extraction flour. A high-protein fraction contained almost 2.4 times as much protein as the original flour and about 3.6 times as much protein as a low-protein fraction. Proteins in the high-protein fraction were low in lysine, arginine, aspartic acid, threonine, glycine, alanine, valine, methionine, and isoleucine; and high in glutamic acid, proline, and cystine. Compared to the high-protein fraction, the low-protein fractions were high in lysine and aspartic acid and low in glutamic acid and cystine.

TABLE 10

Yield, Protein Content,[a] and
Amino Acid Composition[b] of Roller-Milled Barley[c]

Assay	Whole kernel	Flour, 65% extraction	Tailings' flour	Shorts	Bran
Yield (%)	100.0	65.0	17.7	11.9	5.4
Protein	9.3	9.8	11.3	8.8	3.1
Lysine	4.2	4.1	4.1	4.8	5.0
Histidine	2.4	2.4	2.4	2.1	1.4
Ammonia	3.1	3.1	3.0	2.9	3.5
Arginine	5.3	5.5	5.7	5.9	4.6
Aspartic acid	7.4	7.1	7.5	8.2	8.6
Threonine	3.6	3.6	3.6	3.8	4.2
Serine	4.1	4.0	4.1	4.2	4.7
Glutamic acid	22.6	23.3	22.9	21.2	20.6
Proline	11.4	10.1	9.6	9.2	9.9
Cystine/2	1.1	1.4	1.3	1.1	0.3
Glycine	4.5	4.3	4.7	5.1	5.0
Alanine	4.6	4.4	4.7	5.1	5.0
Valine	5.3	5.2	5.2	5.5	6.1
Methionine	2.5	2.7	2.5	2.5	2.3
Isoleucine	3.6	3.7	3.6	3.7	3.7
Leucine	6.8	7.0	6.8	6.9	7.5
Tyrosine	2.7	3.2	3.0	2.9	2.5
Phenylalanine	4.9	5.0	5.2	5.0	5.1

[a]$N \times 6.25$, %.

[b]Grams of amino acid per 100 g amino acid recovered.

[c]From Robbins and Pomeranz (1972).

OATS

Changes in Developing Grain

Changes in protein content and amino acid composition of developing oats have been the subject of few investigations. According to Wiggans and Frey (1958), the relative proportion of prolamines does not increase in developing oats. Sedova and Pleskov (1968) reported only small changes in the content of essential amino acids, including lysine, during the development of oat grains. Brown et al. (1970) showed that proteins of 5-day groats contained more lysine, aspartic acid, threonine, and alanine and less arginine, glutamic acid, proline, phenylalanine, and tyrosine than proteins of mature oats. The differences in amino acid content of 10-day, 15-day, and mature oats were small and rather inconsistent for most amino acids. However, relative lysine content declined slightly with increasing maturity.

Pomeranz et al.(submitted) determined protein content and amino acid composition in groats and hulls of three oat cultivars (*A. sativa*) harvested at four stages of development. The results are summarized in Table 11. Protein content was slightly higher in mature than in immature groats. In the hulls, protein content decreased during development to about one-third the content of immature hulls. The large decrease in protein content of the hulls was accompanied by little change in amino acid composition. In the hulls, however, there were consistent and large decreases in concentrations of lysine, threonine, and aspartic acid and an increase in glutamic acid. The results suggest that in addition to deposition of storage proteins in the groat, amino acids are translocated from the hulls to the groats.

Avena sativa

Frey (1951) found that oat cultivars with a wide range of protein content from 9.3 to 15.8% all had remarkably uniform prolamine: protein ratios of 0.18 to 0.19. Frey (1952) reported that changes

TABLE 11

Protein Content[a] and Concentrations of Certain Amino Acids[b]
in Proteins of Groats and Hulls of Three Oat Cultivars Grown in
Madison, Wisconsin, in 1971 and Harvested at Four Stages of Development[c]

Variety and parameter	Weeks after anthesis			
	1	2	3	4
Groats				
Protein	17.9	18.0	19.1	21.2
Lysine	6.1	5.0	4.4	4.2
Aspartic acid	9.8	8.4	8.2	8.4
Threonine	4.2	3.6	3.3	3.2
Glutamic acid	17.1	20.2	22.1	23.0
Hulls				
Protein	8.2	5.9	3.7	2.5
Lysine	6.1	6.9	7.1	6.3
Aspartic acid	14.1	13.9	12.8	11.6
Threonine	4.8	5.2	5.3	5.2
Glutamic acid	12.3	13.6	13.7	15.6

[a]N x 6.25, %, dry matter basis.

[b]Grams amino acid per 100 g amino acid recovered.

[c]Averages for the three cultivars. From Pomeranz et al.
(submitted).

in protein content of oat groats were accompanied by changes in
lysine, methionine, and tryptophan. Differences in the lysine content of the varieties with varying protein content for any given year
were small. However, when samples from various years were arranged
according to increasing protein content, concentration of lysine in
the protein also increased. McElroy et al. (1949) found that the
lysine content of nine oat samples ranging in protein content from
9.4 to 18.9% was uniform. The samples were of one pure variety.
Thus, variations in protein content reflected environmental effects.
Hischke et al. (1968) determined protein content and amino acid

composition in seven oat cultivars grown under similar environmental conditions. Samples of oat groats ranging in protein content from 18.1 to 22.2% had highly significant differences in lysine, glutamic acid, and glycine content. The content of the other amino acids was uniform in all samples. Rat growth data revealed no significant differences in nutritive value of the oat varieties that were studied. However, Weber et al. (1957) showed that Cimarron, Froke-deer, and Winter Fulghum cultivars produced high body-weight gains when fed to rats, but DeSoto and Selection 4829 produced low gains. There were no associations between lysine or methionine contents of the cultivars and the gains these cultivars produced.

Robbins et al. (1971) recently reported results from a survey of the protein content and amino acid composition of groats from 289 common oat cultivars. This group included cultivars grown commercially in the U.S. and Canada during the period 1900 through 1970, plus some advanced breeding lines with potential for becoming released cultivars or had utility as germplasm. The group of 289 was considered a random sample of the genetic variability available in "common oats" (*Avena sativa*) for protein content and amino acid composition. The samples contained 12.4-24.4% crude protein (average 17.1%). Chemical analyses of the oat hydrolyzates indicated that the amino acid composition was nutritionally superior to that of other cereal grains. More data based on bioassays using animal and/or human subjects are needed to substantiate these findings.

Mean lysine content of the 289 samples was 4.2 g per 100 g protein (Table 12). The correlation coefficient between lysine and protein was low (-0.183). This is encouraging and indicates that increased protein in oats need not be accompanied by a decreased lysine concentration in the protein as in other cereals (i.e., wheat and barley). Unfortunately, the survey has shown that correlations between protein and other limiting amino acids (i.e., threonine) were highly negative. Consequently, the oat breeder must pay strict attention to not only protein content and percent lysine, but also

PROTEINS AND AMINO ACIDS OF BARLEY, OATS, AND BUCKWHEAT

TABLE 12

Mean, Maximum (Max), Minimum (Min), and
Coefficient of Variability (CV) for Crude Protein[a]
and Amino Acid Composition[b] of Groats in 289 Oat Samples[c]

Parameter	Mean	Max	Min	CV
Protein	17.1	24.4	12.4	11.7
Lysine	4.2	5.2	3.2	7.6
Histidine	2.2	3.1	1.2	14.1
Ammonia	2.7	3.0	2.5	2.9
Arginine	6.9	7.8	6.2	3.3
Aspartic acid	8.9	9.9	8.3	3.1
Threonine	3.3	3.5	3.0	2.9
Serine	4.2	4.8	3.8	4.4
Glutamic acid	23.9	26.9	21.9	3.9
Proline	4.7	5.8	3.8	8.7
Cystine/2	1.6	2.6	0.6	26.8
Glycine	4.9	5.5	4.4	4.3
Alanine	5.0	5.5	4.2	3.7
Valine	5.3	5.7	4.9	2.0
Methionine	2.5	3.3	1.0	13.9
Isoleucine	3.9	4.1	3.4	2.2
Leucine	7.4	7.8	4.8	2.8
Tyrosine	3.1	4.4	2.3	7.4
Phenylalanine	5.3	5.7	4.9	2.6

[a]N x 6.25, %, dry matter basis.
[b]Grams amino acid per 100 g amino acid recovered.
[c]From Robbins et al. (1971).

to the maintenance of a satisfactory level of the second and third
limiting amino acids. In fact, levels of threonine may be more critical than levels of lysine. The rather low coefficient of variation
of threonine indicates that a marked increase in threonine through
breeding would be difficult to attain. Genetic variability within a

population is a prerequisite for progress through selection for that characteristic. It was hoped (Pomeranz, 1973) that *Avena* germplasm, other than *A. sativa*, may provide greater opportunity for increase in threonine.

Avena sterilis

These findings prompted amino acid analyses in several *Avena* species. The most extensive studies were conducted on *A. sterilis*, a wild hexaploid oat indigenous to the Mediterranean region. Collections of this species were made originally for disease resistance, particularly to the pathogen causing crown rust of oats (Murphy et al., 1967). *A. sterilis* has since proved to be a veritable storehouse for genes for resistance which can be readily transferred (at least in cases attempted thus far) to our common oats (Frey and Browning, 1973a, b; McDaniel, 1974a, b). *A. sterilis*, on the average, has higher groat protein content than our cultivated oats, but it has poor agronomic traits such as weak straw, kernel pubescence, long, geniculate awn, low kernel weight, and low grain yield. The seed shatters when ripe. Most genotypes are not well adapted to oat growing areas in the U.S. and Canada.

Ohm and Patterson (1973a) crossed six high protein *A. sterilis* collections in a diallel to learn about groat protein percent and total protein yield. The *A. sterilis* parents averaged 25.6% groat protein and two *A. sativa* check cultivars included in the experiment averaged 17.9% groat protein. The two check cultivars yielded twice the amount of seed and more total protein. Level of protein in the F_1 and F_2 generations resembled that of midparent values. Correlation between protein content and yield was generally negative, but not significant.

In another study, Ohm and Patterson (1973b) crossed each of the same six *A. sterilis* collections with five *A. sativa* commercial cultivars for further information on genetic control of protein content and total protein. Again, the *A. sativa* parents averaged twice as much seed yield and produced more total protein. Heterosis was expressed for yield in the F_1, but protein content of the hybrids was lower than the midparental value. The authors suggest that the small reduction in percent protein of the F_1 could be a result of increased yield of the hybrids. General combining ability was highly significant for groat protein content and high percent protein was recessive in all crosses. They also report that groat protein content was highly heritable. Percent groat protein was correlated negatively with yield, but the correlation was insignificant.

Campbell and Frey (1972a) used 10 interspecific crosses of *A. sativa* X *A. sterilis* to study inheritance of crude protein percentage of the groats. They concluded that sufficient genetic variability in protein content existed in progenies from such crosses and that inheritance of the trait was sufficiently simple. Computed heritabilities were high enough to expect progress toward breeding for high protein content in oats. In a subsequent report, Campbell and Frey (1972b) reported on amino acid analyses of 15 F_2 derived lines from an interspecific cross involving "O'Brien" (*A. sativa*) and PI 296255 (*A. sterilis*). Of particular interest are their data on lysine which ranged from 5.3 to 8.2% of protein. They state that two of the lines had more than 8% lysine. Analyses of the seed from the *A. sterilis* parent designated as Iowa B430-3006-1 did not corroborate the high value for lysine (G.S. Robbins and J.T. Gilbertson, unpublished data). The *A. sativa* parent, O'Brien, had a lysine content of 4.3% of the protein (Robbins et al., 1971).

Briggle et al. (in press) determined protein content and amino acid composition in groats from 68 collections of *Avena sterilis*. The data were compared to protein content and amino acid composition in 289 common oat cultivars and in 68 of the 289 cultivars having the smallest kernels and finally with 68 of the 289 cultivars having the largest kernels. *A. sterilis* collections contained from 22.1 to 31.4% protein (mean of 25.9%) compared to 12.4 to 24.4% (mean of 17.1%) for all 289, 14.4 to 22.3% (mean of 17.6%) for 68 small-kernelled, and 12.4 to 24.4% (mean of 17.5%) for 68 large-kernelled cultivars. There were significant differences in protein content and amino acid composition of the two species. *A. sterilis* contains more protein and more histidine, arginine, threonine, proline, valine, isoleucine, and leucine; and less lysine, alanine, glutamic acid, and aspartic acid.

Other *Avena* Species

According to Clark and Potter (1971), the most important varieties of oats are divided into red oats (*Avena byzantina*) and white oats (*Avena sativa*). In general, the red oats have a lower protein and higher fat content than the white oats although subgroup differences may be larger than major class differences. Varietal differences, to the extent that they exist, have little effect on composition and nutritive value of commercially available food products as the latter are made from a blend of many varieties. The authors' data indicated a rather constant amino acid composition over a wide span of protein content. The limiting amino acids in oat groat proteins are lysine, the sulfur amino acids, and threonine. While chemical analyses indicated that threonine was not markedly deficient, biological data indicated such a deficiency (Clark and Potter, 1971).

Pomeranz et al. (1973b) studied the following species of *Avena* from the U.S. Department of Agriculture World Collection: *A. barbata*, *A. pilosa*, *A. brevis*, *A. strigosa*, *A. hirtula*, *A. weistii*, *A. abyssinica*, *A. magna*, *A. fatua*, *A. nuda*, *and A. murphyii*. Samples of all species (except for the hull-less *A. nuda*) were separated into hulls and groats. The above species are not grown in the U.S. because of their poor agronomic characteristics. They were studied as potential donor parents in breeding to increase the protein content and improve the amino acid composition of oat cultivars used as food or feed.

Results of the analyses are summarized in Tables 13 and 14. The protein-rich groats (17.8-37.1%, mean 27.1%) differed substantially and consistently in amino acid composition from the protein-

TABLE 13

Average Protein Content[a] and Amino Acid
Composition[b] of Groats in 289 Cultivars of *A. sativa*,
68 Selections of *A. sterilis*, and 11 Other Oat Species[c]

Protein or amino acid	A. sativa	A. sterilis	11 other oat species
Protein (%)	17.1	25.9	27.1
Lysine	4.2	4.0	3.8
Histidine	2.2	2.4	2.2
Ammonia	2.7	2.9	2.7
Arginine	6.9	7.0	6.7
Aspartic acid	8.9	8.7	8.3
Threonine	3.3	3.3	3.3
Serine	4.2	4.3	4.2
Glutamic acid	23.9	22.6	22.6
Proline	4.7	5.8	6.1
Cystine/2	1.6	1.8	2.3
Glycine	4.9	4.8	4.9
Alanine	5.0	4.4	4.7
Valine	5.3	5.6	5.5
Methionine	2.5	2.4	2.9
Isoleucine	3.9	4.0	3.9
Leucine	7.4	7.5	7.3
Tyrosine	3.1	3.2	3.3
Phenylalanine	5.3	5.4	5.3

[a] Dry matter, N x 6.25.
[b] Grams amino acid per 100 g amino acid recovered.
[c] From Pomeranz et al. (1973b).

low hulls (2.0-8.1%, mean 4.2%); awns resembled hulls in protein
content and amino acid composition. Interspecies differences in
amino acid composition of hulls were greater than interspecies
differences in composition of groats. Groats from the 11 oat species

41

TABLE 14

Protein Content[a] and Amino Acid Composition[b] of
Groats and Hulls from 11 Oat Species and Awns from *A. magna*[c]

Protein or amino acid	Groats		Hulls		Awns
	Mean	Coefficient of variation	Mean	Coefficient of variation	
Protein (%)	27.1	21.8	4.2	56.0	3.9
Lysine	3.8	5.4	5.6	13.8	5.2
Histidine	2.2	4.0	2.1	32.2	2.7
Ammonia	2.7	3.0	4.4	28.7	6.8
Arginine	6.7	4.0	4.1	44.1	6.0
Aspartic acid	8.3	3.6	15.6	46.2	22.8
Threonine	3.3	2.7	4.8	14.3	3.8
Serine	4.2	11.3	4.6	18.5	3.7
Glutamic acid	22.6	7.5	14.5	26.4	12.4
Proline	6.1	9.0	4.8	33.0	4.6
Cystine/2	2.3	8.6	0.2	113.0	0.1
Glycine	4.9	4.5	5.8	19.3	4.2
Alanine	4.7	3.9	7.0	18.3	5.7
Valine	5.5	2.5	6.4	18.6	5.4
Methionine	2.9	11.5	2.3	20.2	1.8
Isoleucine	3.9	2.1	3.9	19.4	3.3
Leucine	7.3	2.1	7.2	19.0	5.9
Tyrosine	3.3	6.6	2.3	49.8	2.0
Phenylalanine	5.3	2.7	4.3	15.2	3.7

[a] Dry matter basis, N x 6.25.

[b] Grams amino acid per 100 g amino acid recovered.

[c] From Pomeranz et al. (1973b).

contained, on the average, more protein than groats from *A. sativa*,
but differences in amino acid composition were small.

These results were, admittedly, disappointing. Two points were
emphasized in reviewing the above results: a) oat groats, on the

average, are highest in protein among cereal grains, and b) the oat
groat proteins have an excellent amino acid balance (as determined
by chemical analyses). Inasmuch as the above results indicated no
readily available genetic stocks to improve the amino acid balance
of oats, it might be advisable, at this stage, at least, to concentrate efforts on increasing protein content (rather than on improving
amino acid balance) by genetic selection and by cultural practices,
provided amino acid composition and balance are not affected adversely. That possibility is investigated extensively. Another possibility would be to select for oat cultivars with unique grain morphology, i.e., large germ or multiple-aleurone layers that are rich
in protein and lysine. The latter possibility has been suggested on
the basis of investigations which determined the protein content and
amino acid composition of oat tissues.

Oat Tissues and Fractions

Youngs (1972) studied five cultivars and two experimental lines
of *A. sativa* with a wide range of protein. Percent groats, groat
and hull proteins, and 1,000 kernel weight and bran thickness of the
groats were measured. The groats were hand-dissected into the embryonic axis, scutellum, bran (including the aleurone layer), and
starchy endosperm. The embryonic axis accounted for 1.1-1.4% of the
total groat weight; scutellum, 1.6-2.6%; bran, 28.7-41.4%; and endosperm, 55.8-68.3%. The endosperm weights varied inversely, and the
bran weights directly, with the groat protein concentrations. Analysis of each groat fraction for protein showed the greatest concentration in the embryonic axis, with a range of 26.3-44.3%; scutellum
next, 24.2-32.4%; followed by the bran, 18.5-32.5%; and endosperm,
9.6-17.0%. Both the bran and endosperm protein concentrations increased as the total groat protein increased. Since most of the
groat weight is in the bran and endosperm, these fractions contained
the greatest part of the total groat protein. However, groats with
higher protein generally contained a greater amount of bran protein
rather than endosperm protein. Bran thickness was measured on 12

43

different varieties (range 0.058 to 0.101 mm) and varied directly
with groat protein.

Results of analyzing hand-dissected oat fractions are summarized
in Table 15 (Pomeranz et al., 1973b). The protein-rich germ tissues
were richer (than the whole groat) in several amino acids, especially
lysine, histidine, arginine, aspartic acid, and threonine. Germ proteins are relatively poor sources of amino acids of storage proteins
(glutamic acid and proline) and of cystine. The bran (including the
aleurone layer) contained almost twice as much total protein and had
a slightly better amino acid balance (more lysine and less glutamic
acid) than the starchy endosperm.

Light oats, which are rich in hulls, contain less protein than
large oats. The relatively higher concentrations in the hulls, than
in the groats, of lysine, aspartic acid, and threonine, and lower
concentrations of glutamic acid, proline, and sulfur-containing amino
acids, were reflected in the differences in amino acid composition
between heavy and light oats (Pomeranz et al., 1973b). Commercial
flakes resembled in protein content and amino acid composition the
groats from which the flakes were produced. Several oat varieties
shed their husk during threshing. There are difficulties in their
cultivation (Jenkins, 1968) but if these difficulties can be overcome, the hull-less varieties could provide a highly nutritious
grain--both in protein and amino acid composition.

Wu et al. (1972) milled groats of four oat cultivars and reported that the shorts and bran fractions had about twice the protein
content of the whole oats. The 1 M NaCl extract accounted for a
large percentage of total nitrogen from all fractions; the 0.1 N
acetic acid extract represented a major part of the proteins from the
flour fractions.

A wet-milling process was developed (Cluskey et al., 1973) to
produce protein concentrates, starch, and residue fractions from dry-
milled oat varieties having moderate- and high-protein contents.
Solvents and pH values were evaluated for their effectiveness in extracting an oat protein concentrate in good yield. The optimum yield

TABLE 15

Protein Content[a] and Amino Acid Composition[b]
of Hand-Separated Fractions of Oat Groats[c]

Protein or amino acid	Whole groats	Embryonic axis	Scutellum	Bran[d]	Endosperm
Protein (%)	13.8	44.3	32.4	18.8	9.6
Lysine	4.5	8.2	6.9	4.1	3.7
Histidine	2.4	3.9	3.6	2.2	2.2
Ammonia	2.7	1.9	1.8	2.5	2.9
Arginine	6.8	8.3	9.0	6.8	6.6
Aspartic acid	8.7	10.2	9.7	8.6	8.5
Threonine	3.4	5.0	4.7	3.4	3.3
Serine	4.6	4.8	5.0	4.8	4.6
Glutamic acid	21.7	14.2	14.9	21.1	23.6
Proline	5.5	3.3	3.6	6.2	4.6
Cystine/2	2.1	0.5	1.0	2.4	2.2
Glycine	5.2	6.3	6.2	5.4	4.7
Alanine	5.0	7.2	6.9	5.1	4.5
Valine	5.5	6.0	6.2	5.5	5.5
Methionine	2.2	2.2	2.1	2.1	2.4
Isoleucine	3.9	3.9	3.8	3.8	4.2
Leucine	7.6	7.1	7.1	7.4	7.8
Tyrosine	3.0	2.9	3.0	3.5	3.3
Phenylalanine	5.2	4.2	4.4	5.1	5.6

[a]Dry matter, N x 6.25.

[b]Grams amino acid per 100 g amino acid recovered.

[c]From Pomeranz et al. (1973b).

[d]Includes aleurone layer.

of protein was obtained in dilute alkali solution (pH 9). Starch and protein were separated from bran by sieving the alkaline dispersion. After the fine suspension was centrifuged to separate pure starch (0.05% nitrogen), the protein solution was adjusted to pH 6 and freeze-dried. The protein content (nitrogen x 6.25) of the concentrate varied between 59 and 89%, depending on the dry-milled fraction and process used, and accounted for up to 88% of total protein in the starting material.

Protein concentrates, starch, and residue fractions produced by the wet-milling process from ground oat groats were analyzed for amino acid composition, protein, starch, fat, fiber, ash, and various neutral carbohydrates (Wu et al., 1973). The concentrates, which had a bland taste, contained from 59 to 75% protein (nitrogen x 6.25) with 3.9-4.1 g lysine and 3.3-4.3 g total sulfur amino acids per 16 g nitrogen. The concentrates were low in fiber (0.1-0.2%), had 3.5-4.5% ash, no starch, and from 2.2 to 23.3% total carbohydrate. Protein concentrate from high-protein groats had 10.1% fat, whereas defatted moderate-protein groats gave a protein concentrate with 0.3% fat. The starch fraction was essentially composed of pure starch without any other carbohydrate. Protein concentrate from defatted groats had a nitrogen solubility of 83% at pH 2.1, a minimum solubility (15%) around pH 5, and 95% solubility at pH 11.4.

Oat groats, as well as first and second flours, from a high-protein variety and from a normal-protein variety were finely ground and air-classified to yield fractions with protein contents (nitrogen x 6.25) ranging from 4 to 88% (Wu and Stringfellow, 1973). Air classification of the oat flours produced a unique fraction (83-88% protein) not previously observed for wheat, rye, corn, sorghum, or triticale flours. This fraction (2-5% by weight) accounted for 14, 16, and 7%, respectively, of the total protein in first and second flours and groats. The next fraction (25-29% by weight) with 15-39% protein accounted for total protein from flours of 38-48%, and with 21-29% protein from groats, 31-33%. The first and second flours gave a better air classification response than ground groats, and the high-protein variety gave better results than normal-protein oats. Amino acid analyses of all fractions indicated high lysine levels from 3.9 to 5.0 g per 16 g nitrogen and adequate total sulfur amino acids. Data showed that air classification of oat flours and ground groats produced protein concentrates of good amino acid composition and could provide a new food ingredient suitable for a variety of uses.

Sedova and Bazhanova (1971) determined the amino acid composition of the protein fractions of oat grains. The water-, salt-, ethanol-, and alkali-soluble fractions of oat seeds were dialyzed and separated by chromatography on TEAE-cellulose columns, by ionic strength, and/or by pH gradient elution. The fractions varied in amino acid composition.

BUCKWHEAT

Buckwheat (*Fagopyrum esculentum* Möench) is not a true cereal. It belongs to the *Polygonaceae* (or buckwheat) family, but like the cereals, the grain of buckwheat is a dry fruit (Winton and Winton, 1945; Marshall, 1969). The black hulls of the triangular fruit are not suited for human food. Structurally, they have little in common with bran coats of the cereals. The seed proper (groat) is similar to that of cereals in that it consists of starchy endosperm and oily embryo.

Feeding experiments of Sure (1955) have shown that the proteins in buckwheat are the best known source of high biological value proteins in the plant kingdom, having 92.3% of the value of nonfat milk solids and 81.4% of whole egg solids. The proteins of buckwheat were shown to have excellent supplementary value to the cereal grains (Sure, 1955; Wyld et al., 1958).

Sokolov and Semikhov (1968) fractionated proteins of diploid and tetraploid forms of buckwheat; globulins were a main component of both. However, seeds of the tetraploid form contained more globulins and less albumins. Polyacrylamide gel electrophoresis showed no qualitative differences in composition of albumin, globulin, and glutelin fractions of diploid and tetraploid seeds. Similarly, Jacko and Pleskov (1968) found little difference in albumins and globulins, separated by chromatography on tetraethylaminoethylcellulose and by

47

electrophoresis in polyacrylamide gel, in diploid and tetraploid buckwheat.

Amino acid composition of whole buckwheat was determined by several investigators, including Lyman et al. (1956), who used a microbiological assay method, and more recently by Tkachuk and Irvine (1969), who used an ion-exchange procedure. Zebrak et al. (1966) found no significant difference in the amino acid composition of the total protein between diploid and tetraploid buckwheat.

Gross composition of milled buckwheat products was reported by Coe (1931) and by Watt and Merrill (1963).

Changes in Developing Grain

Kernel weight, hull:groat ratio, protein content, and amino acid composition were determined in two buckwheat cultivars harvested at four stages of maturity in 1971 and 1973 (Pomeranz et al., 1975). During maturation, a 3.0- to 5.6-fold increase in whole kernel weight was due to an up to 18-fold increase in weight of the groat and correspondingly smaller (less than 2-fold) increase in hull weight. In the groat, the large increase in weight was accompanied by a relatively small decrease in protein concentration. In the hulls of buckwheat, concentrations of total nitrogenous compounds decreased considerably during maturation. During maturation, the main changes in amino acid concentration in the hull proteins were increases in histidine and glycine. In the groat, concentrations of arginine, glutamic acid, and cystine increased; and concentrations of lysine, proline, alanine, valine, isoleucine, and leucine decreased. Whereas there are large changes in amino acid composition of maturing cereals (i.e., wheat, barley, and oats) and legumes (i.e., peas) (Gritton et al., 1975), amino acids of maturing buckwheat are characterized by a remarkable stability. Both with regard to the limiting amino acids (i.e., lysine) and amino acids of storage proteins (i.e., glutamic acid), changes in buckwheat were intermediate between those of true cereals and legumes.

PROTEINS AND AMINO ACIDS OF BARLEY, OATS, AND BUCKWHEAT

Mature Buckwheat

Crude protein and 17 amino acids were determined in ten samples of genetically diverse buckwheats, in buckwheat fractions from a commercial mill, and in the germ and degermed groats (Pomeranz and Robbins, 1972a). The buckwheat proteins were particularly rich in lysine (6.1%) and contained less glutamic acid and proline and more arginine and aspartic acid than cereal proteins (Table 16). About 56% of glutamic and aspartic acids was in the form of amides. Although correlations among basic or neutral and acidic amino acids were positive, those between basic and acidic or neutral amino acids were negative. Dark flour and feed fractions contained more protein than the whole kernel or the groat, but the amino acid patterns differed little (Table 17). Distribution of amino acids in buckwheat tissues differed significantly from distribution in tissues of cereal grains (Table 18). Chemical analyses of buckwheat hydrolyzates indicated that the amino acid composition was nutritionally superior to that of cereal grains.

Effects of Fertilizers

Ganyushina and Lazarchik (1972) studied the effect of ammonium nitrate on the yield and quality of buckwheat. Ammonium nitrate increased the buckwheat grain yield, the content of dry matter, and the chlorophyl content of the plants. In the grain, the contents of total and protein N and of soluble sugars were also increased. Artemeva and Yarosh (1972) studied composition of buckwheat grain and productivity of different varieties. Of 22 buckwheat varieties tested, three were identified as high-protein (16.1-17.0%) varieties. Positive correlations were established between the protein and P concentration, between protein and starch, yield and protein, and weight of 1000 grains and protein content. Application of double doses of N-P-K (80:120:80 kg/ha) increased the average yield of buckwheat by 0.8 quintal/ha and decreased hull content. Fertilization had no significant effect on kernel composition.

49

TABLE 16

Mean, Maximum Value (Max), Minimum Value (Min),
and Coefficient of Variability (CV) for Crude Protein[a]
and Amino Acid Composition[b] of Ten Buckwheat Samples[c]

Parameter	Max	Min	Mean	CV
Protein	15.4	12.6	13.7	6.2
Lysine	7.0	5.0	6.1	7.5
Histidine	3.1	2.3	2.7	7.1
Ammonia	2.3	1.7	2.1	7.8
Arginine	11.6	8.5	9.7	8.6
Aspartic acid	12.1	10.8	11.3	2.9
Threonine	4.1	3.6	3.9	3.5
Serine	5.2	4.5	4.7	4.2
Glutamic acid	19.4	17.8	18.6	2.2
Proline	4.3	3.2	3.9	8.9
Cystine/2	1.8	1.2	1.6	10.1
Glycine	6.5	5.9	6.3	2.9
Alanine	4.7	4.2	4.5	2.9
Valine	5.4	4.8	5.1	3.2
Methionine	3.0	1.8	2.5	13.5
Isoleucine	4.0	3.6	3.8	2.5
Leucine	6.6	6.1	6.4	2.4
Tyrosine	2.5	1.8	2.1	11.1
Phenylalanine	5.0	4.6	4.8	2.6

[a] N x 6.25, %, dry matter basis.
[b] Grams amino acid per 100 g amino acid recovered.
[c] From Pomeranz and Robbins (1972a).

TABLE 17
Protein Content[a] and Amino Acid
Composition[b] of Commercially Milled Buckwheat[c]

Parameter	Whole buck-wheat	Buck-wheat groats	Light flour	Dark flour	Buck-wheat feed	Hulls
Protein	13.8	16.4	7.4	19.0	18.9	4.0
Lysine	6.0	5.9	5.7	5.2	5.2	6.3
Histidine	2.6	2.6	2.7	2.4	2.8	3.9
Ammonia	2.1	1.9	2.2	1.7	2.3	3.0
Arginine	9.2	10.0	7.9	8.7	9.7	5.4
Aspartic acid	11.4	11.4	10.5	11.8	10.8	10.7
Threonine	4.0	3.8	4.1	4.1	3.9	5.4
Serine	4.9	4.6	4.7	5.5	5.0	5.7
Glutamic acid	18.5	19.3	17.6	20.1	19.2	13.3
Proline	3.8	3.8	5.1	4.1	4.0	4.2
Cystine/2	1.6	1.8	1.8	1.5	1.5	0.5
Glycine	6.6	6.2	6.2	6.6	6.2	7.5
Alanine	4.3	4.4	4.5	4.1	4.2	5.0
Valine	5.3	4.9	5.4	5.1	5.1	6.6
Methionine	2.3	2.8	2.8	1.9	2.3	2.9
Isoleucine	4.0	3.7	4.2	3.9	4.0	5.1
Leucine	6.7	6.2	7.0	6.5	6.7	8.3
Tyrosine	2.0	2.1	2.9	2.1	2.3	1.8
Phenylalanine	4.8	4.8	4.8	4.9	4.7	4.3

[a]N x 6.25, %, dry matter basis.
[b]Grams amino acid per 100 g amino acid recovered.
[c]From Pomeranz and Robbins (1972a).

TABLE 18

Protein Content[a] and Amino Acid Composition[b]
of Whole Buckwheat and of Buckwheat Fractions[c]

Parameter	Whole buckwheat	Groats	Hulls	Germ
Protein	13.8	16.4	4.0	55.9
Lysine	6.0	5.9	6.3	5.6
Histidine	2.6	2.6	3.9	2.6
Ammonia	2.1	1.9	3.0	1.9
Arginine	9.2	10.0	5.4	11.9
Aspartic acid	11.4	11.4	10.7	10.9
Threonine	4.0	3.8	5.4	3.7
Serine	4.9	4.6	5.7	5.0
Glutamic acid	18.5	19.3	13.3	19.3
Proline	3.8	3.8	4.2	3.8
Cystine/2	1.6	1.8	0.5	2.2
Glycine	6.6	6.2	7.5	6.0
Alanine	4.3	4.4	5.0	3.6
Valine	5.3	4.9	6.6	4.8
Methionine	2.3	2.8	2.9	2.0
Isoleucine	4.0	3.7	5.1	3.5
Leucine	6.7	6.2	8.3	5.8
Tyrosine	2.0	2.1	1.8	2.8
Phenylalanine	4.8	4.8	4.3	4.7

[a]N x 6.25, %, dry matter basis.
[b]Grams amino acid per 100 g amino acid recovered.
[c]From Pomeranz and Robbins (1972a).

PROTEINS AND AMINO ACIDS OF BARLEY, OATS, AND BUCKWHEAT

Wild Buckwheat

The selling of wheat on the basis of grade necessitates that, after harvesting, it be cleaned in order to segregate broken kernels, weed seeds, chaff, etc. from the whole kernels. The resulting product is known in the grain trade as wheat screenings. Those screenings may contain up to 30% of wild buckwheat. Little is known about the composition and nutritive value of wild buckwheat. Biely and Pomeranz (in press) determined the amino acid composition of wild buckwheat in, and separated from, No. 1 wheat feed screenings.

The amino acid composition of wild and cultivated buckwheat is similar. Proteins of cultivated species contain more lysine than do proteins of wild buckwheat. Both have better amino acid balance than cereal grains. Proteins in wild and cultivated buckwheat contain comparable amounts of glutamic acid plus proline (the main amino acids of storage proteins--prolamines and glutelins--in cereals) and the S-containing amino acids cystine plus methionine. The high wild buckwheat content in No. 1 wheat feed screenings makes the screenings a good source of essential amino acids. The metabolizable energy content of screenings is lower than that of wheat because of the high fiber content of the screenings. The reduced feed efficiency of screenings can be corrected by the addition of fat. No. 1 wheat feed screenings can be used to advantage in formulating balanced poultry rations as they have a high nutritive value and are lower in cost than wheat.

MALTED CEREALS

About two-thirds of the protein of the endosperm undergoes degradation during malting of barley (Pollock, 1962). During malting there is no loss of nitrogen except minor losses in steeping, but substantial changes occur in the distribution of the nitrogenous compounds and in their forms. The main changes involve translocation from the endosperm to the embryo, degradation, and de novo synthesis. In the whole grain, this constancy is apparently the result of a dynamic equilibrium although the total amount of albumin-globulin fractions remains relatively constant during malting. A rather continuous depletion of albumin and globulin contents of the endosperm is accompanied by their rise in the developing embryo. In addition, total amino acid composition of barley and malt clearly reflects that of the storage proteins, especially hordein, as well as of the salt-soluble proteins.

According to Folkes and Yemm (1958), during germination of barley there is a decrease in the whole grain in glutamic acid, proline, and amide nitrogen. One mode of breakdown of glutamic acid is decarboxylation to γ-aminobutyric acid. This is accompanied by several transamination reactions (e.g., between glutamic and oxalacetic acids to form α-ketoglutaric and aspartic acids). Jones and Pierce (1967) studied changes in nitrogen composition in germinating barley under malting conditions. They report that during growth the concentrations of glutamic acid, glycine, and ammonia decreased and of proline, aspartic acid, and lysine increased.

The main by-product of malting barley is called "malt sprouts." These are obtained during the cleaning of malt and amount to 3-5% of the grain. The main component of malt sprouts are rootlets. Malt sprouts are rich in protein and are mostly used as a feed ingredient. The total protein contents of barley malt sprouts are known to depend on the duration of malting and the method by which the sprouts are obtained (Pomeranz and Robbins, 1971).

Robbins and Pomeranz (1971) determined amino acid composition of grain, malt, and malt sprouts of barley, wheat, oats, rye, and triticale, grown and harvested under comparable conditions. The amino acid composition of malt sprouts from barleys malted under laboratory conditions was compared with that of commercially available products. Changes in contents and amino acid composition of two barleys malted for two, five, and eleven days and of rootlets from those malts were also reported.

Although there was little change in the crude protein contents of the grains and malts, the sprouts contained 1.3-2.1 times as much protein as the malts (Table 19). Protein contents were highest in sprouts from wheat and lowest from oats. Malting of the cereal grains resulted in considerable and consistent changes in amino acid composition. The proteins of the malts were higher than proteins of the original grains in lysine, arginine, aspartic acid, alanine, valine, isoleucine, and leucine; malting decreased concentrations of ammonia and glutamic acid; there was no consistent effect on the concentration of the other amino acids, including proline. Compared with the proteins of the malts, the proteins in sprouts were 1.8- to 3.8-fold higher in the concentration of aspartic acid and 1.4-2.2 times lower in glutamic acid. Among the other amino acids, there were significant increases in the concentrations of lysine, ammonia, threonine, alanine, and valine; concentrations of arginine, serine, leucine, tyrosine, phenylalanine, and particularly proline decreased. Assuming that all ammonia is derived from glutamine and asparagine, about 85% of the two amino acids in all tested cereals was in the form of amides. If the same assumption is made for sprouts, up to 85% of aspartic and glutamic acids of the sprouts is in the form of amides.

A comparison of five barley sprouts prepared in the laboratory with seven commercial samples and one sample sold under the name of malt cleanings is shown in Table 20. Laboratory prepared sprouts were higher in protein than the commercial sprouts, and especially higher than the malt cleanings; the latter would be expected to contain substantial amounts of husks that are relatively low in protein. The amino acid composition of the proteins in the commercial sprouts was similar to that of the laboratory product. The somewhat higher lysine and arginine contents and lower glutamic acid and proline contents of the commercial sprouts would indicate more extensive growth and modification than in the samples prepared in the laboratory. With increase in malting time, there was an increase in the malt proteins in lysine, aspartic acid, proline, valine, and leucine; concentrations of glutamic acid decreased. In the rootlets, there was a consistent and large decrease in protein contents with increase

TABLE 19

Nitrogen Contents and Amino Acid Composition[a]
of Grains, Malts, and Malt Sprouts From
Cereals Grown and Malted Under Comparable Conditions[b]

Assay	Barley			Oats		
	Grain	Malt	Sprouts	Grain	Malt	Sprouts
Kjeldahl N (%)	2.38	2.35	4.84	2.70	2.87	3.76
Lysine	2.9	3.5	5.5	3.6	3.8	6.4
Histidine	1.8	2.0	2.2	2.1	2.1	2.5
Ammonia	3.3	3.2	4.3	3.2	3.1	3.6
Arginine	4.9	5.2	5.2	6.9	6.8	5.3
Aspartic acid	6.3	6.9	23.1	9.8	10.1	18.3
Threonine	3.3	3.3	3.9	3.5	3.5	4.2
Serine	4.1	4.1	4.0	4.9	4.8	4.2
Glutamic acid	25.5	23.9	13.1	22.7	21.7	14.8
Proline	14.6	14.5	5.9	6.3	6.7	4.5
Cystine/2	0.3	0.2	0.4	0.7	0.5	0.2
Glycine	3.9	3.9	4.3	4.9	4.9	4.9
Alanine	4.0	4.1	5.2	4.7	5.0	6.2
Valine	4.9	4.9	5.5	5.4	5.6	6.1
Methionine	2.3	2.3	2.0	2.0	2.2	1.8
Isoleucine	3.5	3.6	3.9	4.1	4.2	4.2
Leucine	6.4	6.3	5.8	7.1	7.2	6.8
Tyrosine	2.9	2.9	2.3	2.8	2.7	2.4
Phenylalanine	5.2	5.2	3.6	5.5	5.5	3.7

[a]Grams amino acid per 100 g amino acid recovered.

[b]From Robbins and Pomeranz (1971).

TABLE 19 (cont.)

Assay	Rye			Wheat			Triticale		
	Grain	Malt	Sprouts	Grain	Malt	Sprouts	Grain	Malt	Sprouts
N (%)	2.38	2.36	4.50	3.38	3.36	5.10	3.23	3.35	4.76
Lys	3.1	3.9	4.8	2.4	2.7	5.7	2.6	3.1	4.8
His	2.0	2.2	1.8	2.2	2.2	2.1	2.0	2.1	1.8
Ammonia	3.5	3.2	4.2	3.9	3.7	4.2	3.4	3.3	4.7
Arg	4.9	5.3	4.7	4.1	4.5	5.2	5.0	5.3	5.1
Asp	7.5	8.4	21.5	5.0	6.3	24.1	6.5	7.6	26.2
Thr	3.1	3.4	3.3	2.6	2.7	3.6	2.9	3.2	3.6
Ser	4.2	4.2	3.5	4.2	4.3	3.7	4.2	4.4	3.8
Glu	27.2	22.5	15.3	33.2	30.5	13.6	34.2	29.0	13.2
Pro	13.1	13.3	12.4	10.8	10.8	7.7	10.6	11.1	6.8
Cys/2	0.3	0.2	0.2	1.0	1.1	0.2	0.5	0.7	0.4
Gly	4.1	4.3	4.1	3.8	3.9	4.3	3.8	3.9	4.1
Ala	4.1	4.5	4.6	3.3	3.6	5.0	3.8	4.0	4.9
Val	4.5	4.9	4.7	4.2	4.4	4.6	4.1	4.5	4.7
Met	2.3	2.6	1.8	2.1	1.6	1.8	1.8	1.8	1.7
Ile	3.4	3.7	3.3	3.5	3.6	3.5	3.1	3.4	3.5
Leu	5.7	6.0	4.9	6.4	6.5	5.3	5.4	5.7	5.3
Tyr	2.2	2.5	2.0	2.6	2.7	2.2	2.3	2.6	2.1
Phe	4.7	4.8	3.1	4.7	4.9	3.3	4.0	4.5	3.4

TABLE 20

Nitrogen Contents and Amino Acid Composition[a] of Commercial and Laboratory Barley Malt Sprouts[b]

Assay	Commercial sprouts		Commercial malt cleanings	Laboratory sprouts	
	Range	Average of 7 samples		Range	Average of 5 samples
Kjeldahl N (%)	3.82 – 5.49	4.75	4.24	4.56 – 5.22	4.96
Lysine	5.3 – 6.0	5.7	6.1	4.9 – 5.8	5.4
Histidine	1.8 – 2.4	2.1	1.9	1.7 – 2.3	2.1
Ammonia	3.5 – 4.5	4.0	3.3	3.6 – 4.7	4.1
Arginine	4.9 – 5.8	5.5	5.5	4.5 – 5.2	4.9
Aspartic acid	16.3 – 19.4	18.4	14.9	18.9 – 23.1	22.0
Threonine	4.1 – 4.6	4.3	4.6	3.6 – 3.9	3.8
Serine	4.0 – 4.6	4.3	4.6	3.8 – 4.0	3.9
Glutamic acid	12.0 – 14.0	12.8	12.9	12.3 – 14.6	13.3
Proline	5.9 – 9.1	7.5	8.2	5.9 – 11.8	9.0
Cystine/2	0.1 – 0.3	0.2	0.2	0.2 – 0.4	0.3
Glycine	4.5 – 5.1	4.8	5.3	4.1 – 4.5	4.3
Alanine	5.5 – 6.3	5.9	6.6	4.8 – 5.6	5.2
Valine	5.6 – 6.6	5.9	6.2	5.0 – 5.5	5.2
Methionine	1.9 – 2.2	2.1	2.2	1.7 – 2.0	1.8
Isoleucine	3.8 – 4.7	4.2	4.4	3.5 – 3.9	3.7
Leucine	5.9 – 6.9	6.4	6.9	5.4 – 5.8	5.6
Tyrosine	2.2 – 2.5	2.3	2.2	1.7 – 2.3	2.1
Phenylalanine	3.5 – 4.2	3.9	4.1	3.3 – 3.6	3.4

[a]Grams amino acid per 100 g amino acid recovered. [b]From Robbins and Pomeranz (1971).

in malting time. This decrease was accompanied by a reduction in the concentration (in the proteins) of lysine, arginine, threonine, serine, glutamic acid, glycine, alanine, isoleucine, leucine, tyrosine, and phenylalanine; concentrations of ammonia and aspartic acid were highest after five days of malting and decreased slightly thereafter. Proline was the only amino acid that accumulated throughout the 11-day malting period.

Jones and Pierce (1967) reported that during the germination of barley the amount of lysine increased over a 6-day period by about 40%. Whitehouse (1970) remarked that an increase of this magnitude is probably more than could be achieved by breeding. However, a varietal survey did not confirm the large increase. There was a small increase in only one out of four varieties. Similarly, the data in Table 19 and analyses of the same grain cultivars from a second crop year (unpublished data) and of their malts and sprouts showed consistent but rather small increases in lysine.

It is interesting to compare changes in distribution of amino acids in malted and maturing cereal grains. Such a comparison for barley, oats, and wheat is given in Table 21. The comparison in Table 21 is an oversimplification, as only two extreme stages in development (or malting) are recorded. During maturation increases were largest in glutamic acid, proline, and cystine; and decreases were largest in alanine, lysine, aspartic acid, and threonine. During malting, the main changes were increases in concentrations of lysine and aspartic acid and a decrease in glutamic acid.

SCORING PROCEDURES

The limited information on genetic variation in the nutritional quality of proteins in cereal crops has been due, in part, to lack of adequate measurement techniques (Johnson et al., 1968). The situation has changed with the availability of reliable and rapid methods to determine amino acid composition. The two most useful methods are the microbiological assay procedures and especially

TABLE 21

Amino Acid Composition of Immature and
Mature Oats, Wheat, and Barley; and Malted Barley

| Amino acid | Oats[b] | | Wheat[c] | | Barley[d] | | Barley[e] | |
	5 days after flowering	Mature	Days preripe 23	0	Days preripe 23	0	Malted for 2 days	11 days
Lysine	7.6	4.2	3.8	2.6	6.9	4.1	3.7	4.6
Histidine	2.1	1.9	2.4	2.3	2.4	2.4	2.4	2.7
Ammonia	3.7	3.0	3.5	3.7	2.8	3.0	3.2	3.0
Arginine	5.0	6.5	4.8	4.1	5.7	5.5	5.1	5.7
Aspartic acid	12.0	9.1	7.1	5.0	9.7	7.4	7.0	8.7
Threonine	4.9	3.3	3.6	3.1	5.1	3.7	3.5	3.8
Serine	4.8	4.7	4.7	4.6	5.3	4.1	4.2	4.1
Glutamic acid	16.2	22.0	27.9	33.8	15.1	23.4	24.6	20.3
Proline	4.7	6.1	8.2	10.0	5.2	10.7	11.3	11.9
Glycine	5.3	4.8	5.3	4.2	5.5	4.5	4.1	4.3
Alanine	7.3	5.0	5.2	3.6	8.4	4.6	4.5	4.5

Cystine/2	0.2	1.3	--	--	0.5	1.4	1.2	1.3
Valine	6.4	6.0	5.2	3.9	6.0	5.5	5.2	5.3
Methionine	1.1	1.5	--	--	2.7	2.4	2.3	2.3
Isoleucine	4.6	4.2	4.1	3.9	4.4	3.8	3.7	3.8
Leucine	7.5	8.0	7.3	6.9	7.5	7.1	6.6	6.7
Tyrosine	3.2	3.7	2.0	2.2	2.8	2.8	2.6	2.4
Phenylalanine	4.0	5.2	4.7	4.8	4.4	5.0	5.1	5.1

[a] Grams amino acid per 100 g amino acid recovered.

[b] Average of primary and secondary groats, except for cystine. Calculated from Brown et al. (1970).

[c] Average of two cultivars. Calculated from Pomeranz et al. (1966).

[d] Average of three cultivars, each, from the 1969 and 1970 crops.

[e] Average of two cultivars. Calculated from Robbins and Pomeranz (1971).

chemical separation and determination by ion-exchange column chromatography (Moore et al., 1958). The use of those methods in scoring
procedures is based on the fact that the biological value of a protein depends on the quantitative content of the component amino
acids.

Protein reserves in cereal grains are usually made of 18
α-amino acids. They, and their symbols, are:

1. Alanine (Ala)	10. *Lysine (Lys)*
2. Aspartic acid (Asp)	11. *Methionine (Met)*
3. <u>Arginine</u> (Arg)	12. *Phenylalanine (Phe)*
4. Cysteine (Cys)	13. Proline (Pro)
5. Glutamic acid (Glu)	14. Serine (Ser)
6. Glycine (Gly)	15. *Threonine (Thr)*
7. <u>Histidine</u> (His)	16. *Tryptophan (Trp)*
8. *Isoleucine (Ile)*	17. Tyrosine (Tyr)
9. *Leucine (Leu)*	18. *Valine (Val)*

Major systematic tables covering surveys of amino acid contents
of foods and feeds were prepared by:

a) The U.S. Department of Agriculture (Orr and Watt, 1957),

b) The Commonwealth Bureau of Animal Nutrition (Harvey,
   1958), and

c) Revised Tables of the Food and Agriculture Organization
   of the United Nations (Rao and Odendaal, 1968).

The data in these compilations were reviewed by Bigwood (1972).

The amino acids Ile, Leu, Lys, Met, Phe, Thr, Trp, and Val
(italicized in above list) are essential in the sense that humans
cannot synthesize them in vivo. They must be present in the diet to
maintain an equilibrated nitrogen balance and to maintain steady
normal growth in infant and growing children. If they are not present in sufficient amounts, the body will lose nitrogen and draw on
its protein reserves and growth will be impeded. His and Arg (underlined above) are synthesized only partly in the body tissues, generally in amounts that are insufficient to maintain a healthy growth.
Cys and Tyr are complementary, respectively, to Met and Phe from

which they are formed and insufficient amounts of the former will
deplete the amounts of the latter.

Several scoring procedures have been recommended as preliminary
screening methods for predicting the limiting amino acid or acids
and the approximate amino acid balance of a food. The procedures
are based on the assumption that all the protein is completely hydrolyzed to free amino acids in the digestive tract and that all
those acids are absorbed by the organism.

The chemical score method of Mitchell and Block (1946) is based
on the assumption that the biological value of a protein depends
only on the limiting essential amino acids. This method does not
take into account whether the amino acids are available and whether
some of them are in excess to the requirements of the organism. In
the Essential Amino Acid Index (EAAI) method of Oser (1951), all
essential amino acids are incorporated in the calculations. Hansen
and Eggum (1973) developed, on the basis of N balance experiments
with rats and amino acid analyses of 221 feedstuffs, a model to
estimate total amino acid value (TAAV) from amino acid composition.
The correlation coefficient between biological value and TAAV for
all feedstuffs was 0.74; that coefficient increased to 0.85 if groups
of related feedstuffs were analyzed.

Nutritional values of the proteins of wheat, oats, buckwheat,
barley, and normal and *opaque-2* corn are compared with an egg
reference pattern in Table 22. The data in Table 22 are based on a
scheme proposed by Kasarda et al (1971). The ratio of essential to
total amino acids (E:T) in all cereals is lower than in the egg
reference pattern. The E:T ratio in eggs is actually twice as high
as would be needed for most efficient use of its essential amino
acids. Consequently, the E:T ratio is of limited value in direct
evaluation of nutritional adequacy. A more meaningful evaluation
can be obtained by calculating the ratio of specific essential amino
acids to the sum of the essential amino acids (A:TE).

A comparison of the A:TE ratio with the egg reference pattern
yields a chemical score which indicates the limiting amino acids;

TABLE 22

Nutritional Values of the Proteins of Several
Cereal Grains Compared with Whole Egg Protein as a Reference

Amino acid	Egg reference pattern[a]	Wheat[a]	Oats[b]	Buckwheat	Barley	Corn[c]	
						Normal	Opaque-2
E:T values[d]	3.22	1.99	2.38	2.41	2.19	2.65	2.54
A:TE values[e]							
Isoleucine	129	122(95)[f]	102(79)[f]	99(77)[f]	105(81)[f]	94(73)[f]	93(72)[f]
Leucine	172	213	194	166	197	328	241
Lysine	125	82(66)	110(88)	158	111(89)	66(53)	116(93)
Tyrosine + phenylalanine	195	243	220	179(92)	208	217	206
Cystine + methionine	107	196	107	106	94(88)	76(71)	81(76)
Threonine	99	93(94)	86(87)	101	97	85(86)	96
Tryptophan	31	41	42[g]	60[g]	40	17(55)[h]	32[h]
Valine	141	150	139	132(94)	148	118(84)	135

[a]From Kasarda et al. (1971).
[b]From Robbins et al. (1971).
[c]From Mertz et al. (1965).
[d]Grams essential amino acids per g to total N.
[e]Milligrams specific amino acid per g of total essential amino acids.
[f]Values in parentheses are A:TE for specific amino acid : A:TE for egg reference pattern X 100.
The lowest value under a commodity shows the first limiting amino acid and gives a chemical score.
[g]From Tkachuk and Irvine (1969).
[h]From Johnson et al. (1970).

the lower the value the more limiting the amino acids. Thus, in wheat, lysine is the first limiting amino acid; the next are threonine and isoleucine. In oats, isoleucine, threonine, and lysine are the first limiting amino acids, though the balance between the essential amino acids is much better than in wheat. Similarly, *opaque-2* is superior to normal corn. In agreement with feeding tests of Sure (1955), the chemical amino acid assays indicate that buckwheat has a better balance and better potential than cereal grains for supplementing foods which are low in lysine.

There is presumptive evidence that concentrations of the essential amino acids of egg protein are higher than concentrations required by man. Isoleucine and methionine are particularly high, and the use of egg as a reference may overestimate the extent to which those amino acids are limiting and may underestimate the quality of a protein for human use. Consequently, the nutritional value of *opaque-2* corn, oat, and buckwheat proteins is probably higher than indicated in the data given in Table 22. On the other hand, as mentioned before, amino acid analyses do not measure one of the most important parameters that determine nutritive value of a food--its digestibility. Chemical scores should be considered primarily as a powerful and convenient screening tool.

A release of the Protein Advisory Group of FAO/WHO/UNICEF (PAG Statement No. 3 on Plant Improvement by Genetic Means, October 10, 1969) states: "The PAG recommends that greater attention be given to the important food staples in developing countries other than maize, wheat, and rice." I hope this review has shown that, at least insofar as chemical scores are concerned, the minor cereals have much to offer as potentially excellent sources of high-quality plant proteins.

WHAT ABOUT THE FUTURE?

Cereal grains are a most valuable commodity since they represent a concentrated store of highly digestible material which is in a dehydrated, prepackaged form; they are easy to handle, transport, and store. As mentioned in the introduction, some nutritionists claim that cereal grain crops can contribute most as efficient producers of concentrated energy and that protein needs can be met best by crop plants (i.e., legumes, oilseeds) which are efficient protein producers. However, both the magnitude of the protein malnutrition problem and the recent discoveries of cereal grains with increased protein content and improved amino acid balance prompt increased research efforts to utilize the potential of cereals to satisfy human protein needs.

Much progress, probably, will be made by the conventional methods of screening world collections for new lines with improved chemical composition and incorporating the desirable traits into presently acceptable cultivars. Several recent reviews and articles discuss some novel and rather unorthodox approaches. At present, some of these are ideas which are somewhat in the realm of science fiction. But today's fiction has the habit of becoming tomorrow's fact (Wareing, 1970).

According to Kamra (1971), the most effective way of altering the amino acid composition of seeds with a high concentration of alcohol-soluble proteins is through mutations which reduce the concentration of synthesized prolamines and at the same time increase synthesis of other protein fractions (preferably albumins plus globulins).

Simple changes in grain morphology could be the basis of selection. The embryo of cereal seeds is rich in protein (up to 38%) and the protein may contain about 7% lysine (Whitehouse, 1970). Selection for larger embryos is particularly important if the whole seed (rather than starchy endosperm) is consumed. Variations in the number of aleurone cells of the endosperm exist in rice and barley. The seed aleurone layer is rich in protein which has a good amino acid balance. Selection for a high aleurone cell number could be useful provided the high number is associated with improved nutritional value. Increasing the relative surface area of the seed

66

could lead to an increase in the aleurone layer. Such an increase results from the otherwise undesirable development of long and thin, very small, or shrunken kernels. Both in wheat and in rice, much of the protein is concentrated in the aleurone and outermost sub-aleurone. These tissues are diverted to feed during milling and polishing rice or during the milling of highly refined wheat flour. "Restructuring" cereal grains to obtain a more even distribution of protein throughout the whole endosperm would increase the protein content of milled products.

The hulls are rich in fibrous materials and low in protein. Many hull-less varieties of barley and oats have substantially more protein than the hulled varieties. However, the low yield of the available hull-less varieties discourages their cultivation.

The problem of protein malnutrition is second only to the total food supply problem (Altschul, 1967). Bearing in mind the relationship between yield and protein content it may be best to concentrate on growing the highest-yield varieties. These varieties could be supplemented by legume or oilseed proteins, as suggested before, or fortified by adding synthetic amino acids. Alternatively, the grain can be pulverized and air-classified into a protein-rich fraction (fortified by synthetic lysine, for human consumption) and a protein-poor fraction (for animal feeding).

The improvement in amino acid balance during malting suggests their uses as food and feed. However, the small changes are associated with losses of carbohydrates as a result of metabolism and the cost of wetting the grain and especially subsequent drying make this approach economically prohibitive.

The amino acid balance of immature grain is superior to that of the mature grain. The protein yield and the total amount of amino acids in the mature grain is much larger than in the unde-veloped grain. The changes which take place in selected amino acids during the development of wheat, oats, buckwheat, and peas are compared in Figure 5. The main proteins of the legumes are globulins. Consequently, the amino acid composition of legume seed proteins is

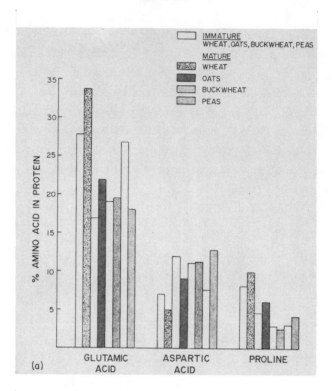

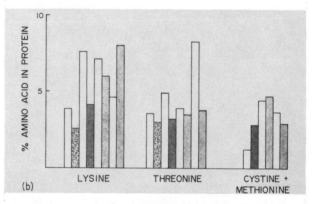

FIG. 5. Amino acids in immature (empty bars) and mature (shaded bars) wheat, oats, buckwheat, and peas.
(a) Glutamic acid, aspartic acid, and proline.
(b) Lysine, threonine, and cystine + methionine.
(c) Valine and tyrosine + phenylalanine.
From Pomeranz et al. (1975).

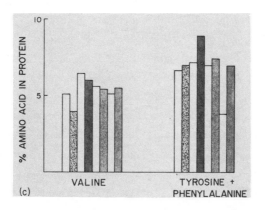

FIG. 5 (cont.)

quite different from those of cereal proteins. If we could continue the high deposition rate of albumins plus globulins throughout the whole grain development cycle, the proteins in the mature grain would have an excellent amino acid balance.

Scientific analysis of crop yields has shown that production of total dry matter and yield of usable crop is lower in cereal grains than in sugar beets, kale, or grass (Wareing, 1970). The material stored in the grain is produced by photosynthesis in only a small part of the total leaf tissue ("flag leaf") during a relatively short period of time (about 6 weeks, from anthesis to maturity). Delaying the senescence of the flag leaf, increasing the supply of assimilates to the ear, or breeding grain in which leaves other than the flag leaf can supply assimilates could increase the yield. More adventurous approaches include improving the photosynthetic rates. In order to accomplish this objective, the rate-limiting processes in photosynthesis under field conditions must be established. Hageman et al. (1967) emphasized that growth and grain yield are the end results of a series of biochemical reactions, each of which is controlled or catalyzed by one or more specific enzymes. Understanding the role of major metabolic enzymes and enzyme systems would enhance the control of producing greater amounts of plant tissue, grain, or specific grain components.

"Genetic engineering," "biochemical genetics," "physiological ecology," and "physiological genetics" were the subject of a thoughtful analysis by Sprague (1969). The significance of recent developments in tissue culture techniques and somatic cell genetics in biochemical genetics was reviewed by Nelson and Burr (1973).

Wareing (1970) lists several recent developments which could have far-reaching effects on plant breeding. They include new methods of chromosome pairing which introduce into cereal grains desirable characteristics of related species, fusion of isolated protoplasts in "vegetative hybridization," production of haploid plants by regeneration from pollen in sterile cultures, and incorporation of foreign DNA into the genome of higher plants. The latter opens the possibility of modifying the plant genome. In line with those findings, Van Overbeek (1969) visualized transferring a block of genetic information from blue-green algae, capable of photosynthetic fixation, to the protoplasts of cereals or putting root nodules on cereal crops so that they can utilize directly atmospheric nitrogen.

Areas which could add significantly to crop productivity are better control of plant pests and diseases; judicious use of plant growth regulators to control crop growth; computerized optimization of such operations as irrigation, fertilizer applications, and harvesting; and better utilization of cereal crops based on recent developments in food science and technology.

I hope that the examples taken from the fascinating review by Wareing (1970) amply demonstrate the many ways in which major contributions can be made to improve productivity of cereal crops. The committee on biological efficiency of the USDA--State Experiment Station Joint Task Force assessed in 1968 the research needs of the small grains for the next ten years and gave this subject its highest priority. The task force recommended:

"The yield, quality, physical traits and other
characteristics of the cereal varieties grown on millions
of U.S.A. acres are the result of a continuing interaction

between the genotype of the plant and its changing total environment; in fact, they are the result of a sequence of biochemical reactions monitored by enzymes, themselves under the control of genes. This whole area of the physiological ecology of the cereals is not well understood; high yielding varieties have been bred without fully understanding why they are superior in performance. For crop scientists to progress in the future it is essential that favorable plant metabolic processes be recognized and used in variety development and crop production.

"Biological efficiency involves a host of important subject areas but the Task Force wishes to stress the need for research on the basic biological processes, morphological traits, response characteristics and genotype--environment interactions in the cereals so that these traits will become as well known and usable in plant improvement as are, for example, genes for height, disease resistance, or stiff straw."

The needs of the hungry world are well recognized; the challenges to meet those needs are great; the scientific possibilities and opportunities are almost unlimited. The question is whether the required scientific talent and resources will be channeled into those high-priority projects to solve the world food problems. If those talents and resources will be organized and made available to solve those problems, many of the "far-out" ideas of today will become tomorrow's reality.

REFERENCES

Altschul, A.M. 1967. Food proteins: new sources from seeds. Science 158:221.

Artemeva, A.E. and N.P. Yarosh. 1972. Biochemical properties of buckwheat grain and productivity of different varieties in Belorussia. Vest. Akad. Navuk Belarus. SSR., Ser. Sel's Kagaspad Navuk 3:61 (Chem. Abstr. 78:28476u).

Biely, J. and Y. Pomeranz. The nutritive value of wild buckwheat in No. 1 wheat feed screenings. (In press).

Bigwood, E.J. 1972. Amino acid patterns of animal and vegetable proteins--common features and diversities. *In* Protein and Amino Acid Function. Pergamon Press, Oxford and New York. Chapter 5, p. 215.

Bishop, L.R. 1928. The composition and quantitative estimation of barley proteins. J. Inst. Brew. 34:101.

Briggle, L.W., R.T. Smith, Y. Pomeranz and G.S. Robbins. Protein content and amino acid composition of *Avena sterilis* L. groats. (In press).

Brown, C.M., E.B. Weber and C.M. Wilson. 1970. Lipid and amino acid composition of developing oats (*Avena sativa* L. cultivar "Brave"). Crop Sci. 10:488.

Campbell, A.R. and K.J. Frey. 1972a. Inheritance of groat protein in interspecific oat crosses. Can. J. Plant Sci. 52:735.

Campbell, A.R. and K.J. Frey. 1972b. Amino acid percentages in the groat protein of oat lines from an interspecific cross. Crop Sci. 12:391.

Carpenter, K.J. 1970. Nutritional considerations in attempts to change the chemical composition of crops. Proc. Nutr. Soc. 29:3.

Clark, W.L. and G.C. Potter. 1971. The composition and nutritional properties of protein from selected oat varieties. Proc. 161st National Meeting Amer. Chem. Soc., Agr. Food Chem. Div., Los Angeles, California. Paper No. 26.

Cluskey, J.E., Y.V. Wu, J.S. Wall and G.E. Inglett. 1973. Oat protein concentrates from a wet-milling process: preparation. Cereal Chem. 50:475.

Coe, W.R. 1931. Buckwheat milling and its by-products. USDA Circ. 190. Washington, D.C.

Danilova, N.N. and B.P. Pleskov. 1968. Amino acid composition of proteins in barley during ripening. DOKL. TSKHA 144:163.

Day, A.D. and A.D. Dickson. 1957. Association between nitrogen percentage and certain morphological characteristics in barley. Agron. J. 49:244.

Eggum, B.O. 1969. Evaluation of protein quality and the development of screening techniques. *In* New Approaches to Breeding for Improved Plant Protein. Panel Proceedings, Joint FAO/IAEA Division of Atomic Energy in Food and Agriculture. STI/PUB/212. International Atomic Energy Agency, Vienna, Austria.

Folkes, B.F. and E.W. Yemm. 1956. Amino acid content of the proteins of barley grain. Biochem. J. 62:4.

Folkes, B.F. and E.W. Yemm. 1958. The respiration of barley plants. X. Respiration and the metabolism of amino acids and proteins in germinating grain. New Phytol. 57:106.

Food and Agriculture Organization, United Nations, Production Yearbook 23. 1969. Rome, Italy.

Foote, W.H. and F.C. Batchelder. 1953. Effect of different rates and times of application of nitrogen fertilizers on the yield of Hannchen barley. Agron. J. 45:532.

Frey, K.J. 1951. The relation between alcohol-soluble and total nitrogen content in oats. Cereal Chem. 28:506.

Frey, K.J. 1952. Variations in the protein and amino acid contents of different oat varieties. Cereal Chem. 29:77.

Frey, K.J. 1973. Improvement of quantity and quality of cereal grain protein. In Alternative Sources of Protein for Animal Production. National Acad. Sci. ISBN 0-309-2114-6. Washington, D.C.

Frey, K.J. and J.A. Browning. 1973a. Registration of E (early) series of isolines of oats as parental lines. Crop Sci. 13:291.

Frey, K.J. and J.A. Browning. 1973b. Registration of M (midseason) series of isolines of oats as parental lines. Crop Sci. 13:291.

Ganyushina, E.V. and V.M. Lazarchik. 1972. Effect of ammonium nitrate on the yield and quality of buckwheat. Vestn. Mosk. Univ. Biol., Pochvoved. 27:95.

Gritton, E.T., Y. Pomeranz and G.S. Robbins. 1975. Protein content and amino acid composition of developing peas. J.Fd.Sci. 50:584.

Hageman, R.H., E.R. Leng and J.W. Dudley. 1967. A biochemical approach to corn breeding. Advan. Agron. 19:45.

Hansen, N.G. and B.O. Eggum. 1973. The biological value of proteins estimated from amino acid analyses. Acta Agr. Scand. 23:247.

Harvey, D. 1958. Tables of the Amino Acids in Foods and Feedingstuffs. Tech. Commun. 19. Commonwealth Bur. Animal Nutr., Rowett Inst. Bucksburn, Aberdeenshire, Scotland (Commonwealth Agr. Bur., Farnham Royal, Slough, Bucks.).

Hischke, H.H., G.C. Potter and W.R. Graham. 1968. Nutritive value of oat protein. I. Varietal differences as measured by amino acid analysis and rat growth responses. Cereal Chem. 45:374.

Howe, E.E., G.R. Jansen and E.W. Gilfillan. 1965. Amino acid supplementation of cereal grains as related to the world food supply. Amer. J. Clin. Nutr. 16:315.

Hughes, B.P. 1960. The composition of foods. Medical Research Council Special Report Series No. 297. HMSO, London, England.

Ingversen, J., B. Koie and H. Doll. 1973. Induced seed protein mutant of barley. Experientia 29:1151.

Ivanko, S. 1971. Changeability of protein fractions and their amino acid composition during maturation of barley grain. Biol. Plant. 13:155.

Jacko, V.P. and B.P. Pleskov. 1968. Studying the proteins of diploid and tetraploid buckwheat by chromatography on tetraethylamino-ethylcellulose and by electrophoresis in polyacrylamide gel. Rep. Timirjazev Agr. Acad. 144:221 (from Plant Breeding Abstr. 39, No. 2203).

Jenkins, G. 1968. Naked oats. NAAS Quarterly Rev. 79:120.

Johnson, V.A., J.W. Schmidt and P.J. Mattern. 1968. Cereal breeding for better protein impact. Econ. Bot. 22:16.

Johnson, V.A., P.J. Mattern and J.W. Schmidt. 1970. The breeding of wheat and maize with improved nutritional value. Proc. Nutr. Soc. 29:20.

Jones, M. and J.S. Pierce. 1967. The role of proline in the amino acid metabolism of germinating barley. J. Inst. Brew. 73:577.

Juliano, B.O., G.M. Bautista, J.C. Lugay and A.C. Reyes. 1964. Rice quality studies on physiochemical properties of rice. J. Agr. Food Chem. 12:131.

Kamra, O.P. 1971. Genetic modification of seed protein quality in cereals and legumes. Z. Pflanzenzucht. 65:293.

Kasarda, D.D., C.C. Nimmo and G.O. Kohler. 1971. Proteins and the amino acid composition of wheat fractions. In Y. Pomeranz (Ed.) Wheat: Chemistry and Technology. Amer. Ass. Cereal Chem., St. Paul, Minnesota.

Kent, N.L. 1966. Technology of Cereals, with Special Reference to Wheat. Pergamon Press, Oxford.

Kent, N.L. 1969. Structural and nutritional properties of cereal proteins. In R.A. Lawrie (Ed.) Proteins as Human Food. Butters-worth, London. p. 280.

Kneen, E. and A.D. Dickson. 1967. Malts and malting. Kirk-Othmer Ency. Chem. Technol. 12:861.

Lykes, A.H. 1970. Grain sorghum in poultry nutrition. Tech. Publ. U.S. Feed Grains Council, 28, Mount Street, London, England.

Lyman, C.M., K.A. Kuiken and F. Hale. 1956. Essential amino acid content of farm feeds. Agr. Food Chem. 4:1008.

Malting Barley Improvement Association. 1971. Malting Barley, Protein Content. Milwaukee, Wisconsin.

Marshall, H.G. 1969. Description and culture of buckwheat. Pennsyl-vania State Univ. Agr. Exp. Station Bull. 754.

McBeath, D.K. and J.A. Toogood. 1960. The effect of nitrogen top-dressing on yield and protein content of nitrogen-deficient cereals. Can. J. Soil Sci. 40:130.

McDaniel, M.E. 1974a. Registration of Tam 0-301 oats. Crop Sci. 14:127.

McDaniel, M.E. 1974b. Registration of Tam 0-302 oats. Crop Sci. 14:128.

McElroy, L.W., D.R. Clandinin, W. Lobay and S.I. Pethybridge. 1949. Nine essential amino acids in pure varieties of wheat, barley, and oats. J. Nutr. 37:329.

Mertz, E.T., O.A. Veron, L.S. Bates and O.E. Nelson. 1965. Growth of rats fed on *opaque-2* maize. Science 148:1741.

Mikaelsen, K. 1972. An erectoides mutant in barley with increased seed protein content. Hereditas 72:201.

Miller, D.F. 1958. Composition of Cereal Grains and Forages. Publ. 585, Nat. Acad. Sci., Nat. Res. Council. Washington, D.C.

Mitchell, H.H. and R.J. Block. 1946. Some relationships between the amino acid contents of proteins and their nutritive value for the rat. J. Biol. Chem. 163:599.

Moore, S., D.H. Spackman and W.H. Stein. 1958. Chromatography of amino acids on sulfonated polystyrene resins. Anal. Chem. 30:1185.

Mosse, J. 1966. Alcohol-soluble proteins of cereal grains. Fed. Proc. 25:1663.

Munck, L. 1971. High lysine barley--a summary of the present research development in Sweden. Barley Genetics Newsletter 2:54.

Munck, L., K.E. Karlsson and A. Hagberg. 1969. Selection and characterization of a high-protein, high-lysine variety from the World Barley Collection. *In* Proc. 2nd Int. Barley Symp. Washington State Univ. Press, Pullman, Washington. p. 544.

Munck, L., K.E. Karlsson, A. Hagberg and B.O. Eggum. 1970. Gene for improved nutritional value in barley seed protein. Science 168:985.

Murphy, H.C., I. Wahl, A. Dinoor, J.D. Miller, D.D. Morey, H.H. Luke, D. Sechler and L. Reyes. 1967. Resistance to crown rust and soilborne mosaic virus in *Avena sterilis*. Plant Disease Rptr. 51:120.

Nelson, O.E. and B. Burr. 1973. Biochemical genetics of higher plants. Ann. Rev. Plant Physiol. 24:494.

News Acad. Sci. Beloruss. S.S.R. 1:133 (from Plant Breeding Abstr. 40, No. 640).

Ohm, H.W. and F.L. Patterson. 1973a. A six-parent diallel cross analysis for protein in *Avena sterilis* L. Crop Sci. 13:27.

Ohm, H.W. and F.L. Patterson. 1973b. Estimation of combining ability, hybrid vigor, and gene action for protein in *Avena* spp. L. Crop Sci. 13:55.

Orr, M.L. and B.K. Watt. 1957. Amino Acid Content of Food. Household Economics Research Div., Inst. Home Economics. Research Dept. No. 4. Agr. Res. Service, U.S. Dept. Agr. Washington, D.C.

Oser, B.L. 1951. Method for integrating essential amino acid content in the nutritional evaluation of protein. J. Amer. Dietetic Ass. 27:396.

Pollock, J.R. 1962. The nature of the malting process. In A.H. Cook (Ed.) Barley and Malt. Academic Press, New York.

Pomeranz, Y. 1973. A review of proteins in barley, oats, and buckwheat. Cereal Sci. Today 18:310.

Pomeranz, Y. and M.M. MacMasters. 1970. Wheat and other cereal grains. Kirk-Othmer Ency. Chem. Technol. 22:253.

Pomeranz, Y. and G.S. Robbins. 1971. Malt sprouts, their composition and use. Brewer's Digest 46(5):58.

Pomeranz, Y. and G.S. Robbins. 1972a. Amino acid composition of buckwheat. J. Agr. Food Chem. 20:270.

Pomeranz, Y. and G.S. Robbins. 1972b. Amino acid composition of maturing barley. Cereal Chem. 49:560.

Pomeranz, Y., K.F. Finney and R.C. Hoseney. 1966. Amino acid composition of maturing wheat. J. Sci. Food Agr. 17:485.

Pomeranz, Y., R.F. Eslick and G.S. Robbins. 1972. Amino acid composition and malting and brewing performance of high-amylose and Hiproly barleys. Cereal Chem. 49:629.

Pomeranz, Y., G.S. Robbins, D.M. Wesenberg, E.A. Hockett and J.T. Gilbertson. 1973a. Amino acid composition of two-rowed and six-rowed barleys. J. Agr. Food Chem. 21:218.

Pomeranz, Y., V.L. Youngs and G.S. Robbins. 1973b. Protein contents and amino acid composition of oat species and tissues. Cereal Chem. 50:702.

Pomeranz, Y., H.G. Marshall, G.S. Robbins and J.T. Gilbertson.1975. Protein content and amino acid composition of maturing buckwheat (Fagopyrum esculentum Möench). Cereal Chem. 52:479.

Pomeranz, Y., G.S. Robbins, R.T. Smith, J.C. Craddock, J.T. Gilbertson and J.G. Moseman. Protein content and amino acid composition of barleys from the world collection. (In press).

Pomeranz, Y., D.M. Wesenberg, G.S. Robbins and J.T. Gilbertson. 1974. Changes in amino acid composition of maturing Hiproly barley. Cereal Chem. Cereal Chem. 51:635.

Pomeranz, Y., H.L. Shands, G.S. Robbins and J.T. Gilbertson. Changes in protein content and amino acid composition in groats and hulls of developing oats (Avena sativa). (Submitted).

PROTEINS AND AMINO ACIDS OF BARLEY, OATS, AND BUCKWHEAT

Rao, K.K. and P.N. Odendaal. 1968. New Revised FAO Tables of Amino Acids Content of Foods and Biological Data on Proteins. Food Consumption and Planning Branch, Nutr. Div., FAO, Rome, NU. IDA/68/1.

Robbins, G.S. and Y. Pomeranz. 1971. Amino acid composition of malted cereals and malt sprouts. Amer. Soc. Brew. Chem. Proc. p. 15.

Robbins, G.S. and Y. Pomeranz. 1972. Composition and utilization of milled barley products. III. Amino acid composition. Cereal Chem. 49:240.

Robbins, G.S., Y. Pomeranz and L.W. Briggle. 1971. Amino acid composition of oat groats. J. Agr. Food Chem. 19:536.

Sedova, E.V. and V.V. Bazhanova. 1971. Amino acid composition of the protein fractions of oat grains. DOKL. TSKHA 162:212 (Chem. Abstr. 75:85163b).

Sedova, E.V. and B.P. Pleskov. 1968. Changes of fractional and amino acid composition of oat grain protein in the course of maturation. Izv. Timiryazev. Sel'skokhoz. Akad. 105 (Chem. Abstr. 70:26366).

Sokolov, O.A. and F.V. Semikhov. 1968. Protein complex of polygonum seeds dependent on ploidy and nutrition conditions. In F.E. Reiners (Ed.) Fiz. Biokhim, Sorta, Tr. Konf. Fiziol. Biokhim. Rast. Sib. Dalnego Vostoka (Chem. Abstr. 74:22196y).

Sprague, G.F. 1969. Germ plasm manipulations of the future. Physiol. Aspects Crop Yield. 16:375.

Standridge, N.N., E.D. Goplin and Y. Pomeranz. 1970. Evaluation of 2-row and 6-row malting barley. Brewer's Digest 45(12):58.

Sure, B. 1955. Protein quality and supplementation. Nutritive value of proteins in buckwheat and their role as supplements to proteins in cereal grains. J. Agr. Food Chem. 3:793.

Thielebein, M. 1969. The world's protein situation and crop improvement. In New Approaches to Breeding for Improved Plant Protein. Panel Proceedings, Joint FAO/IAEA Division of Atomic Energy in Food and Agriculture. STI/PUB/212, 306. International Atomic Energy Agency, Vienna, Austria.

Tkachuk, R. and G.N. Irvine. 1969. Amino acid composition of cereals and oilseed meals. Cereal Chem. 46:206.

Van Overbeek, J. 1969. What botanists can do. All-Congress Symposium on World Food Supply. Int. Bot. Congress, Seattle, Washington.

Viuf, B.T. 1969. Breeding of barley varieties with high-protein content with respect to quality. In New Approaches to Breeding for Improved Plant Protein. Panel Proceedings, Joint FAO/IAEA Division of Atomic Energy in Food and Agriculture. STI/PUB/212, 23. International Atomic Energy Agency, Vienna, Austria.

Wareing, P.F. 1970. Plant science and food production. Adv. Science 27:1.

Watt, B.K. and A.L. Merrill. 1963. Composition of Foods, Agr. Handbook No. 8. USDA, Washington, D.C.

Weber, E.B., J.P. Thomas, R. Reder, A.M. Schlehuber and D.A. Benton. 1957. Protein quality of oat varieties. J. Agr. Food Chem. 5:926.

White, W.C. and C.A. Black. 1954. Wilcox's agrobiology. III. The universal yield--nitrogen ratio. Agron. J. 46:310.

Whitehouse, R.N.H. 1970. The prospects of breeding barley, wheat and oats to meet special requirements in human and animal nutrition. Proc. Nutr. Soc. 29:31.

Whitehouse, R.N.H. 1973. The potential of cereal grain crops for protein production. In J.G.W. Jones (Ed.) The Biological Efficiency of Protein Production. Cambridge University Press.

Wiggans, S.C. and K.J. Frey. 1958. The ratio of alcohol soluble to total nitrogen in developing oat seeds. Cereal Chem. 35:235.

Winton, A.L. and K.B. Winton. 1945. The Analysis of Foods. Wiley, New York.

Woodham, A.A. 1973. The effect of nitrogen fertilization on the amino acid composition and nutritive value of cereals. Qual. Plant. 23:281.

Wu, Y.V. and A.C. Stringfellow. 1973. Protein concentrates from oat flours by air classification of normal and high-protein varieties. Cereal Chem. 50:489.

Wu, Y.V., K.R. Sexson, J.F. Cavins and G.E. Inglett. 1972. Oats and their dry-milled fractions: protein isolation and properties of four varieties. J. Agr. Food Chem. 20:757.

Wu, Y.V., J.E. Cluskey, J.S. Wall and G.E. Inglett. 1973. Oat protein concentrates from a wet-milling process: composition and properties. Cereal Chem. 50:481.

Wyld, M.K., R.L. Squibb and N.S. Scrimshaw. 1958. Buckwheat as a supplement to all-vegetable protein diets. Food Res. 23:407.

Youngs, V.L. 1972. Protein distribution in the oat kernel. Cereal Chem. 49:407.

Zebrak, E.A., N.M. Kolcin and Yu K. Nikolskij. 1966. Amino acid spectrum in seeds of diploid and tetraploid buckwheat. News Acad. Sci. Beloruss. S.S.R. 1:133 (from Plant Breeding Abstr. 40, No. 640).

3

NUTRITIONAL EVALUATION OF HIGH LYSINE BARLEY FED TO PIGS

S. O. S. Thomke and Birgit Widströmer
Department of Animal Husbandry
Agricultural University
Uppsala, Sweden

By screening the world barley collection at the Swedish Seed
Association, Svalöv, on protein quality, high protein and high protein quality (HPHPQ) barley types have been selected. HPHPQ barley
is characterized by an increase in crude protein (CP) content of up
to 50% and a significant increase in essential amino acids (AA)
(lysine 30%) compared with Swedish standard cultivars. The report
gives the results from feeding HPHPQ barley (original Hiproly and
primary crossings) to pigs. Two years HPHPQ material was tested at
suboptimal CP levels to piglets (10-18 kg) and to growing-finishing
pigs (20-90 kg) to evaluate its nutritive value. The determinations
of biological value (BV), net protein utilization (NPU), true digestibility of CP and essential AA to piglets showed a significant
superiority of HPHPQ barley compared with standard cultivars.
According to difference calculations the nitrogen free extract (NFE)
digestibility coefficients were significantly lower for HPHPQ, which
agrees with results on growing-finishing pigs. Comparing primary
crossings with conventional barley to growing-finishing pigs resulted
in significantly ($P < 0.01$) better average daily gains, feed efficiency ratios, and carcass quality. Results indicate that by using
HPHPQ barley considerable parts of the protein supplements may be
saved. The experiments showed significantly higher digestibility
coefficients for CP but unexpectedly lower for NFE.

INTRODUCTION

Cereal protein plays an important role as a protein source in, for instance, pig production. Thus, under Scandinavian conditions, the cereal part of barley-based diets supplies at least 60% of the required amount of limiting amino acids. Improvement in the quality of cereal protein will reduce the need for supplementary protein, as has been experimentally demonstrated with opaque-maize. The work of Mertz et al. (1964) on maize has stimulated the research on increasing protein quality of other cereals and is now in progress at many laboratories (Whitehouse, 1973; Eggum, 1973a). At the Swedish Seed Association, Svalöv, work is concentrated on barley. After screening investigations on 2,500 barley varieties (Hagberg and Karlsson, 1969; Munck et al., 1969), tests with a selected number of barleys on rats and mice confirmed the analytical results that had suggested improved protein quality in Hiproly, a barley type with high protein and high lysine contents (Munck, 1972). There are only a few reports on the nutritional evaluation of high lysine barley. According to Newman et al. (1974), the cultivar Hiproly gave higher PER values with rats, but a lower "apparent biological value." However, the latter was probably a result of systematic differences in feed intake.

Results obtained in experiments with laboratory animals cannot be directly transferred to farm animals. The final evaluation must take place with the species to which the cereal is to be fed. In such investigations not only the protein quality is of interest but also the energy value, since in maize, for instance, it has been shown that high lysine mutants may influence the endosperm structure. The objective of the present work was to use piglets and growing-finishing pigs in tests of the protein quality in high lysine barleys [high protein and high protein quality (HPHPQ) barley] which were chosen with regard to their protein content, AA pattern, and results of experiments with rats and mice. Evaluation of the barleys in the piglet experiments was by means of metabolic studies with determinations of the digestibility of the barley and different parameters of the protein quality. With growing-finishing pigs the feasibility of

HIGH LYSINE BARLEY FOR PIGS

using HPHPQ barley in place of normal barley plus soybean oilmeal (SBOM) was studied. The digestibility of the diets was also determined in these experiments.

MATERIALS

Barleys

Apart from Hiproly the material consisted of two-rowed spring barleys grown in 1972 and 1973. In the former year the material was grown in one place (L = Linköping), in the latter year at two places (S and H = Svalöv and Hammenhög, respectively). In all comparisons the reference used was Ingrid, a cultivar with moderate protein content under Swedish conditions. A total of 4 HPHPQ and 3 reference barleys were tested (Table 1).

TABLE 1
Identification of Barleys

Barley	Growing locale & season	Identifi- cation	Used in experiment no. with
Ingrid	Linköping 1972	IL 72	1 & 3, piglets and growing pigs, respectively
Hiproly	Linköping 1972	HiL 72	1, piglets
Primary crossing	Linköping 1972	PrL 72	1 & 3, piglets and growing pigs, respectively
Ingrid	Svalöv 1973	IS 73	2 & 4, piglets and growing pigs, respectively
Primary crossing	Svalöv 1973	PrS 73	2 & 4, piglets and growing pigs, respectively
Ingrid	Hammenhög 1973	IH 73	2, piglets
Advanced primary crossing	Hammenhög 1973	AdvPrH 73	2, piglets

The 1972 material consisted of Ingrid (IL 72) and two HPHPQ
varieties, namely, the original Hiproly (Cl 3947 in the world list;
here denoted HiL 72) described by Hagberg and Karlsson (1969) and
Munck et al. (1969), and a primary crossing of Hiproly and a selection of the Swedish cultivar Pallas (PrL 72), all grown at L. In
1973 the primary crossing was grown at S with the designation PrS 73.
Genetically more advanced material of primary recrossing type based
on Hiproly x Mona was grown at H and became denoted AdvPrH 73.

In 1972 the barleys were grown at L (58°N) and in 1973 in the
southernmost part of Sweden (56°N) under field conditions; the N
fertilization was in 1972 and 1973, 42 and 70 kg/ha, respectively.
As it was intended that the HPHPQ varieties should give a maximum
seed multiplication rate, lower seed rates (50%) were used in relation to Ingrid. Consequently it was not possible to obtain comparable
yield figures. It was estimated that HiL 72 gave 25-30% of the yield
for IL 72. AdvPrH 73 yielded ca. 90% of that of IH 73 (Persson, personal communication). The 1000-kernel weights of the HPHPQ varieties
tended to be somewhat lower (and consequently the crude fiber content
somewhat higher) than in Ingrid.

The chemical composition of the barleys is given in Table 2.
Apart from differences in the crude protein content--Kjeldahl N x
6.25--the starch content between normal and HPHPQ barleys also was
different. The latter are to some extent caused by differences in
the CP content. Barley HiL 72 had a lower content of crude fiber
owing to the lower husk percentage. Despite the higher CP content of
the HPHPQ barleys these show a favorable AA pattern, in concordance
with the description mentioned earlier. The AA content, on a percentage basis, indicates that the HPHPQ material is considerably
superior to normal type barleys and is intermediate to those of the
parental cultivars.

Large differences were noticed in the time taken to grind the
various batches of barley (hammer mill, 4-mm screen). Ingrid barley was fairly easy to grind. The kernel hardness was determined
by the amount worn off by abrasion milling 20-g samples for 2 minutes

TABLE 2

Chemical Composition and Other Data of Barleys

Item Barley:	IL 72	HiL 72	PrL 72	IS 73	PrS 73	IH 73	AdvPr H 73
Dry matter, %	88.2	87.6	88.8	89.5	90.9	89.7	88.9
Crude protein, %DM	13.1	19.4	15.7	10.8	14.6	16.1	17.1
Ether extract, %DM	5.1	4.7	4.7	2.1	2.4	2.3	2.2
Crude fiber, %DM	5.0	3.8	5.8	4.0	4.6	4.2	4.5
Crude carbo-hydrates, %DM	79.3	73.2	76.6	84.6	80.2	79.1	78.0
Starch, %DM	58.5	48.9	50.9	61.4	54.3	55.9	52.4
Ash, %DM	2.5	2.7	3.0	2.5	2.8	2.5	2.7
1000-kernel wt, g	41	47	39	40	36	43	39
Germination %	98	68	91	85	97	95	96
Abrasion %	36	--	30	42	31	36	29
Amino acids, g/16 g N							
Lys	3.9	3.7	4.2	3.8	4.3	3.4	4.0
His	2.2	2.0	2.2	2.1	2.2	2.0	2.2
Arg	5.3	4.9	5.1	5.2	5.1	4.7	5.0
Asp	6.3	6.1	6.6	6.5	6.9	6.0	6.3
Thr	4.0	3.9	3.4	3.4	3.6	3.3	3.5
Ser	4.4	4.3	4.3	4.2	4.7	4.5	4.8
Glu	24.3	23.4	23.3	20.9	22.5	24.6	24.0
Pro	11.4	12.5	10.8	10.2	10.6	12.1	11.8
Gly	4.2	4.0	4.0	4.1	4.2	3.9	3.9
Ala	4.1	4.1	4.4	4.0	4.6	3.9	4.4
Cys	2.4	2.0	1.9	2.6	2.0	2.5	1.9
Val	5.1	5.0	5.3	5.0	5.5	4.9	5.3
Met	1.6	1.6	1.8	1.6	1.8	1.5	1.7
Ile	3.6	3.9	3.8	3.2	3.7	3.4	3.7
Leu	7.2	7.2	7.1	7.0	7.5	7.1	7.4
Tyr	3.5	3.5	3.3	3.1	3.2	3.2	3.1
Phe	5.0	5.5	5.5	4.8	5.5	5.3	5.8
Trp	1.1	1.2	1.2	1.2	1.4	1.2	1.3

in a Scott-Strong Seedburo mill. The amount worn off is defined as
the abrasion percentage. The results (Table 2) show that the HPHPQ
batches were characterized throughout by a lower abrasion percentage
than the reference barley and that there is a relationship between
the abrasion percentage and the starch content of barleys (r = +0.95).

Other Feedstuffs

Maize starch with a CP content of less than 0.2% was used in
the piglet experiments. The cellulose preparation contained 80%
crude fiber. The ingredients were otherwise of commercial grade,
as in the growing pig experiments.

Animals

Two litters of Swedish Landrace from a health-controlled herd
were used in the piglet experiments. The litter in trial 1 comprised
5 barrows and 3 gilts; that in trial 2 comprised 4 animals of each
sex. They had been weaned at ca. 5 weeks and the experiments started
about a week later when the animals had become accustomed to the
experimental conditions. They then weighed about 10 kg and at the
end of the experiments 17 kg in trial 1 and 18 kg in trial 2. Only
gilts were used in the growing-finishing pig experiments, as they
have a higher protein requirement. Trials 3 and 4 each comprised
5 litters of four individuals taken from health-controlled herds and
were distributed evenly between the four treatments.

METHODS

Feeds, feces, and urine were analyzed according to official
methods. Kjeldahl-N was determined on fresh samples of feces and
urine. Crude fat was determined in feces by petroleum ether extraction following acid hydrolysis in order to include the saponi-
fied fraction of fecal fat. Determinations of AA were made according to Stein and Moore by ion exchange chromatography with a Beckman
automatic amino acid analyzer. Metabolizable energy was determined

HIGH LYSINE BARLEY FOR PIGS

by bomb calorimetry of feed, feces, and urine.

Piglet Experiments

The experiments with piglets were largely conducted according to the method described by Eggum (1973b). Corrections for metabolic N and AA in feces and endogenous N in urine were also calculated according to this author. The piglets were individually kept in metabolism cages which enabled the separate quantitative collection of feces and urine.

Trial 1 comprised three twelve-day periods and trial 2 four periods of fourteen days. For three and five days, respectively, at the start of each period, the piglets were given a starter ration containing 16% protein feeds in order to improve their nutrient status prior to the subsequent feeding with isonitrogenous barley diets. Following this initial period the animals were fed the experimental diets for 9 days. The collections were undertaken the last four days.

Each treatment embraced 8 individuals. The animals were allocated to different treatments period-wise. Trial 1 comprised 24 and trial 2 32 separate metabolic experiments. One of the animals in trial 1 was rejected and thus the number of replicates per treatment became 7 as opposed to 8 in trial 2.

The composition of the formulas is given in Table 3. The diets were composed to be isonitrogenous at 1.5% N. The differences in the CP contents of the barleys were balanced by additions of maize starch and sucrose.

The amount of air dry feed was adjusted to 4% of the live weight at the beginning of each period. The animals were fed twice a day and water was supplied together with the dry feed in the ratio 2:1. No feed was rejected. Feces and urine were collected at least twice a day and were stored at +4°C.

Growing-Finishing Pigs

Trials 3 and 4 were conducted as production experiments with

TABLE 3

Piglet Experiments 1 and 2:
Ingredients and Chemical Composition of Diets

Item	Expt:	1			2			
	Barley:	IL 72	HiL 72	PrL 72	IS 73	PrS 73	IH 73	AdvPr H 73
Ingredients, %								
Barley		72.1	48.8	58.6	91.3	70.5	64.7	61.7
Maize starch		14.0	32.3	24.1	--	20.8	26.6	29.6
Sucrose		4.7	10.1	8.1	3.0	3.0	3.0	3.0
Vegetable oil		3.0	3.0	3.0	2.0	2.0	2.0	2.0
Cellulose powder		4.0	4.0	4.0	0.7	0.7	0.7	0.7
Minerals and vitamins[a]		2.2	2.2	2.2	3.0	3.0	3.0	3.0
Chemical analyses, %DM								
Crude protein		9.7	9.2	9.2	9.9	10.4	10.4	10.4
Ether extract		5.1	4.7	4.9	4.1	4.0	3.8	3.6
Ash		4.1	3.5	3.9	5.7	5.3	5.0	5.0

[a]According to Eggum (1973b).

control of weight gain, feed efficiency ratio, carcass quality and
with the determination of the digestibility. The compositions
of the diets are given in Table 6. The protein supplements A and B
in trial 3 was only 2%. The feed composition in treatments D and H
corresponds to that used in practice and are positive controls. The
diet analyses show that the feed-mixture with HPHPQ barley gave the
same lysine content per kg feed as the reference barley supplemented
with 5.2% SBOM. This means that at corresponding production results
of the two treatments the use of HPHPQ barley could save 5.2% SBOM.

The same composition of diets was used from the start of the
experiments until the animals were slaughtered. The energy intensity from the start was somewhat lower than the one earlier used
(Thomke, 1972) in order to avoid feed rejects owing to the relatively

limited amount of protein. During the latter half of trial 3 and
for all trial 4 the energy level was increased to the weight standard given in the above publication.

The animals were housed individually. Wood shavings were used
as bedding. The pigs weighed 22-23 kg at the start of the experiments. Trial 3 ended when the pigs weighed about 93 kg. An acci-
dent forced the termination of trial 4 at the end of the digestibility experiment when the pigs weighed 55 kg. Consequently, the
latter trial only covers a gain of 32 kg and lacks the carcass
evaluation. The carcass evaluation in trial 3 was conducted according to a standard procedure (Thomke, 1972).

In trials 3 and 4 the digestibility of the diets was determined
according to the Cr_2O_3 technique. A given amount of the marker was
daily mixed into the feed for 14 days. Feces were collected during
the last 5 days. At termination all samples for each individual
were homogenized. Organic matter and CP were determined on each
sample while crude fat and fiber were determined only on a pooled
sample for each treatment. Consequently, individual observations
are lacking for the other nutrients.

RESULTS

Piglets (Trials 1 and 2)

The true digestibility (TD) of the protein was higher (Tables
4 and 5) for the barleys containing higher levels of CP. Significant differences (P < 0.001) in BV were found between the barleys
in trial 1, owing to the HPHPQ variety PrL 72 differing from IL 72.
Despite the former's higher CP content compared with the reference
barley (IL 72) its BV was also found to be higher. HiL 72 was
characterized by a somewhat lower BV than the primary crossing,
which is explained by its very high CP content. The 1973 barleys
showed highly significant differences between growing localities,
primarily an effect of the large differences in CP contents. By
considering the general effect of the barleys' N content on the

TABLE 4

Piglet Experiment 1:
True Digestibility (TD), Biological Value (BV),
Net Protein Utilization (NPU) of Crude Protein,
Utilizable Nitrogen (UN), True Digestibility of Some
Amino Acids (AA), and Digestibility of Nutrients in the Barleys

Item	Barley: IL 72	HiL 72	PrL 72	F-values	$LSD_{0.05}$
No. of observations	7	7	7		
TD	78.0	82.0	81.8	4.5^b	3.7
BV	55.4	57.9	60.6	4.7^b	4.3
NPU	43.0	47.5	49.6	7.7^c	4.4
UN, %DM	0.90	1.47	1.40	81.6^d	0.12
Digestibility of AA[a]					
Lys	62	69	73	13.6^c	6.8
Arg	84	85	87	3.2	3.6
Thr	71	76	74	2.4	6.2
Glu	89	91	91	11.9^c	1.7
Met	74	78	80	5.8^b	5.7
Cys	82	81	81	5.2^b	1.5
Ile	71	78	78	13.0^c	4.7
Trp	71	76	77	7.3^b	5.0
Digestibility of nutrients					
Organic matter	86.3	87.8	84.2	1.0	6.4
NFE	90.8	87.9	86.4	6.9^c	3.0
Crude carbohydrates	88.9	92.6	86.4	1.6	8.8
Mcal ME/kg DM	3.14	3.21	3.08	1.1	0.22

[a]AA determinations carried out for each treatment on 3-4 pooled feces samples, each from two individuals.

[b]$p < 0.05$.

[c]$p < 0.01$.

[d]$p < 0.001$.

TABLE 5

Piglet Experiment 2:
True Digestibility (TD), Biological Value (BV),
Net Protein Utilization (NPU) of Crude Protein,
Utilizable Nitrogen (UN), True Digestibility of Some
Amino Acids (AA), and Digestibility of Nutrients in the Barleys

Item	Barley				Analyses of variance			
	IS 73	PrS 73	IH 73	AdvPr H 73	Simple F-values	LSD 0.05	2-fact., F-values between	
							I-Pr	Locales
No. of observations	8	8	8	8				
TD	73.6	75.4	76.9	78.0	1.7	5.7	1.1	4.1
BV	71.6	70.7	59.2	66.1	20.4^d	4.8	5.8^b	45.7^d
NPU	52.6	53.2	45.5	51.6	9.0^c	4.6	8.0^c	13.8^d
UN, %DM	0.91	1.24	1.17	1.41	53.8^d	0.11	10.4^d	57.1^d
Digestibility of AA[a]								
Lys	54	61	55	61	0.9	14.8	2.8	0.0
Arg	80	83	81	81	1.1	6.3	1.4	0.4
Thr	66	69	70	69	0.4	11.2	0.2	0.5
Glu	86	87	90	89	2.2	4.6	0.0	5.5^b
Met	70	75	73	74	0.7	10.7	1.3	0.3
Cys	85	81	86	81	4.6^b	4.5	13.4^c	0.3
Ile	67	72	73	74	1.6	10.5	1.7	2.6
Trp	73	75	74	78	1.2	6.9	2.7	1.0
Digestibility of nutrients								
Organic matter	83.2	79.2	82.0	80.5	6.5^c	2.6	16.4^d	0.1
NFE	89.9	86.2	88.9	86.8	19.4^d	1.5	54.5^d	0.0
Crude carbohydrates	86.0	81.3	84.9	82.2	17.0^d	2.1	48.0^d	0.2
Mcal ME/ kg DM	3.27	2.99	3.13	3.11	7.2^c	0.13	13.8^d	1.1

[a]AA determinations carried out for each treatment on 4 pooled feces samples, each from two individuals.

[b]$p < 0.05$.　　　[c]$p < 0.01$.　　　[d]$p < 0.001$.

protein quality, the superiority of the HPHPQ over the reference barley is even more pronounced. The net protein utilization (NPU = TD x BV) of the HPHPQ varieties significantly differed in trial 1 (P < 0.05) and trial 2 (P < 0.01) from Ingrid in favor of the former type. Finally, utilizable N (UN = NPU x CP, exclusively an index of quantity) shows a clear superiority (20-35%) for HPHPQ varieties in relation to the reference barley.

The true digestibility of AA was determined, despite awareness of the limitations of the method used. The results for some AA are given in Tables 4 and 5. It is interesting to note that in both trials some of the limiting AA in the HPHPQ varieties were digested better than in Ingrid. This fact partly explains the higher BV in the former barleys. For cystine, however, the availability was significantly lower for HPHPQ barleys in both trials.

The digestibility of the other nutrients in the barleys was determined by difference calculations. In contrast to the high digestibility of CP, lower digestibility values throughout were found for organic matter, NFE, and crude carbohydrates in the HPHPQ varieties. This phenomenon is supported by a high degree of significance in trial 2 (P < 0.001). This also influences the barleys' content of metabolizable energy. Figure 1 demonstrates the relationships between the barleys' content of different carbohydrate fractions, abrasion percentage, and digestibility of organic matter. The lines are only drawn for auxiliary purpose.

Growing-Finishing Pigs (Trials 3 and 4)

The experimental design is given in Table 6. The results of trial 3 are given in Table 7. Daily weight gains and feed efficiency ratios show that diet A with HPHPQ barley gave results comparable with the combination of standard barley plus 5.2% SBOM (C), i.e., supplementation with SBOM to the same level of limiting AA. Significantly poorer results (P < 0.01) were obtained when the reference barley was used without the SBOM supplement. The high protein supply in diet D gave the best results, as expected. The carcass evaluations

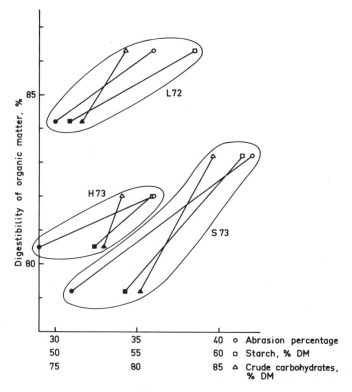

FIG. 1. Relationships between the barleys' content of starch and crude carbohydrates and abrasion percentage on one side and the digestibility of organic matter on the other, Trials 1 and 2. Open marks = HPHPQ barleys; filled marks = reference barley.

also suggest that diets A and C gave similar production results. In trial 4 the figures for gain and feed efficiency ratio are uncertain because of the shortness of the experimental period. The figures indicate, however, a clear superiority of PrS 73 over IS 73.

The figures in Table 8 refer to the digestibility of the entire diets. Apart from the barley, the alterations in composition between A and C in trial 3 and between E and G in trial 4 are relatively small and cannot explain the effects observed concerning the digestibility of the crude carbohydrates. The poorer digestibility of carbohydrates observed in the piglet experiment (2-4 percent units in

TABLE 6

Growing Pig Experiments 3 and 4:
Ingredients and Chemical Composition of Diets

| Experiment: | | 3 | | | | 4 | | |
Item / Diet:	A	B	C	D	E	F	G	H
Ingredients, %								
Ingrid (IS 72)	--	95.1	89.9	88.1	--	--	--	--
Ingrid (IS 73)	--	--	--	--	--	92.2	89.3	88.1
Primary crossing (PrS 72)	95.1	--	--	--	--	--	--	--
Primary crossing (PrS 73)	--	--	--	--	95.1	--	--	--
Protein concentrate[a]	2.0	2.0	2.0	10.0	2.0	2.0	2.0	10.0
Soybean oilmeal	--	--	5.2	--	--	2.9	5.8	--
NaCl	0.4	0.4	0.4	0.4	0.4	0.4	0.4	0.4
Ca-Carbonate	0.8	0.8	0.8	0.5	0.8	0.8	0.8	0.5
Di-Ca-Phosphate	0.7	0.7	0.7	--	0.7	0.7	0.7	--
Vitamins[b]	1.0	1.0	1.0	1.0	1.0	1.0	1.0	1.0

Chemical analyses[c]

Crude protein, %	14.8	12.6	14.5	16.7	13.9	11.5	12.6	15.5
Mcal ME/kg (calcd)[d]	2.90	2.92	2.92	2.98	2.96	2.94	2.94	3.01
Ash, %	4.8	4.5	4.7	4.8	5.5	4.7	4.4	4.0
Lys, g/kg	6.7	5.3	6.9	8.2	6.2	5.3	6.1	7.8
Met + Cys, g/kg	5.7	5.4	5.8	6.7	5.2	4.5	4.9	5.6
Thr, g/kg	5.6	4.7	5.8	6.7	5.1	4.2	4.6	6.0
Trp, g/kg	1.9	1.5	1.9	1.8	1.9	1.5	1.6	1.9

[a]Fish meal 70%, SBM 30%.

[b]Vitamins and trace minerals, see Thomke (1972).

[c]Air dry basis.

[d]Calculated according to Eriksson et al. (1972).

TABLE 7

Growing Pig Experiment 3:
Growth Rates, Feed Efficiency Ratios, and Carcass Measurements

Item	Diet: A	B	C	D	F-values	$LSD_{0.05}$
Number of animals	5	5	5	5		
Initial weight, kg	23.3	23.4	23.4	23.1		
Average daily gain, g	523	461	497	538	7.3^c	51
Mcal ME/kg w.g.	10.3	12.1	10.8	10.3	5.9^c	1.4
Fat measurements, mm						
Mean, back	24.8	28.3	23.2	23.8	4.2^b	4.5
Mid back	13.0	17.6	12.0	12.0	6.4^c	4.3
Slight of lean	21.0	28.0	20.4	19.0	9.6^d	5.3
Meatiness score[a]	13.8	11.9	13.7	14.7	7.5^c	1.7
Eye muscle area, cm^2	31.1	27.6	29.7	33.2	1.9	7.0
Density of hind quarter	1.048	1.040	1.049	1.051	9.5^d	0.006

[a]High value = increasing leanness.

[b]$P < 0.05$.

[c]$P < 0.01$.

[d]$P < 0.001$.

TABLE 8

Growing Pig Experiments 3 and 4:
Digestibility of Nutrients in the Diets

Experiment: 3

Item Diet:	A	B	C	D	F-values	$LSD_{0.05}$
No. of observations	5	5	5	5		
Organic matter	77.6	79.6	80.0	80.7	13.8[b]	1.6
Crude protein	69.8	65.2	69.5	74.0	8.3[a]	3.4
NFE	86.6	88.8	89.0	89.7		
Crude carbohydrates	81.2	84.2	84.1	84.8		

Experiment: 4

Item Diet:	E	F	G	H	F-values	$LSD_{0.05}$
No. of observations	5	5	5	5		
Organic matter	78.8	81.1	82.1	81.2	10.1[b]	1.8
Crude protein	73.4	68.2	71.7	69.6	6.9[a]	3.5
NFE	86.3	89.2	90.3	89.3		
Crude carbohydrates	81.0	84.8	85.6	84.9		

[a] $p < 0.01$.
[b] $p < 0.001$.

the HPHPQ material) is also confirmed in these trials with 50-kg animals. Certain conclusions may also be drawn concerning the CP digestibility. The results fully confirm the observation made in the piglet experiments that the CP in the HPHPQ diets had a better digestibility than in the diets based on the reference barley.

DISCUSSION

Evaluation of the barley protein quality in piglet experiments was shown to be valuable since these results correlate well with the growing-finishing pig trials. The determination of a cereal's nutritive value with piglets is also advantageous with regard to the relatively limited amount of material required.

The HPHPQ barleys showed throughout higher N digestibility, BV, NPU, and UN than the reference barley. The higher protein quality is most likely dependent on the more favorable AA pattern of the barley protein and to an improved availability of certain limiting AA. The higher digestibility of the protein appears to be a result of the increased protein content of the HPHPQ barleys being localized in subaleurone cells in the form of protein bodies (Munck, 1972).

It is well known that the protein quality of barley decreases with increased N content. For normal type barley this has been demonstrated under Scandinavian conditions by, among others, Eggum (1970) and Thomke (1970). Similar changes in HPHPQ material were reported by Munck (1972). The quality of different types of barley should be compared at the same protein content. At present there is no suitable base for the correction of BV for barley with varying N contents to pigs. As there appears to be a fairly good relationship for BV between pigs and rats (Eggum, 1973b) it might be justified to base a correction procedure on experiments with rats. With reference to the investigations of Eggum (1970) and Schiller and Oslage (1970) the following values are obtained (Table 9). After a correction has been made a more marked difference appears, favoring the HPHPQ material.

TABLE 9

Comparison of Biological Values (BV) for Barley

Item	CP mean % DM	Biological value (BV)		
		Obtained	After correction according to	
			Eggum (1970)	Schiller and Oslage (1970)
Regression coefficient of BV on CP of barley			1.04	2.23
IL 72	14.4	55.4	54.0	52.5
PrL 72		60.6	62.0	63.5
IL 73	12.7	71.6	69.6	67.4
PrS 73		70.7	72.7	74.9
IH 73	16.6	59.2	58.7	58.1
AdvPrH 73		66.1	66.6	67.2

The barleys tested here have also been evaluated on other animal species. The results of rat experiments performed by Eggum (personal communication) are given in Table 10. These results are in good agreement with the present observations on piglets and confirm that HPHPQ barleys have a higher protein quality and a lower energy value than the reference barley. In Denmark Madsen et al. (1973) tested PrL 72 and PrS 73 on growing-finishing pigs in a rather more extensive trial than ours. Results of these experiments also confirm that HPHPQ barley can save about 5% SBOM. HPHPQ barley has been tested on broilers by Elwinger (to be published). These experiments again suggest that this type of barley allows marked savings of protein supplements when fed to broilers.

In the calculations of carbohydrate digestibility in the piglet experiments it was assumed that added maize starch and sucrose were digested to 100%. This assumption is based on investigations by Eggum (1973b) and is indirectly confirmed by the present experiments where significant differences in the digestibility of carbohydrates were observed despite approximately similar contents of

TABLE 10

Nutritional Evaluation of Barleys Using Rats[a]

Item	Barley:	IL 72	HiL 72	PrL 72	IS 73	PrS 73	IH 73	AdvPrH 73
TD		86.8	88.0	87.4	84.0	87.8	89.5	89.2
BV		72.7	79.9	81.6	76.9	81.7	73.7	75.3
NPU		63.1	70.3	71.3	64.6	71.7	66.0	67.2
UN, %DM		1.33	2.18	1.75	1.12	1.68	1.70	1.84
Digestibility of energy		--	--	--	79.3	76.5	80.6	78.9

[a]Carried out by Eggum, 1973-1974 (personal communication).

maize starch in the diets (IH 73 as opposed to Adv PrH 73). The digestibility values for barley nutrients calculated according to the difference technique seem, therefore, to be reliable.

In both the trials with piglets and those with growing pigs a lower digestibility was noted for organic matter in HPHPQ barleys than in the reference barley, despite significantly higher digestibility of CP. Small systematic differences in the crude fiber content could be noticed between HPHPQ and reference barley which must have influenced the digestibility of nutrients. The present results, however, cannot fully be explained by the differences in the crude fiber content. The HPHPQ barleys were characterized by a starch content varying between 66 and 68% of the crude carbohydrate content while the variation for Ingrid barley was 71-74%. The HPHPQ varieties thus had both a lower absolute starch content and a decrease in the proportion of starch in the crude carbohydrates. It is assumed that this resulted in a decrease in the digestibility of the carbohydrates. It is interesting to note that this effect was not only limited to 15-kg piglets but was also found in 50-kg growing-finishing pigs.

Macroscopically, none of the tested HPHPQ varieties differed from the reference barley. However, there were considerable differences in milling properties, manifested in lower abrasion values in

HPHPQ barley. Information is lacking on the existence of a general relationship between abrasability of barley and the digestibility of organic matter and whether this only applies to HPHPQ barleys.

The results motivate further work with HPHPQ barley and a widening of the scope of the investigations to include larger production trials permitting economic comparisons. Future work should also be directed at explaining, and if possible, eliminating the reasons for the poorer digestibility of carbohydrates. A feasibile approach in this work might be genetical control, as pointed out by Whitehouse (1970).

NOTES

The different experiments have been performed at the Department of Animal Husbandry by Claes-Göran Claesson, Anders Malm, and Margareta Rundgren in qualifying for their degrees. Economical support has been provided by the Swedish Council for Forestry and Agricultural Research.

REFERENCES

Eggum, B. 1970. Über die Abhängigkeit der Proteinqualität vom Stickstoffgehalt der Gerste. Z. Tierphysiol., Tierernährg. u. Futtermittelkde. 26:65.

Eggum, B. 1973a. Kornarternes värdi som proteinkilde. Tolvmandsbladet 45:2:2.

Eggum, B. 1973b. A study of certain factors influencing protein utilization in rats and pigs. Landhusholdningsselskabets forlag, Copenhagen. 173 pp.

Eriksson, S., S. Sanne and S. Thomke. 1972. Fodermedlen, LT:s förlag, LTK. Boras. 296 pp.

Hagberg, A. and K.E. Karlsson. 1969. Breeding for high protein and quality in barley. In New Approaches to Breeding for Improved Plant Protein. IAEA/FAO, STJ/PUB 212, Vienna. p. 23.

Madsen, A., H.P. Mortensen, A.E. Larsen and B.T. Viuf. 1973. Byg med forskelligt proteinindhold og proteinkvalitet. Landøkonomisk Forsøgslaboratoriums efterarsmøde, Arbog, p. 75.

Mertz, E.T., L.S. Bates and O.E. Nelson. 1964. Mutant gene that changes protein composition and increases lysine content of maize endosperm. Science 145:279.

Munck, L. 1972. Improvement of nutritional value in cereals. Hereditas 72:1.

Munck, L., K.E. Karlsson and A. Hagberg. 1969. High nutritional value in cereal protein. J. Swed. Seed Ass. 79:194.

Newman, C.W., R.F. Eslick and R.C. Rasmuson. 1974. Effect of barley variety on protein quality and nutritional value for rats. J. Animal Sci. 38:1:71.

Schiller, K. and H.J. Oslage. 1970. Untersuchungen über die Variabilität von Futtergerstenprotein. 1. Mitt. Über den Einfluss ökologischer Faktoren auf den Proteingehalt in Gersten und dessen ernährungsphysiologische Qualität. Lantwirtsch. Forsch. 23:317.

Thomke, S. 1970. Über die Veränderung des Aminosäurengehaltes der Gerste mit steigendem Stickstoffgehalt. Z. Tierphysiol., Tierernährg. u. Futtermittelkde. 27:23.

Thomke, S. 1972. Über den Futterwert von Gerste für Mastschweine. 3. Mitt. Schätzung der Wertes von Mehrprotein. Z. Tierphysiol., Tierernährg. u. Futtermittelkde. 28:148.

Viuf, B.T. 1972. Varietal differences in nitrogen content and protein quality in barley. Kgl. Vet. Landbohojs. Arskrift. p. 37.

Whitehouse, R.N.H. 1970. The prospects of breeding barley, wheat oats to meet special requirements in human and animal nutrition. Proc. Nutr. Soc. 29:31.

Whitehouse, R.N.H. 1973. The potential of cereal grain crops for protein production. In J.G.W. Jones (Ed.) The Biological Efficiency of Protein Production. Cambridge University Press. p. 83.

4

NUTRITIONAL QUALITY OF RICE ENDOSPERM

B. M. Kennedy

Department of Nutritional Sciences
University of California at Berkeley

Starch in 12 lots of milled rice subjected to abrasive milling was least concentrated in the perifery of the kernel, 54 to 65%, and increased toward the center which contained 93%. All other constituents studied--protein, fat, ash, seven minerals, four vitamins, and phytic acid--were most concentrated in the outer portion of the kernel and decreased in concentration as the center was approached. The steepness of the gradient, however, varied greatly with the different constituents. The most evenly distributed was sodium for which the concentration in the outer 2% of the kernel was 150% that of the original rice and in the residual kernel (88% of the whole), 70%, while phytic acid concentration in the perifery was 23 times that of the whole kernel with only a trace in the residual.

INTRODUCTION

That the various parts of food plants differ in chemical composition is well known. The unequal distribution of nutrients was recognized as early as 1900-1911 when it was first suggested that beriberi was a nutritional disease produced by the consumption of rice from which the outer layers had been removed by milling (Hinton and Shaw, 1953).

Although much information is available concerning the content of nutrients in the various anatomical parts of seed kernels--particularly the endosperm, bran, and germ, e.g. wheat and rice (MacMasters et al., 1971; Juliano, 1966), much less has been reported on the distribution within the endosperm which constitutes from 80 to 90% of the edible kernel.

For rice, one of the major cereal grains of the world, only scant data were published before 1960. Subrahmanyan and Sreenivasan (1938) noted that both nitrogen and phosphorus progressively decreased as more of the polishings were removed. Hinton (1948) reported differences of vitamin B_1, by a micro-thiochrome method, in two fractions of endosperm obtained by hand dissection from a white variety of rice. One fraction containing the outer layers comprised 18.8% of the original kernel, the other containing the inner portion, 73.1%. Values for the outer endosperm were 4.5 times as great as for the inner portion, 0.45 international units (i.u.) per gram as compared with 0.10 i.u. Later Hinton and Shaw (1953) published data on the distribution of nicotinic acid determined by microbiological assay also on hand dissected samples. The inner endosperm in each of two samples of rice contained 3.7 μg nicotinic acid per gram while the outer portion, about 6% of the whole endosperm, contained 93.8 μg in one sample and 87.0 in the other. Thus the concentration in the outer layers averaged 24 times as great as that of the inner layers so that about two-thirds of the nicotinic acid of the endosperm was found in the outer 6%.

Microscopic studies

In addition to vitamins this concentration of nutrients in the outer portions of the endosperm was reported for protein and fat using histological techniques. Little and Dawson (1960) published excellent photographs of stained sections of rice kernels. They observed that protein was most concentrated in the peripheral-lateral and peripheral-ventral cells where starch granules were fewest, was least concentrated in peripheral-dorsal cells, and was often rather sparse in central, dorsal, and ventral cells. They also noted that protein material lined endosperm cell walls and encased all starch granules and that starch granules were fewest in lateral and ventral peripheral cells, forming tiny clusters well separated by the surrounding dense protein material. Numerous fatty globules appeared in appropriately treated sections and their position suggested that fats occur in combination with the proteins.

This uneven distribution of protein has since been confirmed by the electron-micrograph studies of protein bodies in rice endosperm by Mitsuda et al. (1967) and with photomicrographs of histological sections by Del Rosario et al. (1968).

Abrasive milling

About the same time the removal of successive peripheral layers of rice by abrasive milling, using experimental mills as well as existing commercial machinery, made possible the quantification of a number of constituents (Primo et al., 1963; Hogan et al., 1964; Houston et al., 1964). In these and later works the distribution of protein was studied the most extensively, but fat and ash were included in several reports (Casas et al., 1963; Hogan et al., 1968; Houston et al., 1964; Houston, 1967; Normand et al., 1966) while starch, sugars, fiber, B-vitamins, amylases, phosphorus, calcium and amino acid composition of the protein were each included in one or in two studies (Barber et al., 1967; Hogan et al., 1968; Normand et al., 1966; Houston, 1967; Houston et al., 1964, 1969). In most reports data were presented only for one or two varieties of rice. These studies showed that the concentration of the constituent, except for the starch, was greatest in the peripheral layers and decreased as the center of the kernel was approached (Barber, 1972). The concentration of starch, however, was least in the periphery and increased toward the center.

Because of the limited information on many of the constituents and of the small number of varieties of rice analyzed, we undertook a comprehensive study of several different lots of commercially milled rice which we submitted to further milling. The concentrations of about twenty different constituents were determined in each of the milled samples.

EXPERIMENTAL

Approximately a half ton each of 12 different lots of commercially milled rice was obtained (Kennedy et al., 1974). Included in these were six varieties, two each of long-, medium-, and short-grain rices, and two of parboiled. Each lot was passed three times through a Japanese rice polishing machine (CeCoCo), removing with each pass 3 to 4% of the outer portion of the kernel as a coarse flour. When sieved, from 50 to 75% of the flour passed through a 40-mesh sieve. Thus seven samples were obtained from each lot: the original kernel, the coarse and the fine portions of the flours from each of the three milling passes, and the residual kernel. Concentrations of moisture, protein, ash, fat, starch, amylose, phytic acid, calcium, phosphorus, sodium, potassium, iron, magnesium, silicon, thiamine, riboflavin, niacin, and pyridoxine, and amino acid composition of the protein were determined on all samples except the flours over 40-mesh. For the latter, moisture, protein, fat, and ash only were determined in six lots. Biological evaluation of the proteins, physical properties storage stability, cooking characteristics and acceptability of the flours and residual kernel were also studied.

RESULTS AND DISCUSSION

Protein

In agreement with previous work (Primo et al., 1963; Houston et al., 1964, 1967; Normand et al., 1966; Hogan et al., 1964, 1968), protein content was highest in the peripheral layers of the rice and decreased toward the center of the kernel (Table 1). Values

TABLE 1

Protein Content of Original Kernel and Milled
Samples of 12 Lots of White Rice[a]

Sample	Protein[b]	Ratio with Respect to Original Kernel[b]
	(% of dry matter)	
Original kernel	7.5 + 1.3	1.00
First-pass flour	14.5 + 2.7	1.92 + 0.15
Second-pass flour	14.0 + 3.0	1.84 + 0.15
Third-pass flour	13.2 + 3.1	1.74 + 0.17
Residual kernel	7.0 + 1.1	0.93 + 0.03

[a]Kennedy et al., 1974.

[b]Mean and standard deviation.

for the first-, second-, and third-pass flours progressively decreased in all lots except for one lot of Belle Patna. For this
rice, values of 20.0 and 19.5% protein for the second- and third-
pass flours were slightly higher than for the first-pass, 19.2%.
Houston et al. (1968) found that both albumins and globulins were
concentrated in proteins at the surface of the rices, and concentrations decreased toward the kernel center.

Long-grain varieties with the highest protein content, 10% of
the dry matter, yielded first-pass flours which were also highest
in protein--18 to 19%, nearly twice that of the original rice--
while a medium-grain Calrose with a much lower percent protein,
6.0%, gave a first-pass flour with only 10.9% protein, the lowest
for the 12 lots studied. Variation was greatest among the lots
for the third-pass flours but very small for the residual kernels.

Considerable variation in values among lots was observed for
all of the constituents, including protein. Such variation has
been reported by other investigators (Juliano, 1973). In the normal

milling of rice the amount of aleurone, sub-aleurone layers and scutellum retained will vary. Thus, since commercially milled rice was used as the starting material this, as well as genetic and environmental factors, will affect the quantity of nutrients in the milled grain.

Amino Acid Composition and Biological Evaluation of the Protein

The amino acid composition of the protein in the various milling samples of any particular lot of rice was remarkably uniform (Table 2). Differences for any given amino acid were greater

TABLE 2

Amino Acids in Samples from the Overmilling of Milled Rice[a]

Amino Acid	Mean[b] St. Dev.	Amino Acid	Mean[b] St. Dev.
	g a.a./16g N		g a.a./16g N
Lysine	3.9 + 0.2	Alanine	5.6 + 0.2
Histidine	2.7 + 0.1	Cystine	1.7 + 0.2
Arginine	9.4 + 0.2	Valine	5.8 + 0.3
Aspartic acid	9.2 + 0.4	Methionine	2.2 + 0.3
Threonine	3.5 + 0.2	Isoleucine	4.1 + 0.3
Serine	5.1 + 0.2	Leucine	8.2 + 0.3
Glutamic acid	18.0 + 0.8	Tyrosine	5.2 + 0.3
Proline	4.7 + 0.4	Phenylalanine	5.1 + 0.2
Glycine	4.6 + 0.3	Tryptophan	1.7 + 0.3

[a]Kennedy and Schelstraete, 1974.

[b]Sixty samples; five samples, original and residual kernels and first-, second-, and third-pass flours, from each of 12 lots of rice.

among lots than among milling samples of the same lot. The greatest varietal differences were found in tryptophan, methionine, and cystine where the differences between the highest and lowest values in the original kernel were 73, 61, and 31%, respectively (Kennedy and Schelstraete, 1974).

This similarity in amino acid composition of proteins within the rice endosperm agrees well with results of biological evaluation. Average protein efficiency ratio (PER, grams gain in body weight per gram protein intake) with standard deviation for 12 test diets containing rice protein from first-pass flours, when adjusted to casein at 2.5, was 2.10 ± 0.20 for a 14-day experimental period (Kennedy and Schelstraete, 1974). For Bluebonnet 50 the average PER for the original and residual kernels and three flours was 2.00 ± 0.10 and for Colusa, 1.90 ± 0.15.

Starch

Starch was the only constituent studied for which, as compared with the original rice, the content was lower in the flours, increased toward the center of the kernel and was highest in the residual kernel (Table 3, Figure 1). There was relatively little variation among the six lots analyzed.

Amylose content showed a similar trend and averaged 25% of the total starch with only small differences among the milled samples. Amylose content of the two long-grain varieties, both 31%, was higher than for the others, 18 to 24%.

Fat

The petroleum-ether extract for the 12 lots of rice averaged 0.49% in the original rices and 7.5% in the first-pass flours, 17 times as much (Table 3, Figure 1). Residual kernels contained only 0.1 to 0.2% fat.

TABLE 3

Proximate Composition of Samples from the Overmilling of Milled Rice[a]

Constituent	Rices No.	Whole Kernel	Flour Through 40-Mesh Screen			Residual Kernel
			First Pass	Second Pass	Third Pass	
			Mean and standard deviation, % dry basis			
Starch	6	91.9 ± 1.3	60 ± 3	71 ± 7	82 ± 3	93.2 ± 0.6
Amylose	6	24 ± 5	15 ± 5	18 ± 4	20 ± 5	24 ± 7
Ash	10	0.54 ± 0.13	4.8 ± 2.3	2.7 ± 1.4	1.8 ± 1.2	0.30 ± 0.05
	2[b]	0.76 ± 0.05	5.8 ± 0.9	3.7 ± 0	2.3 ± 0	0.60 ± 0.05
Fat	12	0.49 ± 0.23	7.5 ± 2.9	4.4 ± 2.1	2.6 ± 1.4	0.12 ± 0.06
Phytic acid	6	0.13 ± 0.02	3.0 ± 0.8	1.7 ± 0.5	1.0 ± 0.4	0

[a]Kennedy et al., 1974.

[b]Parboiled rices.

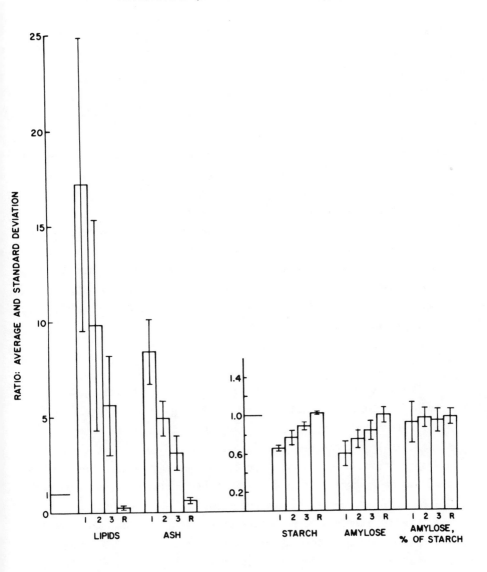

FIG. 1. Average and standard deviation of the ratios of the concentration of constituents in flours through 40-mesh and in residual kernel, with respect to that of the original whole-kernel milled rice. Ash and fat from 12 lots of rice; starch and amylose from six lots. 1, first-pass flour; 2, second-pass flour; 3, third-pass flour; R, residual kernel after third milling pass. (Kennedy et al., 1974).

Minerals and Phytic Acid

In the original kernel as well as the milled samples, the
concentration of mineral elements relative to each other was
similar, that is, phosphorus and potassium, the highest; silicon,
lowest (Table 4). Silicon, the third highest in concentration in
the original rice and the flours, was among the lowest in the residual kernel while the calcium concentration in the residual kernel
*was the third highest. Sodium was the most evenly distributed in
the kernel while iron had the steepest gradient of the mineral
elements analyzed (Figure 2).

Phytic acid was highly concentrated in the first-pass flour,
an average of 3.0%, 23 times as much as in the original rice which
contained 0.13%. The gradient from the periphery to the center of
the kernel was the steepest of any of the constituents studied
(Figures 1 and 2). Only traces of phytic acid could be detected
in the residual kernel.

Vitamins

The distribution of B-vitamins in the endosperm followed the
trend of the other constituents (Table 5, Figure 3). Concentrations were highest in the first-pass flour, 14 times as much as
the original untreated rice for niacin, eight times for thiamine
and pyridoxine, and five for riboflavin, decreasing from the periphery to the interior. Riboflavin was the vitamin most evenly
distributed throughout, niacin the least.

For the two lots of parboiled rice, riboflavin concentration
was essentially the same as for the untreated rices while the
gradient for thiamine was much less than in the untreated. The
highest concentration of niacin, however, was found in the second-
pass flour. Concentration in the first-pass flour averaged 7.5
times that of the original rice while in the second-pass flour,
about 17 times. The steaming process may have released free niacin
from the bound form so that it could diffuse into the inner layer.

TABLE 4

Mineral Content of Samples from the Overmilling of Milled Rice[a]

Mineral	Rices No.	Whole Kernel	Flour Through 40-Mesh Screen			Residual Kernel
			First Pass	Second Pass	Third Pass	
		Mean and standard deviation, mg per 100 g, dry basis				
Phosphorus	6	126 ± 26	1,103 ± 294	670 ± 174	422 ± 134	81 ± 16
Potassium	6	128 ± 36	764 ± 207	451 ± 88	310 ± 80	80 ± 28
Silicon[b]	6	46 ± 30	642 ± 651	323 ± 438	166 ± 315	4 ± 2
Magnesium	6	28 ± 21	297 ± 150	198 ± 140	123 ± 109	8 ± 5
Calcium	6	25 ± 8	168 ± 109	74 ± 41	54 ± 26	17 ± 6
Sodium	6	8.1 ± 2.2	12 ± 4	10 ± 3	8 ± 3	6 ± 2
Iron	12	0.6 ± 0.4	12 ± 6	7 ± 5	5 ± 5	0.2 ± 0.1

[a]Kennedy and Schelstraete, 1975.

[b]Unpublished data.

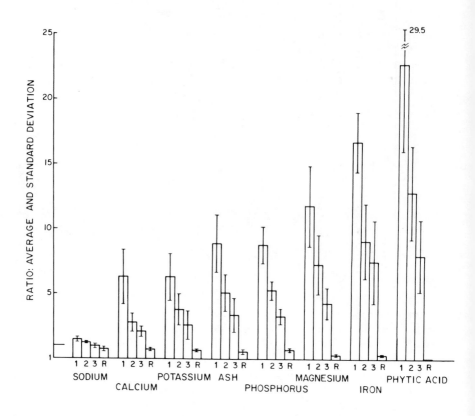

FIG. 2. Ratio and standard deviation of contents of sodium, calcium, potassium, ash, phosphorus, magnesium, iron, and phytic acid in flours and residual kernel of six varieties of rice, with respect to those of the original whole-kernel milled rice: 1, first-pass flour; 2, second-pass flour; 3, third-pass flour; R, residual kernel. For iron, $n = 5$. (Kennedy and Schelstraete, 1975.)

TABLE 5

B-Vitamin Content of Samples from the Overmilling of Milled Rice[a]

Vitamin	Rices No.	Whole Kernel	Flour Through 40-Mesh Screen			Residual Kernel
			First Pass	Second Pass	Third Pass	
Niacin	10	1.5 ± 0.6	20 ± 7	10 ± 5	6 ± 3	0.7 ± 0.3
	2[b]	3.2 ± 0.1	24 ± 1	56 ± 0.4	10 ± 1	2.1 ± 0.2
Pyridoxine	6	0.14 ± 0.02	1.08 ± 0.16	0.74 ± 0.15	0.53 ± 0.13	0.09 ± 0.02
Thiamine	8	0.13 ± 0.03	0.89 ± 0.33	0.56 ± 0.21	0.42 ± 0.21	0.07 ± 0.04
Riboflavin	8	0.041 ± 0.004	0.20 ± 0.04	0.14 ± 0.03	0.10 ± 0.03	0.032 ± 0.002

[a]Kennedy et al., 1975.

[b]Parboiled rices.

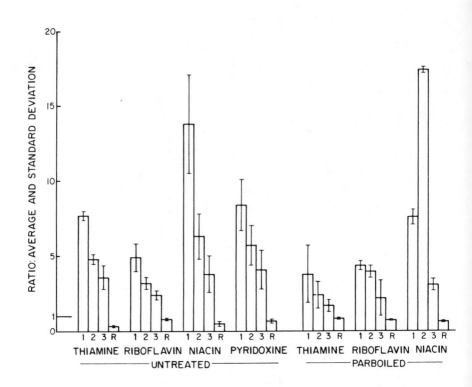

FIG. 3. Ratio, with respect to the original whole-kernel milled rice, and standard deviation of contents of thiamine, riboflavin, and niacin in flours and residual kernel in six varieties of untreated rice and in two varieties of parboiled rice, and of pyridoxine in six varieties of rice;1, first-pass flour; 2, second-pass flour; 3, third-pass flour; R, residual kernel. (Kennedy et al., 1975.)

NUTRITIONAL QUALITY OF RICE ENDOSPERM

Other Constituents

In our studies the sum of the protein, fat, starch, ash, and phytic acid for milling samples of six lots of rice averaged 100 ± 1%, except for the first- and second-pass flours which averaged 91 and 94% respectively.

A few analyses of substances not included in our work have been made by other investigators. Barber et al. (1967) reported 2.9% total sugars in the outer 5% of a milled rice which had 0.4% sugar in the whole kernel and 0.2% in the residual. Houston (1967) found about 3% fiber in the outer 3% of the kernel in two lots of rice for which the original rices had 0.4 to 0.5% fiber and the residual, 0.2 to 0.3%. Although only small amounts of sugar and fiber occurred in the original and residual kernels, their concentration in the outer portions is considerable, together about 6%. It is probable that other minor constituents might also be concentrated in the outer layers.

CONCLUSIONS

Our work, as well as that of previous investigators, shows that the distribution of constituents throughout the endosperm is far from uniform. Although the trend, except for starch, is for a high concentration in the outer portion of the kernel decreasing toward the center, the degree of concentration varies widely. As compared with the whole kernel, the outer 2% contained about twice as much protein but 23 times as much phytic acid. While the residual kernel, 88% of the original rice, had 95% as much protein as did the whole kernel, it contained only a trace of phytic acid.

The relatively high concentration of protein in the outer portions of the rice kernel has attractive possibilities for the use of the high-protein flours. Associated with the doubling of the protein, as compared with that of the whole kernel, are the increases in fat, B-vitamins, and minerals and these outer portions have been considered for use as an infant weaning food, particularly in rice-eating areas. However, due to the high content of silicon and phytic acid, bioavailability of the minerals should be determined to ensure proper mineral nutrition.

REFERENCES

Barber, S. 1972. Milled rice and changes during aging. *In* Rice, Chemistry and Technology, D. F. Houston (Editor). American Association of Cereal Chemists, Inc., St. Paul, Minnesota.

Barber, S., C. Benedito de Barber, J. L. Guardiola y J. Alberola. 1967. Composicion quimica del arroz. IV. Distribucion de los azucares en el grano elaborado. Rev. Agroquim. Tecnol. Alimentos. 7(3): 346.

Casas, A., S. Barber and P. Castillo. 1963. Factores de calidad del arroz. X. Distribucion de grasa en el endospermo. Rev. Agroquim. Tecnol. Alimentos. 3(3): 241.

Del Rosario, A. R., V. P. Briones, A. J. Vidal and B. O. Juliano. 1968. Composition and endosperm structure of developing and mature rice kernel. Cereal Chem. 45: 225.

Hinton, J. J. C. 1948. The distribution of vitamin B_1 in the rice grain. Brit. J. Nutr. 2: 237.

Hinton, J. J. C. and B. Shaw. 1953. The distribution of nicotinic acid in the rice grain. Brit. J. Nutr. 8: 65.

Hogan, J. T., H. J. Deobald, F. L. Normand, H. H. Mottern, L. Lynn and J. W. Hunnell. 1968. Production of high-protein rice flour. Rice J. 71(11): 5.

Hogan, J. T., F. L. Normand and H. J. Deobald. 1964. Method for removal of successive surface layers from brown and milled rice. Rice J. 67(4): 27.

Houston, D. F. 1967. High-protein flour can be made from all types of milled rice. Rice J. 70(9): 12.

Houston, D. F., M. E. Allis and G. O. Kohler. 1969. Amino acid composition of rice and rice by-products. Cereal Chem. 46: 527.

Houston, D. F., T. Iwasaki, A. Mohammad and L. Chen. 1968. Radial distribution of protein by solubility classes in the milled rice kernel. J. Agr. Food Chem. 16: 720.

Houston, D. F., and G. O. Kohler. 1970. Nutritional Properties of Rice. National Research Council, National Academy of Sciences.

Houston, D. F., A. Mohammad, T. Wasserman and E. B. Kester. 1964. High-protein rice flours. Cereal Chem. 41: 514.

Juliano, B. O. 1966. Physicochemical Data on the Rice Grain.

Intern. Rice Res. Inst. Tech. Bull. No. 6. Los Banos, Laguna, Philippines.

Juliano, B. O., A. A. Antonio and B. V. Esmama. 1973. Effects of protein content on the distribution and properties of rice protein. J. Soc. Food Agric. 24: 295.

Kennedy, B. M. and M. Schelstraete. 1974. Chemical, physical, and nutritional properties of high-protein flours and residual kernel from the overmilling of uncoated milled rice. II. Amino acid composition and biological evaluation of the protein. Cereal Chem. 51: 448.

Kennedy, B. M. and M. Schelstraete. 1975. Chemical, physical, and nutritional properties of high-protein flours and residual kernel from the overmilling of uncoated milled rice. III. Iron, calcium, magnesium, phosphorus, sodium, potassium, and phytic acid. Cereal Chem. 52: 173.

Kennedy, B. M., M. Schelstraete, and A. R. Del Rosario. 1974. Chemical, physical, and nutritional properties of high-protein flours and residual kernel from the overmilling of uncoated milled rice. I. Milling procedure and protein, fat, ash, amylose, and starch content. Cereal Chem. 51: 435.

Kennedy, B. M., M. Schelstraete and K. Tamai. 1975. Chemical, physical, and nutritional properties of high-protein flours and residual kernel from the overmilling of uncoated milled rice. IV. Thiamine, riboflavin, niacin, and pyridoxine. Cereal Chem. 52: 182.

Little, R. R. and E. H. Dawson. 1960. Histology and histochemistry of raw and cooked rice kernels. Food Res. 25: 611.

MacMasters, M. M., J. J. C. Hinton and D. Bradbury. 1971. Microscopic structure and composition of the wheat kernel. In Wheat, Chemistry and Technology, 2nd Edition, Y. Pomeranz (Editor). American Association of Cereal Chemists, Inc., St. Paul, Minnesota.

Mitsuda, H., K. Yasumoto, K. Murakami, T. Kusano, and H. Kishida. 1967. Studies on the proteinaceous subcellular particles in rice endosperm: Electron-microscopy and isolation. Agr. Biol. Chem. (Tokyo) 31: 293.

Normand, F. L., D. M. Soignet, J.T. Hogan and H. J. Deobald. 1966. Content of certain nutrients and amino acids pattern in high-protein rice flour. Rice J. 69(9): 13.

Primo, E., A. Casas, S. Barber y C. Benedito de Barber. 1963. Factores de calidad del arroz. IV. Distribucion del nitrogeno en el endospermo. Rev. Agroquim. Tecnol. Alimentos 3(1): 22.

Subrahmanyan, V., A. Sreenivasan and H. P. Das Gupta. 1938. Studies on quality in rice. I. Effect of milling on the chemical composition and commercial qualities of raw and parboiled rices. Indian J. Agric. Sci. 8(4): 459.

5

PULSE PROTEINS

Horace K. Burr

Western Regional Research Laboratory
U.S. Department of Agriculture
Berkeley, California

Pulses, the dry edible seeds of various leguminous plants, are
used for human food throughout most of the world. The principal
species belong to the genera *Phaseolus*, *Pisum*, *Cicer*, and *Vicia*.
Compared to the cereal grains, pulses are relatively rich in protein, most containing from 20 to 25%. However, the quality of the
proteins is only fair because they are deficient in the sulfur-
containing amino acids, methionine and cystine. Furthermore, their
digestibility is somewhat limited since not all their nitrogen is
absorbed from the intestine into the bloodstream. Supplementation
of pulses with methionine and the use of pulses in a mixed diet
containing animal or cereal proteins improves their protein quality.
Raw pulses may contain a wide variety of toxic substances but most
of these are destroyed by the heat of ordinary cooking or are
generally present in too small quantities to cause adverse effects.
Excessive cooking, on the other hand, reduces the biological quality
of the protein. Long storage of common beans at high moisture
contents and temperatures lowers their value as a source of dietary
protein. The observed wide genetic variability in yield, protein
and methionine content will hopefully enable plant breeders to develop improved varieties that will help alleviate protein undernutri-
tion.

PRODUCTION

   Pulses, the dry, edible seeds of various species of leguminous plants, are an important source of dietary protein in many parts of the world. Table 1 shows world production of different pulses on a total and *per capita* basis. The oilseed pulses, such as soybeans (*Glycine max*) and peanuts (*Arachis hypogea*), are not included in these figures. A substantial part of the world-wide peanut crop is crushed for oil and the protein-rich presscake is used in most countries for animal feed or for fertilizer. Similarly, about two-thirds of all soybeans are grown in the United States and of those not exported nearly all the protein-containing fraction

TABLE 1

World and Per Capita Production of Non-Oilseed Pulses, 1972[a]

Type	Production	
	10^6 Metric Tons	Grams Per Capita
Dry beans (*Phaseolus spp.*)	10.90	2900
Dry peas (*Pisum sativum, P. arvense*)	10.22	2720
Chick-peas (*Cicer arietinum*)	6.72	1790
Dry Broad beans (*Vicia faba*)	5.33	1420
Vetch (*Vicia sativa*)	2.04	540
Pigeon peas (*Cajanus spp.*)	1.72	460
Cow peas (*Vigna sinensis*)	1.26	340
Lentils (*Lens esculenta*)	1.18	310
Lupines (*Lupinus spp.*)	0.75	200
Other Non-Oilseed Pulses	3.57	950
Total	43.69	11,630

[a]Based on data in FAO/UN (1973).

goes into non-food uses. In the countries of eastern Asia, on the other hand, soybeans are used almost entirely for human food either directly or as fermented or unfermented products.

Table 2 gives the *per capita* production of non-oilseed pulses in a number of countries where such production is high. China and the United States are included for comparison. It must be emphasized that these figures do not necessarily reflect human consumption in a given country. This may be augmented by imports or decreased by exports, storage losses, and the use of pulses for

TABLE 2

Per Capita Production and Principal Types of Non-Oilseed Pulses in Selected Countries, 1972[a]

Country	Principal Genera	Production kg/capita
U.S.S.R.	*Pisum, Vicia, Lupinus*	28.7
Brazil	*Phaseolus*	25.1
Honduras	*Phaseolus*	21.4
Mexico	*Phaseolus, Cicer*	20.7
India	*Cicer, Cajanus, Phaseolus*	18.9
Turkey	*Cicer, Vicia, Phaseolus*	17.4
Paraguay	*Phaseolus, Pisum*	16.7
Ecuador	*Phaseolus, Pisum*	14.6
Greece	*Phaseolus, Vicia, Cicer*	14.0
China	*Pisum, Vicia, Phaseolus*	10.4
U.S.A.	*Phaseolus, Pisum, Lens*	4.8

[a]Based on data in FAO/UN (1973).

animal feeding. The type of pulses produced varies widely from country to country. For example, Brazil and Honduras grow common beans almost exclusively, while two-thirds of the pulses grown in the U.S.S.R. are dry peas, vetches and lupines making up most of the remainder.

From Table 1 we can estimate that production of non-oilseed pulse protein amounts to between 7 and 8 grams *per capita* per day worldwide. This is based on a figure of 23% as the average protein content of the principal pulses. In the U.S.S.R. pulses could provide nearly 24 grams of protein *per capita*. These figures may be compared with the U.S. Recommended Daily Allowance (U.S. RDA) of 65 grams for "proteins in general."

NUTRITIONAL QUALITY

The nutritional quality of a food protein depends in large measure on the relative proportions of the essential amino acids it contains. The pattern of essential amino acids for a given food can then be compared against that for a reference protein to arrive at a "chemical score" based on the most limiting amino acid. In many cases this score will approximate the Biological Value (BV) determined in feeding studies with rats. The BV is the percentage of nitrogen (N) absorbed from the intestinal tract that is actually retained in the body for maintenance and growth. The Joint FAO/WHO Expert Group on Protein Requirements in 1965 adopted a reference pattern of essential amino acids based on that of whole hen's egg (FAO/WHO 1965). For most foods there was fair but not good agreement between chemical scores based on this pattern and BV's. Eight years later a new provisional pattern was adopted (FAO/WHO 1973). The new pattern was not selected for its ability to predict BV's in rats but rather was based on existing knowledge of human amino acid requirements.

In Table 3 are presented the average amino acid contents of various pulses expressed as percentages of the 1973 provisional pattern. It can be seen that in all but the peanut, the sulfur-containing amino acids are first limiting. Threonine and valine are most often second limiting. When the 1965 reference pattern was used for these calculations, the sulfur-containing acids were first limiting in all 12 pulses and tryptophan was second limiting in more than half.

TABLE 3

Amino Acid Contents of Pulses as Percentage of Provisional Amino
Acid Scoring Pattern (FAO/UN 1970; FAO/WHO 1973)

	Isoleucine	Leucine	Lysine	S-Containing[a]	Aromatic[b]	Threonine	Tryptophan	Valine	E/T[c]
Common Bean	105	108	132	54°	127	99	105	93°°	2.39
Broad Bean	100	101	119	44°	124	84°°	90	89	2.20
Chick-Pea	111	106	126	63°	142	94	90°°	92	2.43
Cowpea	96	100	126	64°	128	90°°	113	91	2.31
Lentil	108	108	132	49°	140	99°°	100	101	2.46
Lima Bean	124	116	137	64°	153	104°°	105	104°°	2.65
Lupine	110	102	97	61°	119	91	105	81°°	2.18
Pea	107	97	138	58°	121	102	93°°	95	2.35
Pigeon Pea	78	90	141	42°	169	73	58°°	73	2.25
Vetch	91	98	106	59°	101	84	--	80°°	1.99
Peanut	84	90	65°	68	146	65°	108	84	2.03
Soybean	114	110	118	74°	133	96°°	133	97	2.46

[a]Methionine + cystine.

[b]Phenylalanine + tyrosine.

[c]Grams of total essential amino acids per gram of N.

°First limiting amino acid.

°°Second limiting amino acid.

The values in Table 3 were calculated from data in FAO/UN
(1970) but small differences should not be regarded as significant.
For example, the amino acid contents given for *Phaseolus vulgaris*
were based on 49 to 60 samples reported by various workers, all

of whom used column chromatographic methods. However, the coefficient of variation (100 x standard deviation/mean) ranged from 4.4%
for isoleucine to 37.4% for cystine and 55.7% for methionine. This
variability can be attributed to differences between types of beans
within the species and those due to cultural differences as well as
to errors in analysis.

The E/T ratio for each type of pulse is given in the last
column. This value is the ratio of grams of total essential amino
acids to grams of nitrogen in the sample. For comparison, E/T
ratios for some other proteins are as follows: casein, 3.25; egg,
3.22; beef muscle, 2.85; rice, 2.61; oats, 2.30; wheat gluten, 1.99;
and gelatin, 1.05 (FAO/WHO 1965). The FAO provisional pattern
proposed in 1973 calls for an E/T value of 2.25. This is about the
ratio estimated to be required by infants and somewhat higher than
that needed by older children or adults. If the ratio is high,
essential amino acids will be converted in the body to "nonessential"
amino acids and this would be wasteful in a hungry world. Much
more needs to be learned about optimum E/T ratios for human beings
in various physiological states.

The chemical score, based on a comparison of the amino acid
pattern of a given protein with some reference pattern, is at best
a first approximation of the value of the protein in human feeding.
A truer evaluation of protein quality requires biological testing
in experimental animals, usually rats. Among many measures of
biological quality, three will be considered here. "Biological
Value" (BV) was defined above. "Digestibility" (D) is the percentage of the N ingested in food that is actually absorbed. "Net
protein utilization" (NPU) is the percentage of ingested N that is
retained in the body. It follows that NPU = BV x D. In measuring
any of these quantities account must be taken of "endogenous N,"
the loss of N from the body when N intake is zero.

Table 4 gives average BV, D, and NPU values and chemical scores
for various pulses (FAO/UN 1970). The digestibility values for
many of the pulses are rather low in comparison with those for whole

TABLE 4

Chemical Score, Biological Value, Digestibility, and Net Protein
Utilization of Various Pulses

Pulse	Chemical Score	BV	D	NPU
Bean[a]	54	58	73	42
Broad Bean	44	55	87	48
Chick-Pea	63	68	86	58
Cowpea	64	57	79	45
Lentil	49	45	85	38
Lima Bean	64	66	78	51
Pea	58	64	88	56
Pigeon Pea	42	57	78	44
Peanut	65	54	87	47
Soybean	74	73	90	66

[a]*Phaseolus* spp. excluding *P. lunatus*.

wheat (91%), rice (98%), cow's milk (97%), or beef and veal (99%),
These results suggest that a considerable portion of pulse protein
is not hydrolyzed in the digestive tract into amino acids for
absorption into the bloodstream. Since the chemical score does not
take into account digestibility, the former should approximate BV
more closely than NPU. This is seen to be the case in Table 4,
where the algebraic sum of CS-BV = -20, while that of CS-NPU = +82.
The chemical score is evidently a better predictor of NPU in foods
with higher digestibility values.

AMINO ACID SUPPLEMENTATION

If the biological value of a protein is largely fixed by its
content of the first limiting amino acid, why not fortify it by the
addition of that amino acid? For example, the common "bean" shown
in Table 3 has a chemical score of 54 because it contains only 119 mg

of sulfur-containing amino acids per g of N compared to 220 mg in
the present provisional pattern (FAO/WHO 1973). If we were to fortify beans with 101 mg of methionine per g N to bring the level up
to that of the provisional pattern, valine would become first
limiting and the score would be increased only to 93. Nothing
would have been gained from adding more than 85 mg unless valine
was also added.

These theoretical considerations have been amply confirmed
by experiments both with laboratory animals and with human beings.
For example, Kakade and Evans (1965) studied the protein efficiency
ratio (PER, grams of weight gain per gram of protein ingested) in
rats under standardized conditions. Casein as the protein source
in the diet gave a PER of 3.18. With cooked beans the PER was 1.90.
Supplementing the beans with methionine alone raised the value to
3.13. Supplementing with methionine and other amino acids to bring
each up to the level found in casein gave a PER of 3.20.

Thus fortification of pulses with methionine improves their
value as a source of protein in the diet. However, whether it is
feasible to do this in those countries where protein malnutrition
is common and where pulses are an important dietary item remains
to be shown.

PULSES IN MIXED DIETS

Fortunately, man does not live by beans alone; in a mixed diet
the biological value of bean protein may be effectively increased.
Since many foods of animal origin are relatively rich in methionine,
inclusion of a relatively small amount of meat, fish, milk, or eggs
enables the body to utilize a larger proportion of pulse protein
than would otherwise be the case. In many of the poorest countries,
of course, little animal protein is available and the diet consists
largely of cereal grains or roots and tubers. Most of the cereals
have amino acid patterns that complement those of the pulses. For
example, they are generally fairly rich in the sulfur-containing

amino acids and low in lysine, whereas in pulses the opposite is true. Protein quality of mixed diets has been studied by many workers. Results reported by Bressani (1973) will be cited as an illustration. PER values in rats were determined where the sole source of protein was a cereal and again where common beans were substituted for 10% of the cereal, the total amount of protein being held constant. The PER was 2.15 on a straight rice diet. The PER was increased to 2.32 on the rice-bean diet. Corresponding figures for other grains were as follows: maize, 0.87 and 1.40; sorghum, 0.88 and 1.39; wheat, 1.05 and 1.73; and oats, 1.60 and 2.37 (casein in this experiment gave a PER of 2.71).

Bressani (1973) also reported PER assays in which maize, beans and various mixtures of these supplied the protein. The level of total protein was maintained constant. Corn, itself, gave a PER of about 0.9. As beans were substituted for an increasing part of the corn, the PER rose to a maximum of approximately 2.0 and then fell to a level of 0.3 for 100% beans. The maximum occurred when maize and beans each supplied half the protein in the mixture, the ratio by weight being 2.6 parts maize to one part beans.

These results show that while the protein quality of beans alone is not high, in effect it is much better in the mixed diets that are usually consumed.

In the mixed diet studies mentioned above, the two protein sources were eaten simultaneously. It is noteworthy that when two proteins with complementary amino acid patterns are ingested separately, at times a few hours apart, they do not supplement each other in the same way. Geiger (1948, 1950) found that neither wheat gluten nor blood protein would support the growth of rats, the former protein being deficient in lysine and the latter in isoleucine. When a 50:50 mixture of both was used, good growth was obtained. However, no growth occurred when the two protein sources were fed alternately for 10-hour periods separated by a 2-hour fast. Essentially similar results were obtained with two other pairs of incomplete but complementary proteins, gluten-yeast, and yeast-blood.

The time of eating of complementary proteins is also important for humans (Leverton and Gram, 1949). Fourteen college-age women were fed the same standardized diet for two successive 18-day periods. The only source of protein at breakfast during the first period was wheat bread, which is deficient in lysine. Sixteen ounces of milk was consumed at dinner. During the second period 8 ounces of milk was ingested with breakfast and 8 ounces at dinner. The only difference was in the distribution of animal protein between the meals. Leverton and Gram (1949) found that significantly more N was retained and less N excreted in the urine during the second period than during the first.

TOXIC SUBSTANCES IN PULSES

A wide variety of toxic and potentially toxic substances are found among the pulses. These include trypsin inhibitors, phytohemagglutinins, goiterogens, cyanogenetic glycosides, antivitamin factors, metal-binding constituents, estrogenic factors, toxic amino acids, lathyrogens, favogens, and unidentified growth inhibitors (Liener, 1973; see also Liener, this volume). Despite this formidable list, pulses have been used for food for thousands of years. Fortunately, cooking destroys many of the toxicants. Others are present in small concentrations so that they are not deleterious in a varied diet. Only a relatively small proportion of the world population is strongly susceptible to favism from *Vicia faba*. "Nevertheless," as Liener (1973) points out, "there is the ever-present possibility that the prolonged consumption of a particular legume that may be improperly processed could bring to the surface toxic effects that otherwise would not be apparent."

EFFECT OF COOKING

Many raw pulses will not support growth, or life of rats if they are the sole source of protein in the diet. However, a relatively

short period of cooking is sufficient to overcome this difficulty
and the PER rises from zero to some maximum value. Presumably this
is due to the destruction of heat-labile toxic factors. As cooking
is prolonged, the PER slowly declines and may eventually reach zero
again. Kakade and Evans (1965) ground raw navy beans and, autoclaved
part of them for various times at 121°C. Four-week rat feeding
studies gave the following PER values: raw beans, 0 (all rats died);
5 min, 1.57; 15 min, 1.26; 30 min, 1.09; 1 hr, 0.67; 4 hr, 0. The
casein control gave a PER of 3.41. Bresanni et al. (1963) obtained
similar results with a variety of black beans although the decline
in PER with cooking time was somewhat less rapid. Bressani (1973)
reported a PER of 1.24 for plain boiled beans (casein = 2.73);
1.43 for beans boiled, then strained to remove part of the seedcoat;
and 0.87 for boiled, strained, and fried beans. The extra heat of
the frying step evidently caused a decrease in protein quality.

Finally, Tannous and Ullah (1969) found that common beans,
chick-peas, lentils, and broad beans autoclaved at 121°C for 5
minutes gave higher PER values than those fed raw or autoclaved for
20 minutes.

EFFECTS OF IMPROPER STORAGE

Improper storage of pulses, i.e., storage at elevated moisture
contents and/or temperatures, results in progressive changes in a
number of characteristics. These include darkening in color, impairment of flavor, destruction of thiamine, and an increase in
required cooking time. It also causes a lowering of protein quality
and digestibility. Mitchell and Beadles (1949) stored soybeans for
34 months at 25.5 C and the low moisture content of 6.6%. The
biological value of the protein fell from 69.1% to 56.0% and the
nitrogen digestibility decreased from 85.3% to 75.0% during this
period. This corresponds to a 29% drop in NPU. Note that this took
place even at a very low moisture content. Schuphan (1963) followed
the amino acid contents of dry peas stored in a ventilated warehouse.

129

During a twelve-month period, the sum of 10 essential amino acids fell 20%, methionine decreased by 32%, and lysine by 21%. Unfortunately, the author did not specify the temperatures encountered or the moisture content of the peas. The present author (Burr, 1975) reported that pinto beans stored 9 years at 21°C and 13.5-13.9% moisture had a significantly (P < 0.01) lower PER value than beans which had been held at 8.3-8.6% moisture. However, this appeared to be due entirely to the much longer cooking time required by the higher moisture beans. Current experiments (unpublished data) tend to confirm this conclusion.

The effect of storage on cooking time is markedly dependent on the moisture content during storage (Burr et al., 1968). Beans are frequently held at moisture levels considerably higher than those mentioned above. For example, the U.S. Standards for Dry Beans (USDA 1969) permit a maximum of 18% moisture without special labeling. Ritchey et al. (1973) obtained from local markets three lots or brands of each of 10 types of pulses. The *average* moisture content of the navy beans was 18.2% and that for the chick-peas, 18.6%.

IMPROVEMENT OF VARIETIES

On the basis of the material presented above it is apparent that pulses contribute substantially to the dietary protein supply in many parts of the world but that the protein quality is not high. High-yielding varieties of rice have been developed in recent years and the deficiency of maize in lysine and tryptophan has been overcome by plant breeders. The question arises as to whether plant breeders can develop new varieties of pulses with higher yields, increased protein content, and improved protein quality. The answer appears to be yes because agronomists have found wide genetic variability in these characters within several important species of pulses.

PULSE PROTEINS

Rutger (1971) has presented data that give an indication of the variation in yield of lines of common beans grown in a single location in a single year. For ten lines having unusually high protein content the range varied from 400 to 1960 lb/ac (450 to 2200 kg/ha). Not all this variation can be attributed to variety alone. In another experiment, the average yield of 8 varieties grown in 6 environments (two locations, three years) ranged from 1400 to 2480 lb/ac (1570-2780 kg/ha). Year and variety effects and variety x year interaction were all significant at $P = 0.01$.

The same report demonstrates the variability that can be expected in protein content. The average for the 8 varieties ranged from 22.5 to 36.2%. Variety, year, and location effects and variety x year and year x location interactions were all significant at $P = 0.01$. Unfortunately there was a fairly strong inverse relationship between yield and protein content and the range in average yield of protein per acre was somewhat narrower, 400-560 lb protein/ac (450-630 kg/ha). Seeds of *P. vulgaris* representing 343 collections from around the world were grown in one location in one year. Protein content ranged from 19 to 31%. Late maturity, small seed size, and low fat content were all positively correlated with high protein content at $P = 0.01$. Interestingly, beans from Central America and Mexico showed a disproportionately large number of high-protein lines.

Singh et al. (1973) studied 14 genotypes of pigeon pea grown during two years in India. They found that the heritability in the broad sense (genotypic variance/phenotypic variance) was 57% for protein, 71% for methionine, and 79% for tryptophan content. These high values suggest that substantial improvement in both protein content and protein quality might be achieved in this species by plant breeding.

Kelly (1971) determined the microbiologically available methionine, total methionine, and nitrogen contents of a large number of cultivars, lines, and single plant selections of common beans. Commercial cultivars showed a high degree of uniformity in their available methionine but he found sufficient variability in this character within the species to conclude that very considerable improvement could be obtained through selection and hydridization.

A high degree of variability in protein quality was also found in peas; the PER's of 28 breeding lines ranged from 14% to 79% that of casein (Bajaj et al., 1971).

Yohe and Poehlman (1972) analyzed 321 strains of mung beans and found high variability in the protein content and in the percentages of lysine and methionine.

A symposium sponsored by the Protein Advisory Group of the United Nations (PAG/UN 1973) offers additional evidence that the yield, protein content, and protein quality of pulses could, indeed, be improved by breeding. The consensus of the participants was that intially efforts should be directed toward increasing yields since this is likely to have the greatest and most rapid effect in relieving protein malnutrition in those areas of the world where it is serious.

If rapid progress is to be made in such breeding programs, there is a need for quick, simple, and reliable methods for assaying protein content and protein quality. For preliminary screening purposes nondestructive tests adaptable to small samples are highly desirable. The rather unsatisfactory state of the art has recently been the subject of an excellent critical review by McLaughlan and Campbell (1974). See also, Part 1.

REFERENCES

Bajaj, S., O. Mickelsen, L. R. Baker, and D. Markarian. 1971. The quality of protein in various lines of peas. Brit. J. Nutr. 25: 207.

Bressani, R. 1973. Legumes in human diets and how they might be improved. *In* PAG/WHO 1973, pp. 15-42.

Bressani, R., L. G. Elias, and A. T. Valiente. 1963. Effect of cooking and of amino acid supplementation on the nutritive value of black beans (*Phaseolus vulgaris* L.). Brit. J. Nutr. 17: 69.

PULSE PROTEINS

Burr, H. K. 1975. Effect of storage on cooking qualities, processing, and nutritive value of beans. *In* Jaffe, W. G. (Editor). Nutritional Aspects of Common Beans and Other Legume Seeds as Animal and Human Food. Archivos Latinoamericanos de Nutricion, Caracas.

Burr, H. K., S. Kon, and H. J. Morris. 1968. Cooking rates of dry beans as influenced by moisture content and temperature and time of storage. Food Technol. 22(3): 88.

FAO/UN. 1970. Amino-acid content of foods and biological data on proteins. Food and Agriculture Organization of the United Nations, Rome.

FAO/UN. 1973. Production Yearbook, 1972, Volume 26. Food and Agriculture Organization of the United Nations, Rome.

FAO/WHO. 1965. Protein requirements. FAO Nutrition Meetings Report Series #37, Rome.

FAO/WHO. 1973. Energy and Protein Requirements. FAO Nutrition Meetings Report Series #52, Rome.

Geiger, E. 1948. The role of the time factor in feeding supplementary proteins. J. Nutr. 36: 813.

Geiger, Ernest. 1950. The role of the time factor in protein synthesis. Science 111: 594.

Kakade, M. L. and R. J. Evans. 1965. Nutritive value of navy beans. (*Phaseolus vulgaris*). Brit. J. Nutr. 19: 269.

Kelly, J. F. 1971. Genetic variation in the methionine levels of mature seeds of common bean (*Phaseolus vulgaris* L.). J. Amer. Soc. Hort. Sci. 96: 561.

Leverton, R. M. and M. R. Gram. 1949. Nitrogen excretion of women related to the distribution of animal protein in daily meals. J. Nutr. 39: 57.

Liener, I. 1973. Antitryptic and other antinutritional factors in legumes. *In* PAG/WHO 1973, p. 239.

McLaughlan, J. M. and J. A. Campbell. 1974. Methodology for evaluation of plant proteins for human use. *In* Hulse, J. H. and E. M. Laing (Editors) Nutritive Value of Triticale Protein. International Development Research Center, Ottawa.

Mitchell, H. H. and J. R. Beadles. 1949. The effect of storage on the nutritional qualities of the proteins of wheat, corn, and soybeans. J. Nutr. 39: 463.

PAG/UN. 1973. Nutritional Improvement of Food Legumes by Breeding. Protein Advisory Group of the United Nations, New York.

Ritchey, S. J., C. R. Meiners, N. L. Derise, H. C. K. Lau, and E. W. Murphy. 1973. Yield, proximate, and mineral composition of commonly consumed legumes. *In* Report of Bean Improvement Cooperative and Natl. Dry Bean Research Assn. Conference, Rochester, N.Y., Nov. 6-8.

Rutger, J. N. 1971. Variation in protein content and its relation to other characters in beans (*Phaseolus vulgaris* L.). Report of 10th Dry Bean Research Conference held at Davis, California, August 12-14, 1970.

Schuphan, W. 1963. Essentielle Aminosaeuren und B-Vitamine als Qualitaetskritieren bei Nahrungspflanzen unter besonderer Beruecksichtigung tropischer Leguminosen. Qual. Plant. et Mat. Veg. 10: 187.

Singh, L., D. Sharma, A. Daodhar, and Y. Sharma. 1973. Variation in protein, methionine, tryptophan and cooking period in pigeon pea (*Cajanus cajan* (L.) Millsp.). Indian J. Agric. Sci. 43: 795.

Tannous, R. I. and M. Ullah. 1969. Effects of autoclaving on nutritional factors in legume seeds. Trop. Agriculture, Trin. 46: 123.

USDA. 1969. The United States standards for beans. U.S. Dept. of Agriculture, Consumer and Marketing Service, Washington, D.C.

Yohe, J. M. and J. M. Poehlman. 1972. Genetic variability in mungbean, *Vigna radiata* (L.) Wilczek. Crop Sci. 12: 461.

6

BIOLOGICAL QUALITY AND FUNCTIONAL PROPERTIES
OF LIMA BEAN PROTEIN FOR BREAD ENRICHMENT

B. S. Luh, Saipin Maneepun, and R. B. Rucker
Department of Food Science and Technology and Department of Nutrition
University of California
Davis, California

A protein-rich fraction from large lima beans (*Phaseolus lunatus*, L. var BC_6) was obtained by extraction with a 0.1 M phosphate buffer (pH 7.2) and then precipitation after acidification with phosphoric acid and heating at 100°C for 10 minutes. This fraction, designated as lima bean protein concentrate (LPC), contained 54.3% protein as the freeze-dried product. Its amino acid content as well as that of whole large lima beans was determined.

In relation to protein quality, LPC is low in methionine and lysine, and perhaps phenylalanine and valine. In feeding trials using rats the nutritive value of the LPC was found to be as good as that of casein after fortification with 0.5% methionine, 0.3% lysine, 0.5% phenylalanine, and 0.3% valine in the diet. The freeze-dried LPC has a protein efficiency ratio (PER) of 1.68 ± 0.07, feed efficiency ratio (FER) of 5.94 ± 0.25, and net protein utilization (NPU) value of 48.41 ± 1.97. Fortification of the LPC with essential amino acids as described above increased the PER to 3.04 ± 0.09, decreased the FER to 3.42 ± 0.03, and increased the NPU to 72.70 ± 3.38.

Freeze-dried LPC and precooked lima bean powder (LBP) were used to increase the protein content of white bread. The loaf volume and

texture of the enriched bread were improved by adding 1% sodium
stearoyl-2-lactylate (SSL) to the flour mixture as a conditioner.
The characteristics and sensory quality of the enriched breads are
presented.

INTRODUCTION

As the population of the world grows there is a sense of
urgency springing from the stark reality that the demand for food
exceeds the supply. In order to meet the food needs of the world's
population it is necessary to expand the use of plant sources.
Though certain vegetable proteins are low in some essential amino
acids (Orr and Watt, 1957), they are the main source of protein intake in certain parts of the world where availability of animal
protein is scarce. The legumes are an important source of plant
proteins for human consumption.

Bressani and Elias (1968) have reviewed the literature on the
use and processing of plant proteins as human food. Rockland et al.
(1974) have reviewed the literature dealing with the chemical, physical, and biological properties of dry beans. A variety of procedures appear successful in the isolation of protein from beans. For
example, Hang et al. (1970) have shown that the solubility of nitrogenous constituents of mung beans, pea beans, and red kidney beans
in solutions of disodium phosphate, trisodium citrate, or sodium
carbonate increases when the concentrations of these salts are increased. Pant and Tulsiani (1969) succeeded in extracting nitrogenous constituents from seed meals (*Phaseolus mungas*) to the extent
of 74-80 percent.

The methods for biological evaluation of proteins have been
discussed by Bender and Doell (1957b). Bender (1972) reported on
the beneficial effects of heating to improve the nutritive value of
beans. Moderate heat treatment usually improves the nutritive value
of many legume proteins by inactivating heat labile compounds which
are deleterious; however, overheating often causes a decrease in

LIMA BEAN PROTEIN FOR BREAD ENRICHMENT

nutritive value. Whitaker and Feeney (1973) have reviewed the
literature on enzyme inhibitors in foods. With respect to lima
beans, Haynes and Feeney (1967) have separated six chromatograph-
ically distinct trypsin and chymotrypsin inhibitors.

In this report, the amino acid composition and protein efficiency ratio of freeze-dried lima bean protein concentrate are compared with those of casein and soy bean proteins. The effect of
fortification with essential amino acids on PER of LPC is presented.
Freeze-dried LPC and precooked lima bean powder were used to increase the protein content of bread. The enriched breads were compared for their chemical and physical properties and sensory quality.

MATERIALS AND METHODS

Dry Lima Beans

One hundred pounds of dry lima beans (*Phaseolus lunatus* L.) were
supplied by Dr. Carl Tucker of the Department of Agronomy at the
University of California, Davis. The dry beans were ground prior to
extraction in a MIAG Braunschweig hammer mill with an 8-mesh sieve.
The ground beans were kept in airtight jars and used promptly for
extraction of proteins.

Preparation of Lima Bean Protein Concentrate (LPC)

Two kilograms of ground dry lima bean powder were soaked in 6
liters of distilled water at 22°C for 12 hours. The pH of the slurry
was initially 6.8 and was adjusted to pH 7.2 by the addition of 0.1 M
Na_3PO_4. The resulting product was mixed in a large Waring blender
for 10 minutes and then allowed to stand for an hour with frequent
stirring. Coarse particles were removed by passing the solution
through cheesecloth. The protein extract was then passed through an
80-mesh sieve and centrifuged at 600 g for 15 minutes in an International Centrifuge to remove the residues. The supernatant fraction was adjusted to pH 5.0 with 0.2 M H_3PO_4. The mixture was heated
at 100°C in a steam jacketed kettle for 10 minutes to coagulate the

proteins and to inactivate the trypsin and chymotrypsin inhibitors. The coagulated proteins were separated from the supernatant fraction by centrifugation. The coagulated product was adjusted with 0.1 N NaOH to pH 6.4, deep frozen, and then freeze-dried in a Stokes freeze-drier, Model 2004L, at 1.1 x 10^{-1} Torr for 48 hours. The dried LPC contained 8.66% moisture, 9.73% starch, 0.82% fat, 54.3% protein, and 10.18% ash. It was stored in tightly covered glass bottles at room temperature (Maneepun et al., 1974).

Precooked Lima Bean Powder (LBP)

Five kilograms of dry large lima beans were soaked for 12 hours at 22°C in 15 liters of water. The soaked beans were drained, blanched in water at 100°C for 15 minutes, and then cooled in ice water. After removal of the seed coats, the beans were spread on stainless steel trays and frozen at -26°C for seven hours. The frozen beans were dried in a Stokes freeze-drier, Model 2004, at 1.10 x 10^{-1} Torr for 48 hours. The freeze-dried product (3.2% moisture) was ground in a roller grinder, passed through a 20-mesh sieve, and stored in airtight glass bottles.

Water Absorption Study

The amount of water which had to be added to the wheat flour-LPC or flour-LBP mixture to make a smooth dough was determined. The procedure involved the gradual addition of water to the flour-LBP mixture followed by kneading to give a satisfactory dough. One hundred gram samples of all-purpose wheat flour and LPC (0-12%) or LBP (0-30%) were used. The amount of water absorbed by the mixture of flour and bean powder to form a smooth dough was determined.

The ingredients for making the bread were as follows:

	Weight (g)
Wheat flour [blend all purpose (Gold Medal) with or without the addition of LPC or LBP]	780.0
Dry yeast (Red Star)	7.09

Sucrose	20.0
Sodium chloride	14.0
Shortening (Crisco)	30.0
Non-fat dry milk (Carnation)	52.0
Water	438.0

Addition of LPC or LBP to wheat flour caused an increase in the water absorption capacity of the blends. Thus, the calculated amount of water required to make a smooth dough was added during kneading. The average increase in water absorption was approximately 1.5% for each percent of added LBP. Sodium stearoyl-2-lactylate was also added for some of the studies (see Results).

For the preparation of breads, 52 g of non-fat milk were dissolved in 375 ml of water. Twenty grams of sugar, 14 g of salt, and 10 g of shortening were added. The mixture was then heated to 45°C with stirring and mixed with 250 g of flour in a Hobart stainless mixing bowl (Model N-50) using a mechanical kneader for two minutes. The activated yeast (7.09 g dry yeast in 63 ml water at 45°C) was then added, plus the remaining flour and shortening. A moderately stiff dough was obtained. It was put on a lightly floured board, kneaded for 8-10 minutes until smooth, placed in a greased bowl, and kept in the fermentation cabinet at 38°C for 90 minutes. The dough was kneaded well, covered with a towel, and was again allowed to rise at 38°C for approximately 45 minutes. It was divided into two equal portions, shaped into loaves, placed in greased pans (8.5 x 4.5 x 2.5 inches) for an hour. Baking was carried out in a rotary oven at 204°C for 15 minutes. The pan was covered with aluminum foil and baked at 204°C for another 20 minutes. The bread was removed from the pan, cooled on a wire rack at room temperature, and used for quality evaluation 24 hours after baking.

Chemical Analysis

The Kjeldahl method was used for determination of total nitrogen in the dry bean and the freeze-dried LPC (AOAC, 1970). The sample sizes were 0.5-0.6 g for LPC and 1.0-2.0 g for LBP. The protein content was obtained by multiplying percent N by 6.25, since this value applies for many protein fractions from beans and appeared to be an adequate conversion factor for lima bean protein based on its amino acid composition.

The moisture content of LPC and LBP (2-g samples) was determined by the difference in weight before and after drying at 130°C in an oven for 1 hr (AOAC, 1970). Crude fiber, ash, and fat were also determined (AOAC, 1970). Starch was measured by the anthrone colorimetric procedure described by McCready et al. (1950).

Amino Acid Analysis

Approximately 250 mg of the ground sample was weighed accurately into a 500-ml round bottom flask. The sample was refluxed with 250 ml 6 N HCl for 20 hr on an electrical heater, cooled, and filtered through a sintered glass filter. The filtrate was evaporated almost to dryness in a flask evaporator. The residue was dissolved in a 50-ml volumetric flask and diluted to volume with distilled water. The Technicon amino acid analyzer was used for quantitative determination of amino acids (Hamilton, 1963; Roach, 1966).

Biological Evaluation of Protein Quality

Forty male albino rats at the age of 28 days (weight range 41-54 g) were randomized into five groups. Each group (8 rats) was fed a different assay diet. Rats were housed individually in stainless steel cages in an air-conditioned room at 23°C and 45-55% relative humidity. Assay diet and water were offered ad libitum. The animals were weighed every other day and their food intake was measured every 4 days. The total test period was 21 days. The protein efficiency ratio method recommended by AOAC (1970) was followed except that glucose was replaced by corn starch. The material under test was fed as the sole source of protein at the 10% level. The basal diet was composed of the following: protein, 10%; corn oil, 8%; cellulose, 2%; choline chloride, 0.3%; vitamin premix, 0.3%; mineral premix, 5%; and enough corn starch to make 100%. Vitamins were added so that each

LIMA BEAN PROTEIN FOR BREAD ENRICHMENT

100 g of diet contained: niacin, 20 mg; Ca pantothenate, 10 mg; riboflavin, 1.5 mg; thiamine-HCl, 0.91 mg; pyridoxine-HCl, 1.5 mg; fola-
cin, 0.3 mg; biotin, 0.1 mg; B_{12}, 0.02 mg; vitamin A palmitate, 1000
I.U.; vitamin D_3, 200 I.U.; DL-α-tocopherol acetate, 10 mg; menadione,
0.06 mg; and butylated hydroxyltoluene, 10 mg. Minerals were added so
that each 100 g of diet contained: $CaCO_3$, 1.5 g; K_2HPO_4, 1.625 g;
$CaHPO_4$, 0.3 g; NaCl, 0.5 g; $FeSO_4 \cdot 7H_2O$, 0.125 g; $MgSO_4$, 0.324 g; KI,
0.013 g; $ZnCO_3$, 0.004 g; $CuSO_4 \cdot 5H_2O$, 0.0014 g; and $MnSO_4 \cdot H_2O$, 0.0115 g.
The following diets comprised the five experimental groups:

Group A. Protein-free diet. Starch (10%) was substituted for
protein in the basal diet.

Group B. Casein diet. Casein (superior grade--87% protein)
obtained from Nutritional Biochemical Corp., Cleveland, Ohio, was
added at 11.5% in the basal diet.

Group C. Soybean diet. RP-100. Soy protein (90%) from Purina
Company was added at 11.1% in the basal diet.

Group D. Lima bean concentrate diet. Lima bean protein concentrate (54.31% protein) was added at 18.41% in the basal diet.

Group E. Supplemented lima bean concentrate diet. The basal
diet with lima bean protein concentrate was used, but L-lysine (0.3%),
L-phenylalanine (0.5%), L-methionine (0.5%), and L-valine (0.3%) were
added so that all of the essential amino acids would be present in the
diet at the recommended dietary requirements (NRC, 1962).

The five diets were fed separately to each group of rats for 21
days. From the gain in weight and feed consumption data, the protein
efficiency ratio and feed efficiency ratio were calculated. For net
protein utilization, the method recommended by Miller and Bender
(1955) was used. The method is based on constancy of the ratio of
N/H_2O in the rat. The total N of the body can be determined from
the water content. Body water was determined after killing the
rats with ether, opening the body cavities, and drying the carcasses
(100°C for 48 hr) to a constant weight in a Freas oven, Model 845-A.
The equation for the calculation is:

$$\log (4.8 - y) = 0.437 - 0.0123x$$

where x = age of the rats in days and y = N/H_2O x 100.

By using the equation, the N-content value can be used to calculate the net protein utilization by applying the equation:

$$NPU = (B - B_k + I_k)/I$$

where B and B_k represent values for the total body N (g) of the
animals fed the test or nonprotein diet, respectively, and I and I_k
are the values for N intake (g) for the two groups, respectively.

Properties of the Bread

Moisture Content. The method described by the American Association of Cereal Chemists (AACC, 1962) was used.

One hour after removal from the oven, the bread loaves were
placed on a large sheet of smooth paper and cut into slices 2-3 mm
thick. The cut slices were allowed to dry on the paper at room
temperature until they were in approximate equilibrium with the
moisture of the air. Usually 15-20 hours was sufficient. The dried
slices and crumbs were weighed. The moisture loss in air drying was
computed. The air-dried bread was then ground with a wooden rolling
pin, passed a 20-mesh sieve, mixed thoroughly, and stored in an airtight container.

Two grams of air-dried bread was weighed accurately onto a tared
dish which had been dried previously at 130 ± 3°C. The sample was
dried in an oven at 130°C for 1 hour, starting the timing after the
oven reached 130°C. The dish was covered, transferred to a desic-
cator, and weighed soon after room temperature was attained.

For percent total moisture in the fresh loaf, the following
formula was used for calculation:

$$TM = A + \frac{(100 - A)B}{100}$$

where TM represents moisture, % (w/w), A represents moisture lost
on air drying, and B represents moisture in the air-dry sample, as
determined by the oven-drying method.

Loaf Volume. The volume of each loaf of bread was examined one hour after baking. It was measured by putting the loaf in a box of known volume (size 27 x 15 x 11 cm). After putting the loaf in the box, the remaining space was filled with cellulose powder. The volume of the cellulose powder was measured with a graduated cylinder. The loaf volume was calculated as the difference between total volume and that of the cellulose powder.

Color of Bread. The bread slices containing various levels of LPC or precooked, freeze-dried LBP were evaluated for color using a Gardner automatic color difference meter. A light yellow porcelain plate (LYI) was used as a reference (RD = 60.7, a = -2, b = +22.3). The bread was sliced just prior to color evaluation.

Sensory Evaluation. A panel composed of 19 members evaluated the bread samples 24 hours after baking. The color, aroma, flavor, and texture of each set of breads (4-6 samples) enriched with LPC or LBP were scored by the panel using a 1-10 hedonic scale as follows: excellent, 9-10; good, 7-8; fair, 5-6; poor, 3-4; and very poor, 1-2. The samples were cut into ¼-inch slices of 2 x 2" square. The scores were analyzed for variance (Larmond, 1970). The least significant difference (LSD) at the 5% probability level was calculated (Alder and Roessler, 1968).

RESULTS

Chemical Analyses of Various Fractions

Chemical analyses of whole dry lima beans, the various fractions prepared from them, and wheat flour for comparison, are presented in Table 1. The dry beans contained 12.17% moisture and 21.37% protein. Compared to wheat flour, dry lima beans contained twice as much protein.

The results from amino acid analyses are presented in Table 2. Expressed as g/16 g N, the differences in the individual amino acid content of whole lima bean compared to LPC were not great, with the exception of threonine and cystine which were increased approximately 3 and 1.5 times, respectively. Tryptophan was not determined because

TABLE 1

Chemical Analyses of Various Fractions Prepared from
Lima Beans (*Phaseolus lunatus* L. var BC_6) and Wheat Flour

Sample	Moisture %	Total solids %	Starch %	Fat %	Protein %	Crude fiber %	Ash %
Whole dry lima beans	12.17	87.83	47.67	3.24	21.37	7.35	4.46
Freeze-dried protein preparation	8.66	91.34	9.73	0.82	54.31	0	10.18
Residue	4.20	95.80	36.12	1.25	6.62	8.49	3.24
Starch preparation	3.60	96.40	80.66	1.12	4.62	0.83	1.38
Precooked, freeze-dried lima bean powder	3.20	96.80	50.72	3.12	20.67	5.25	2.56
Wheat flour	9.15	90.85	77.20	1.00	9.47	0	0.50

of destruction during acid hydrolysis. If similar to other bean protein, however, tryptophan is probably present in the order of 1.0-1.5 g per 16 g N. For comparison, the amino acid content of a wheat flour sample is also presented in Table 2. The most nutritionally limiting amino acids in lima bean protein, based on analytical evidence, appear to be the sulfur-containing amino acids.

Biological Evaluation of Protein Quality

Results of the feeding tests using lima bean protein concentrate, isolated soybean protein, and casein are presented in Figure 1 and Tables 3 and 4. The weight of rats fed the nonprotein diet (Group A) decreased during the entire experimental period (-0.54 ± 0.1 g/rat/day). This group was used as a control to calculate the difference between the weight and nitrogen content of the test groups (Bender and Doell, 1957a, b). The rats fed a 10% casein protein diet (Group B) gained 3.23 ± 0.26 g/rat/day. This group was

TABLE 2

Amino Acid Contents[a] of Whole Large Lima Beans,
Freeze-Dried Protein Concentrate, and Wheat Flour

Amino acid	Whole lima bean		Freeze-dried protein concentrate		Wheat flour
	g/100 g of dry bean	g/16 g N	g/100 g dry basis	g/16 g N	g/16 g N
Aspartic acid	3.63	17.51	8.93	17.06	4.17
Threonine	0.71	3.43	2.21	9.84	2.41
Serine	1.55	7.48	3.74	7.15	4.52
Glutamic acid	2.96	14.78	7.41	14.15	34.24
Proline	0.73	3.67	2.21	4.22	13.21
Glycine	1.09	5.26	2.08	3.97	3.64
Alanine	0.90	4.34	2.48	4.74	2.77
Valine	0.79	3.81	2.17	4.15	2.87
Cystine	0.32	1.54	0.55	2.65	2.94
Methionine	0.19	0.92	0.59	1.13	0.79
Isoleucine	0.74	3.57	2.35	4.49	2.65
Leucine	1.55	7.48	4.09	7.81	6.41
Tyrosine	0.74	3.57	2.03	3.88	2.96
Phenylalanine	0.97	4.68	2.47	4.72	4.71
Lysine	1.36	6.56	3.46	6.61	2.13
Histidine	0.57	2.75	1.53	2.92	1.89
Arginine	0.90	4.34	2.62	5.01	3.50

[a]Tryptophan was not determined because it was destroyed during acid hydrolysis of the proteins.

used as the primary reference for comparison of FER, NPU, and PER values. The PER was determined to be 2.93 ± 0.08 and the FER 3.37 ± 0.14. The value for net protein utilization was $62.5 \pm 0.25\%$.

Group C was fed a soybean protein diet. As expected the rate of growth was retarded. For the rat, soybean protein is deficient particularly in methionine when administered at 10% in the diet (Block and Mitchell, 1946; Guggenheim and Friedmann, 1960). The

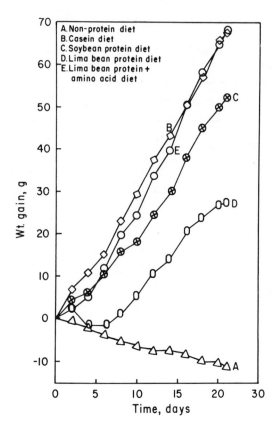

FIG. 1. Weight gain of albino rats fed with various protein sources up to 21 days.

PER and FER values for soybean protein were 2.34 ± 0.08 and 4.30 ± 0.20, respectively, and the NPU value was 50.97 ± 2.19%. These values are similar to those previously reported by Mustakas et al. (1964). Mustakas et al. evaluated 10 commercial products of soy flours by feeding them to rats. They obtained PER values in the range of 2.09-2.46 and NPU values ranging from 55 to 62%. In the present investigation, the weight gain for the soybean diet was 2.5 ± 0.3 g/rat/day. Soybean protein is one of the legume proteins that can be used in dietary foods and for protein fortification.

TABLE 3

Determination of Protein Efficiency Ratio (PER)
and Feed Efficiency Ratio (FER) of Lima Bean
Protein Concentrate by Feeding to Albino Rats

Group	Type of diet	Average initial weight (g) [a]	Gain in weight (g) 21 days [a]	Food consumption g/rat/day [a]	PER [a]	FER [a]
A	Nonprotein	48.13 ± 4.13	-11.25 ± 2.09	4.73 ± 0.38	--	--
B	Casein	45.88 ± 3.52	68.00 ± 5.49	10.91 ± 1.36	2.93 ± 0.08	3.37 ± 0.14
C	Soybean	48.25 ± 3.49	52.50 ± 6.31	10.74 ± 1.66	2.34 ± 0.08	4.30 ± 0.20
D	Lima bean protein	46.75 ± 3.93	26.88 ± 4.15	7.61 ± 0.82	1.68 ± 0.07	5.94 ± 0.25
E	Lima bean protein + methionine, lysine, phenyl-alanine, valine	46.75 ± 3.60	68.38 ± 10.43	10.72 ± 1.99	3.04 ± 0.09	3.42 ± 0.03

[a]Mean ± standard error.

TABLE 4

Net Protein Utilization (NPU) Values
for the Various Protein Preparations[a]

Group	Type of diet	Net protein utilization (%)[b]
A	Nonprotein	--
B	Casein	62.50 ± 0.25
C	Soybean	50.97 ± 2.19
D	Lima bean protein	48.41 ± 1.97
E	Lima bean protein + methionine, lysine, phenylalanine, valine	72.70 ± 3.38

[a]Correlation between the ratio of body N to body H_2O, the equation is $\log (4.8 - y) = 0.437 - 0.0123x$ where x = age of rats = 28 days (weaning period) + 21 days (feeding period).

[b]Mean ± standard error.

In Group D, the rats were fed diets containing 10% LPC as protein. The average weight gain for the lima bean protein concentrate was 1.28 ± 0.2 g/rat/day. The PER and FER were 1.68 ± 0.07 and 5.94 ± 0.24, respectively; the NPU value was 48.41 ± 1.97% (Tables 3 and 4). Previously, Rockland and Metzler (1967) studied the nutritional value of precooked and freeze-dried lima beans. They obtained a PER value of 1.83 which is very close to the value for LPC.

In Group E, the rats were fed with the same freeze-dried LPC but fortified with essential amino acids. The addition of the supplemented amino acids was based on the minimum amounts of these nutrients required for rat growth. All of the essential amino acids (methionine, phenylalanine, valine, and lysine) that were limiting were added so that growth and other parameters would be maximized. This was done primarily to test for the presence of growth inhibitors, such as trypsin inhibitors.

It is clear that addition of the essential amino acids resulted in a significant increase in growth which was similar to that of rats fed the casein diet (Figure 2). In this regard, methionine and lysine were probably most important in stimulating growth. The growth

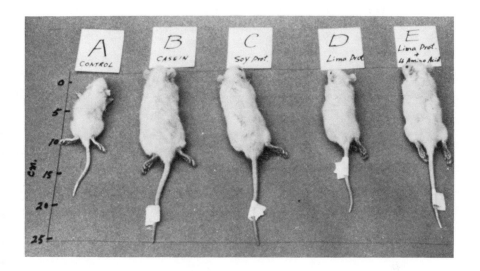

FIG. 2. Photograph of male albino rats after feeding with various protein diets for 21 days.
  A. Nonprotein diet.
  B. Casein diet.
  C. Soybean protein diet.
  D. Lima bean protein concentrate.
  E. Lima bean protein concentrate fortified with methionine, lysine, phenylalanine, and valine.

rate for rats fed diet E was 3.28 ± 0.48 g/rat/day. The PER and FER values of diet E were 3.04 ± 0.09 and 3.42 ± 0.03, respectively, and the NPU value was 72.70 ± 3.38%. The nutritional quality of lima bean protein thus can be improved by fortification with the appropriate amino acids.

Characteristics of Bread Enriched with Lima Bean Protein Concentrate

Freeze-dried LPC containing 54.31% protein was used to increase the protein content of white bread. The amount of LPC added to the wheat flour in the baking formula was 0, 3, 6, 9, and 12%, respectively. The characteristics of the enriched breads are presented in Table 5. The changes in moisture content of the sliced breads after exposure to air at room temperature (25°C) for 20 hours and

TABLE 5

Characteristics of Breads Enriched with Lima Bean Protein Concentrate

Sample No.	Lima bean protein concentrate (%)	Weight after mixing (g)	Weight after baking (g)	Loaf volume (cc)	Moisture lost in air drying[a] (%) (A)	Moisture air-dried sample[b] (%) (B)	Total moisture[c] (%) (C)	Protein on dry basis (%)
1	0 (control)	628	597	1,965	18.15	15.06	30.37	9.43
2	3	633	561	1,698	18.13	15.28	30.64	11.70
3	6	642	569	1,662	17.85	16.79	31.23	13.04
4	9	648	578	1,483	16.42	19.64	32.83	14.31
5	12	650	535	1,258	15.01	21.71	33.26	15.43

[a]The air-dried sample was obtained by exposing the sliced breads to air for 20 hours at room temperature (25°C).

[b]Determined by oven drying: 130 ± 3°C for 1 hour.

[c]Total moisture (C) = A + $\dfrac{(100 - A)B}{100}$. From AACC (1962).

after oven drying at 130°C for one hour are presented. The control
sample (No. 1) lost more moisture on exposure to air for 20 hours
than those enriched with LPC. As the percentage of LPC increased,
the loss of moisture during the air-drying period decreased. It is
apparent that the LPC contributes to the ability of the bread to
hold moisture. The total moisture increased from 30.37% in the
control sample (No. 1) to 33.26% in the sample enriched with 12%
LPC (No. 5). The protein level in the bread increased progressively
from 9.43% in the control (No. 1) to 15.43% in the sample with 12%
LPC (No. 5).

Characteristics of Bread Enriched with Lima Bean Powder (LBP)

When precooked and freeze-dried lima bean powder was added to
the wheat flour at 0, 10, 20, or 30%, respectively, there was also
a progressive increase in total moisture content and a decrease in
loaf volume (Figure 3). The characteristics of the enriched breads
are presented in Table 6. The protein content increased from 9.43%
in the control (No. 1) to 14.22% in the one enriched with 30% LBP
(No. 4).

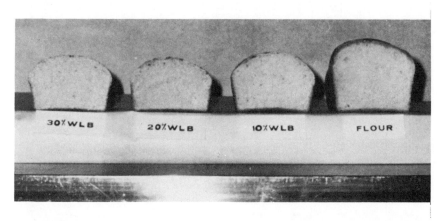

FIG. 3. Bread fortified with 10, 20, or 30% whole lima bean
powder.

TABLE 6

Characteristics of Breads Enriched with Precooked Lima Bean Powder (LBP)

Sample No.	Lima bean powder added to wheat flour (%)	Weight after mixing (g)	Weight after baking (g)	Loaf volume (cc)	Moisture lost in air drying (%) (A)	Moisture air-dried sample[a] (%) (B)	Total moisture[b] (%) (C)	Protein on dry basis (%)
(A) Control								
1	0	638	557	1,926	14.19	15.99	27.91	9.43
2	10	632	558	1,617	11.46	20.06	29.22	12.06
3	20	696	614	1,000	11.42	26.03	34.48	13.11
4	30	737	644	951	11.38	29.02	37.10	14.22
(B) With 1% sodium stearoyl lactylate as conditioner								
1	0	638	557	1,926	14.19	15.99	27.91	9.43
2	10	691	581	2,003	14.52	18.63	30.44	11.83
3	20	715	615	1,907	12.31	25.36	34.56	12.20
4	30	723	629	1,080	13.46	29.16	38.70	14.50

[a]Determined by oven drying.

[b]Total moisture (C) = A + $\dfrac{(100 - A)B}{100}$. From AACC (1962).

152

LIMA BEAN PROTEIN FOR BREAD ENRICHMENT

Effect of Sodium Stearoyl-2-lactylate (SSL) on Loaf Volume

Since the addition of LPC to the flour in the baking formula
reduced the loaf volume of the white bread considerably, sodium
stearoyl-2-lactylate (SSL), a dough conditioner, was used to increase the loaf volume of the bread. SSL is permitted by the Food
and Drug Administration for use in bakery products; it is widely
used in the production of standardized bread and bread type products
to provide additional dough strength, tolerance, and uniformity.
The sodium form of this ingredient is more easily dispersed than the
calcium form and therefore is more effective in the batter. Addition
of the SSL conditioner up to 1% of the weight of flour-LBP mix resulted in a definite improvement in loaf volume. Belshaw (1971) has
recommended addition of SSL to dough as a conditioner to improve
dough tolerance to soy flours or other high protein materials. Alternatively, lecithin added at 1% to flour containing 6% soy bean protein improves loaf volume (Mizrahi et al., 1967).

SSL is the reaction product of two naturally occurring food
components, stearic acid and lactic acid, neutralized to the sodium
salt. The product is marketed under the trade name of Emplex (Patco
Products, Kansas City, Missouri). It is available commercially as
a free-flowing powder with the following molecular structure:

$$C_{17}H_{35} - \overset{\overset{\displaystyle O}{\|}}{C} - O - \overset{\overset{\displaystyle CH_3}{|}}{\underset{\underset{\displaystyle H}{|}}{C}} - \overset{\overset{\displaystyle O}{\|}}{C} - O - \overset{\overset{\displaystyle CH_3}{|}}{\underset{\underset{\displaystyle H}{|}}{C}} - \overset{\overset{\displaystyle O}{\|}}{C} - ONa$$

The SSL can act not only as a dough conditioner but also as an
emulsifier. It has the unique ability to bond with proteins and
starches, resulting in better tolerance to ingredient and processing
variations in baking. The functional characteristics of SSL uniquely
stabilize many food systems containing protein, starch, oil, and
water.

Gardner Color Difference Meter Reading

Color is an important factor affecting the consumer preference for bread. The effect of adding LPC or LBP to the wheat flour on color of breads was evaluated with a Gardner color difference meter. The results are presented in Table 7.

The Gardner b value of the sliced breads appears to be influenced by the addition of LPC to the wheat flour. As the quantity of LPC increased, the Gardner b value (yellowness) increased. Addition of 10% LBP to the wheat flour also increased the Gardner b value from +15.82 to +17.32. A further increase in the LBP content to 20 or 30% did not result in a further increase in the Gardner b value.

Addition of the bread conditioner (SSL) at 1% level seems to have no significant effect on the color of the bread.

TABLE 7

Gardner Color Difference Meter Readings
of Sliced Bread Enriched with LPC and LBP

Sample	Rd	a	b
(A) Enriched with lima bean protein concentrate (LPC)			
Wheat flour	53.47	-1.05	+14.30
Flour + 3% LPC	49.25	-0.85	+16.22
Flour + 6% LPC	50.07	0	+18.10
Flour + 9% LPC	52.85	-0.77	+19.10
Flour + 12% LPC	54.20	0	+21.22
Flour + 10% LBP	55.37	-0.75	+16.45
(B) Enriched with precooked lima bean powder (LBP)			
Wheat flour	52.52	-1.37	+15.82
Flour + 10% precooked LBP	57.04	-0.80	+17.32
Flour + 20% precooked LBP	54.62	-0.40	+17.37
Flour + 30% precooked LBP	54.54	-0.60	+17.50
Flour + 10% precooked LBP + 1% SSL	55.10	-1.10	+17.52
Flour + 20% precooked LBP + 1% SSL	54.28	-0.90	+17.80
Flour + 30% precooked LBP + 1% SSL	55.60	-0.97	+17.10

LIMA BEAN PROTEIN FOR BREAD ENRICHMENT

Sensory Evaluation of Bread Quality

The sensory quality of the bread was evaluated 24 hours after baking by a panel of 19 members. Results on the effect of LPC on color, aroma, flavor, and texture of the breads are presented in Table 8. The color score was lowered from 8.00 to 6.80 when 6% LPC was added. The results were significant at the 95% probability level. The color score was further lowered when the LPC content was increased.

Addition of precooked freeze-dried LBP up to 30% of weight of wheat flour resulted in no significant change in visual color as compared with the control (Table 8).

When precooked freeze-dried LBP was added at the 10, 20, or 30% levels, the resulting breads were equally acceptable to the panel (Table 9). Addition of precooked LBP to the formula did not cause a significant difference in aroma between the control and treated samples even when 30% by weight of the LBP was added.

The effect of adding 1% SSL as a conditioner on quality of the enriched breads is presented in Table 10.

Addition of 1% SSL conditioner can improve texture of bread. The panel did not detect any difference in texture between the control and the treated samples at 95% probability level. Beans are known to contain a trypsin inhibitor which can be inactivated by cooking. The precooked LBP was freed from trypsin inhibitor in the present investigation. Based on the sensory quality of the enriched bread, it appears feasibile to enrich white bread with precooked LBP to yield a product of high protein content.

DISCUSSION

Studies of the biological and functional properties of vegetable proteins are indispensible to the evaluation of new processes for preparing dry bean products and development of new products from commercial varieties of legumes. One of the problems with the vegetable proteins is that they are deficient in one or more of the sulfur-containing amino acids, especially lysine and methionine. Soy bean and

155

TABLE 8

Sensory Evaluation of Bread Enriched with
Lima Bean Protein Concentrate (LPC) and Precooked Lima Bean Powder (LBP)

Quality attribute	Organoleptic mean score						Least significant difference (LSD) P = 0.05
	Wheat flour (control)	Wheat flour + 3% LPC	Wheat flour + 6% LPC	Wheat flour + 9% LPC	Wheat flour + 12% LPC	Wheat flour + 10% LBP	
Color	8.00	7.58	6.80	5.70	5.00	7.32	0.77
Aroma	7.74	7.89	6.68	5.63	5.16	7.31	0.79
Flavor	7.63	7.63	6.74	5.47	5.11	7.21	0.80
Texture	7.21	7.21	6.58	5.68	4.89	7.05	0.89

156

LIMA BEAN PROTEIN FOR BREAD ENRICHMENT

TABLE 9

Sensory Evaluation of Bread Enriched with
Precooked, Freeze-Dried Lima Bean Powder (LBP)

Quality attribute	Organoleptic mean score				Least significant difference (LSD) P = 0.05
	Wheat flour (control)	Wheat flour + 10% LBP	Wheat flour + 20% LBP	Wheat flour + 30% LBP	
Color	7.68	7.47	7.31	7.29	1.41
Aroma	7.63	7.37	7.47	7.79	1.03
Flavor	7.37	7.26	7.57	7.47	0.96
Texture	7.11	7.00	7.79	7.42	1.08

peanut proteins are deficient in methionine while wheat and rice proteins are deficient in lysine. The methionine content of soybean is only 42% that of egg. The lysine content of wheat and rice is only 39 and 46%, respectively, that of egg. The present investigation indicates that the most nutritionally limiting amino acids in lima bean protein, based on analytical evidence, appear to be the sulfur-containing amino acids. Fortification of LPC with the essential amino acids methionine and lysine along with phenylalanine and valine results in a significant increase in growth when fed to rats.

The nutritional quality of bean protein is an important subject to be considered in the utilization of legumes as food. The protein efficiency ratio (PER) is an accepted, although somewhat arbitrary, measure of protein quality. The milk protein, casein, is used as a primary standard for comparison. It is well known that raw beans do not promote growth of weanling rats used in PER studies. This was largely due to the presence of trypsin and chymotrypsin inhibitors (Haynes and Feeney, 1967; Whitaker and Feeney, 1973) which can be inactivated by heating. The precooked lima bean powder (LBP) as well as the lima bean protein concentrate (LPC) used in the present investigation were free of trypsin and chymotrypsin inhibitory activity.

TABLE 10

Sensory Evaluation of Breads Enriched with Precooked, Freeze-
Dried Lima Bean Powder (LBP) and 1% Sodium Stearoyl-2-lactylate (SSL)

| Quality attribute | Organoleptic mean score | | | | Least significant difference (LSD) P = 0.05 |
	Wheat flour (control)	Wheat flour + 10% LBP	Wheat flour + 20% LBP	Wheat flour + 30% LBP	
Aroma	7.26	6.53	6.63	6.53	0.84
Flavor	6.84	6.95	6.89	6.89	0.93
Color	8.11	7.68	7.47	7.21	0.73
Texture	6.68	6.47	6.63	6.11	1.09

Although the PER values for LPC and cooked lima beans are low [1.68 (Table 3) and 1.9 (Rockland et al., 1974), respectively], supplementation with essential amino acids is possible. The use of lima bean protein in combination with other plant protein represents another possibility.

As described here, it is feasible to use lima bean as a fortifying agent and protein source in flour. Enrichment of bread with precooked lima bean powder appears to be adequate and perhaps more desirable than with the protein concentrate because of the lower cost, higher yield, and better color.

REFERENCES

AACC. 1962. Cereal Laboratory Methods (7th Ed.) AACC Method 44-15 pp. 1-2. Amer. Assoc. Cereal Chemists, St. Paul, Minnesota.

Alder, H.L. and E.R. Roessler. 1968. Introduction to Probability and Statistics. W.H. Freeman and Co., San Francisco, California.

AOAC. 1970. Official Methods of Analysis (11th Ed.). Association of Official Agricultural Chemists, Washington, D.C.

Belshaw, F. 1971. Bread has 30-40% more protein, same cost. Food Processing 32:24.

Bender, A.E. 1972. Processing damage to protein foods. In Protein Advisory Group Bulletin. United Nations, New York. Vol. II, p. 10.

Bender, A.E. and B.H. Doell. 1957a. Note on the determination of net protein utilization by carcass analysis. Brit. J. Nutr. 11:138.

Bender, A.E. and B.H. Doell. 1957b. Biological evaluation of proteins: a new aspect. Brit. J. Nutr. 11:140.

Block, R.J. and H.H. Mitchell. 1946. The correlation of the amino acid composition of proteins with their nutritive value. Nutr. Rev. 16:249.

Bressani, R. and L.G. Elias. 1968. Processed vegetable protein mixtures for human consumption in developing countries. Adv. Food Res. 16:1.

Guggenheim, K. and N. Friedmann. 1960. Effect of extraction rates of flour and of supplementation with soy meal on the nutritive value of bread proteins. Food Technol. 14:298.

Hamilton, P.B. 1963. Ion-exchange chromatography of amino acids. A single column, high resolving, fully automatic procedure. Anal. Chem. 35:2055.

Hang, Y.D., K.H. Steinkraus and L.R. Hackler. 1970. Comparative studies on the nitrogen solubility of mung beans, pea beans and kidney beans. J. Food Sci. 35:318.

Haynes, R. and R.E. Feeney. 1967. Fractionation and properties of trypsin and chymotrypsin inhibitors from lima beans. J. Biol. Chem. 242:5378.

Larmond, E. 1970. Methods for Sensory Evaluation of Food. Canada Department Agriculture.

Maneepun, S., B.S. Luh and R.B. Rucker. 1974. Amino acid composition and biological quality of lima bean protein. J. Food Sci. 39:171.

McCready, R.M., J. Goggolz, V. Silviera and H.S. Owen. 1950. Determination of starch and amylose in vegetables. Anal. Chem. 22:1156.

Miller, D.S. and A.E. Bender. 1955. The determination of the net utilization of proteins by a shortened method. Brit. J. Nutr. 9:382.

Mizrahi, S., G. Zimmermann and Z. Berk. 1967. The use of isolated soybean proteins in bread. Cereal Chem. 44:193.

Mustakas, G.C., E.L. Griffin, L.E. Allen and O.B. Smith. 1964. Production and nutritional evaluation of extrusion-cooked full fat soybean flour. J. Amer. Oil Chem. Soc. 41:607.

NRC. 1962. Nutrient requirements of laboratory animals. NRC Pub. 990. National Academy of Sciences--National Research Council, Washington, D.C.

Orr, M.C. and B.K. Watt. 1957. Amino acid content of foods. USDA Home Econ. Res. Report. No. 4.

Pant, R. and D.R.P. Tulsiani. 1969. Solubility, amino acid composition, and biological evaluation of proteins isolated from leguminous seed. J. Agr. Food Chem. 17:361.

Roach, A.G. 1966. The preparation of feedstuffs and samples for amino acid analysis. *In* Technique in Amino Acid Analysis. Technicon International Din. S.A. Geneva, Switzerland.

Rockland, L.B. and E.A. Metzler. 1967. Quick cooking lima and other dry beans. Food Technol. 21(3a):26a.

Rockland, L.B., E.M. Zaragosa and D.M. Hahn. 1974. New information on the chemical, physical and biological properties of dry beans. *In* M.H. Dickson (Ed.) Report of Bean Improvement Cooperative and National Dry Bean Research Association Conference. Rochester, New York, November 6-8, 1973. New York State Agr. Experiment Station, Geneva, New York.

Whitaker, J.R. and R.E. Feeney. 1973. Enzyme inhibitors in foods. *In* Toxicant Occurring Naturally in Foods. ISBN 0-309-02117-0 National Academy of Sciences, Washington, D.C.

7

PROTEIN NUTRITIVE VALUE OF SELECTED
PRESENT AND POTENTIAL MEAT EXTENDERS

Muriel L. Happich

Eastern Regional Research Center
Agricultural Research Service
U.S. Department of Agriculture
Philadelphia, Pennsylvania

The high nutritive value of lean beef protein was used as the criterion for evaluating the relative quality of mixtures of meat and other animal and/or plant proteins. The nutritive value of selected animal and plant proteins, present or potential meat extenders, and their combinations with lean beef is under study. Available data from this study are reported here.

The protein nutritive value of partially defatted chopped beef and partially defatted beef fatty tissue is reviewed (Happich et al., 1975), and analytical data on bovine blood and its fractions, beef by-products that have possible uses in meat products, are discussed.

Protein efficiency ratios (PER) were determined for the proteins of whey, fish, soy, and liquid cyclone process cottonseed protein concentrates individually and in combinations with lean beef. All of the combinations had PER values equal to or higher than 2.5, the assigned PER for casein, a protein standard of high quality.

The use of soy proteins in meat products is expanding rapidly. The PER values and amino acid analyses of samples of textured

161

vegetable protein, meat patties with textured vegetable protein, and a soy protein concentrate were determined. Combinations of lean beef and a soy protein concentrate in 80:20, 70:30, or 60:40 protein ratios, respectively, had PERs that were not significantly different from each other or from the PER of casein.

Cattlehide collagen, a potential food texturizing and binding agent, has little nutritional value when fed as the only source of protein. PER values of collagen in combinations with lean beef and of lean beef-collagen combinations with either a whey or soy protein concentrate indicate parameters for adding collagen as a texturizing agent in designing new meat products with a PER of 2.5. The data also indicate that the whey concentrate proteins supplemented the lean beef-collagen proteins to a greater degree than the soy proteins did. PER values of lean beef-collagen-whey protein combinations were 2.4 or higher.

INTRODUCTION

The protein nutritive value, palatability, and consumer acceptance of red meat are high and these factors have made red meat the chief source of animal protein food in this country. At present, about two-thirds of food-grade protein used in the United States comes from animal sources (Bird, 1974). Currently there is a growing use of plant proteins as extenders in ground meat and meat products. It has been predicted that in the next several decades we will obtain one-half to two-thirds of our food-grade protein from plant-derived sources (Bird, 1974). Blending lean beef with other animal and/or plant proteins that have supplementary amino acid compositions can produce nutritious, economical, and palatable meat products. One of our research objectives is to develop the best possible of such products that will have consumer acceptance.

A second objective is to utilize cattlehide collagen as a texturizer. We believe that small amounts will improve commonly encountered textural deficiencies in some plant protein-meat products.

NUTRITIVE VALUE OF MEAT EXTENDERS

These investigations involve nutritional, processing, and organoleptic aspects. This paper will be limited to the protein nutritional aspects.

Presently we are studying a number of animal and plant proteins as potential meat extenders and obtaining data on the protein
nutritive value of these proteins individually and in combination
with lean beef proteins to obtain parameters for designing new
nutritious meat products.

EXPERIMENTAL PROCEDURES

Preparation of Samples

Lean beef, the semitendinous muscle, commonly called eye of
the round, was selected as the meat to be blended with meat extenders and as a reference protein in our studies. The lean beef,
partially defatted chopped beef, partially defatted beef fatty
tissue, and collagen, were freeze-dried and ground for use in rat
feeding studies as described by Happich et al. (1975).

Bovine whole blood was obtained from a nearby slaughterhouse.
Approximately 8 gallons were collected in a stainless steel milk
can containing a solution of 66 g of citric acid (0.2% on blood
volume) in 100 ml of water and mixed well to prevent clotting. The
blood was cooled immediately and held in a cold room at 2-3°C until
the following day. About 6 lb of whole blood were weighed into
each of 6 stainless steel drying trays which were covered with
plastic wrap and stored in a freezer. The frozen blood was freeze-
dried in a Stokes shelf dryer at a vacuum of about 0.5 mm mercury
and a shelf temperature of 100°F. Drying time of 24-32 hr was
necessary. About 2850 g of dried whole blood was obtained. There
was some loss because blood foamed out of the pans as the dryer was
evacuated. The dried whole blood was ground in a Wiley Mill to
pass a 2-mm screen, mixed well, and sampled for analysis and rat
feeding studies.

A second sample of bovine blood, about 8 gallons, was collected

and allowed to clot. It was cooled and held overnight at 2-3°C.
The following day the serum was removed from the clot by first
separating the clot into large pieces, hanging the clotted material
in a cheesecloth bag, and allowing the serum to drain. The serum
was pink to light red in color. It was frozen in 8 stainless steel
dryer trays (about 3 lb per tray) and freeze-dried in about 16 hr
as described above for whole blood. The yield of dried serum was
807 g, 7.3% of the serum processed. The dried serum was ground to
pass a 2-mm screen with a mortar and pestle to keep losses minimal.
It was well mixed and sampled for analysis and rat feeding tests.

Dried commercial samples of textured vegetable protein and
meat patties with textured vegetable protein were received from the
Food and Nutrition Service of USDA for amino acid analyses. These
samples of meat patties with textured vegetable protein were extracted with petroleum ether to reduce residual lipids and thoroughly dried before amino acid determinations. Ash, moisture, and
nitrogen were determined on these aliquots and on the aliquots of
the 4 samples of textured vegetable protein used for amino acid
analysis.

Commercial samples of a whey protein concentrate (Enrpro 50),
a soy protein concentrate (Promosoy-100), and a whole fish protein
concentrate were obtained. A sample of fish protein concentrate
prepared from whole hake was obtained from National Marine Fisheries
Service, U.S. Department of Commerce (Sidwell, 1970). A sample of
liquid cyclone process cottonseed protein flour, a deglanded cottonseed protein concentrate, was obtained from the Southern Regional
Research Center (Vix, 1971). Proximate analyses were determined on
all the above samples. Amino acid analyses were determined on the
whey and soy protein concentrates.

Chemical Analyses

Official methods of the AOAC (1970) were used to determine
moisture, ash, fat (petroleum ether extraction), and Kjeldahl
nitrogen. Percentage protein was calculated from the total nitrogen

using the factor for the protein(s) analyzed, i.e., N x 6.25 for
meat, partially defatted products, blood, fish, soy, and cottonseed
protein and N x 6.38 for whey protein.

Amino acid analyses were determined in duplicate using the
Piez-Morris system (1960) in collaboration with Dr. Stephen
Feairheller and Miss Maryann Taylor of the Eastern Regional Research
Center unless otherwise indicated. In preparation for amino acid
analyses, samples containing more than 1% fat were extracted with
petroleum ether. The residual solvent was removed from the sample
by evaporation at room temperature and finally under vacuum. The
samples were then dried in a vacuum oven at 50°C followed by hydrolysis with 6 N HCl for 24 hr. Tryptophan was determined on separate
samples of meat, partially defatted products, or collagen after
hydrolysis with methanesulfonic acid (Liu and Chang, 1971). Samples
of textured vegetable protein, meat patties with textured vegetable
protein, whey, and soy protein concentrates containing appreciable
amounts of carbohydrates were hydrolyzed with barium hydroxide
(Knox et al., 1970) in preparation for analysis of tryptophan.
Each amino acid was calculated as grams of amino acid residue per
100 grams of total amino acid residues.

Protein Efficiency Ratios

PER values, unless otherwise indicated, were determined in
collaboration with Dr. Albert Booth at the Western Regional Research
Laboratory, ARS, USDA, on the partially defatted products, lean
beef, collagen, and on the whey, soy, fish, and liquid cyclone process cottonseed protein concentrates individually, and on combinations of these proteins, using the method of Derse (1965). PER
values were determined by feeding rats a diet containing 10% protein (N x 6.25, except N x 6.38 for whey and N x 5.32 for collagen),
supplied by the test protein only, for 4 weeks. Rats of the
Sprague-Dawley strain (5 per group) were used. Casein was fed as
the protein in the control diet. The PER values were corrected to
that of casein at 2.5 using the following equation:

$$\text{Corrected PER} = \frac{\text{determined PER of test protein x 2.5}}{\text{determined PER of reference standard casein}}$$

Standard deviation was determined and Duncan Multiple Range tests were calculated on the actual PER values before correction to 2.5.

RESULTS AND DISCUSSION

The proximate composition of lean beef, the reference protein, is shown in Table 1. It is high in protein and low in fat. Meat also contains essential minerals and vitamins and an analysis is included in Table 1 for beef with low fat (Watt and Merrill, 1963). The PER was 2.8 when corrected to casein at 2.5 for two separately prepared freeze-dried samples (see Tables 3 and 9). The casein PER test is the only official method available for regulatory purposes.

Protein content, probable first limiting amino acid, and PER value of four animal and three plant proteins that are present or potential meat extenders are listed in Table 2. Included are two beef by-product proteins that have possible value as human food, bovine blood plasma and partially defatted beef fatty tissue, a protein-fat residue from low temperature rendering (under 120°F). These by-products will be discussed in more detail.

Alfalfa white leaf protein concentrate, a new research product of the Western Regional Research Laboratory, is a white protein concentrate from the expressed juice of alfalfa leaves (Edwards et al., 1973).

Partially Defatted (PD) Chopped Beef and PD Beef Fatty Tissue

A study in cooperation with Animal and Plant Health Inspection Service, USDA, related to our collagen investigations, yielded new protein nutritional data on PD chopped beef and PD beef fatty tissue (Happich et al., 1975). They are now used to a limited extent as food components and have the potential for much greater use. Partially defatted beef fatty tissue is allowed in meat

166

NUTRITIVE VALUE OF MEAT EXTENDERS

TABLE 1

COMPOSITION OF LEAN BEEF
100 GRAMS, EDIBLE PORTION

Component, g		Mineral, mg[a]		Vitamin, mg[a]	
Water	72.6	Calcium	12	Thiamine	0.09
Protein	21.8	Phosphorus	203	Riboflavin	0.18
Fat	4.6	Iron	3	Niacin	4.80
Ash	1.1	Magnesium	22	Vitamin A value[b]	20

[a]Mineral and vitamin values taken from Watt and Merrill, 1963, p. 15, No. 352.

[b]International units.

products in limited quantities. The nutritional value of these relatively new commercial food components was evaluated measuring the protein quality individually and in combination with other food proteins (Happich et al., 1975) and is reviewed here. Two PD chopped beef, 1 PD cured cooked chopped beef, and 3 PD beef fatty tissue residues were analyzed. They came from six different establishments. The residues were approximately 90% digestible and contained all of the essential amino acids although tryptophan was present only in traces in the beef fatty tissue residues. Collagen is the principal protein of the beef fatty tissue residues.

The essential amino acid composition of typical samples of lean beef, a PD chopped beef, a PD beef fatty tissue, and collagen is given in Table 3. The data are amino acid residues per 100 grams of total amino acid residues. The variation in the percent of each amino acid in the samples of lean beef, the partially defatted products, and collagen is evident, with lean beef containing the highest quantities and collagen the lowest.

Cystine and tyrosine are not essential in the diet but are included because they can replace part of the methionine and phenylalanine requirement, respectively (Rose and Wixom, 1955b; Rama Rao et al., 1961).

TABLE 2

PER Data on Selected Animal and Vegetable Protein Products

Product	Protein %[c]	Probable first limiting amino acid	PER[d]
PD beef fatty tissue[a,b]	48.3-51.5	TRP	1.1-1.7
Cattle blood plasma		MET or ILEU	2.2[e]
Protein concentrates:			
Whey[b]	58.0	TRP	2.7
Fish	96.0	MET	2.8
Whole fish[b]	91.5	MET	2.6
Soy[b]	67.4	MET	2.2
LCP cottonseed[a]	65.0	ILEU or MET	2.0
Alfalfa, white leaf	90.0	MET	2.5[f]

[a]Product code: PD, partially defatted; LCP, liquid cyclone process.

[b]Commercially available.

[c]Moisture-free basis.

[d]All PER values, except cattle blood plasma, corrected to that of casein at 2.5.

[e]Young et al., 1973.

[f]Kohler, private communication, 1974.

The protein efficiency ratio of lean beef and each partially defatted product is directly proportional to and correlates with the total essential amino acids in the protein. The correlation coefficient for this relation in lean beef and the 6 partially defatted products is 0.97. In all products each essential amino acid, except valine, and tryptophan which could not be calculated, shows a correlation with the PER values. These correlation coefficients range from 0.92 to 0.98. The quality of the protein in the PD beef fatty tissue residues is surprisingly high, PERs range from 1.1 to 1.7, and the data indicate that small amounts of tryptophan had a strikingly beneficial effect.

TABLE 3

Essential Amino Acid Composition and PER Value of Proteins of Lean Beef, Partially Defatted Chopped Beef, Partially Defatted Beef Fatty Tissue, Collagen, and a Whey Protein Concentrate[a]

Amino acid	Lean beef	Partially defatted		Collagen	Whey
		Chopped beef	Beef fatty tissue		
Histidine	3.6	3.0	1.9	0.8	2.1
Isoleucine	5.0	4.1	2.7	1.6	6.1
Leucine	8.3	7.2	5.7	3.0	10.4
Lysine	8.8	7.9	5.2	3.7	7.7
Methionine	2.6	1.9	1.2	0.7	1.5
1/2 cystine	1.3	1.0	1.1	0.0	2.2
Phenylalanine	4.9	4.2	3.6	2.1	3.9
Tyrosine	3.9	3.1	2.2	0.9	3.7
Threonine	4.4	3.8	3.2	1.9	6.4
Tryptophan	1.3	0.6	Trace	0.0	0.9[c]
Valine	5.5	4.6	4.9	2.3	5.7
Total	49.6	41.4	31.7	17.0	50.6
PER[b]	2.8	2.4	1.7	0	2.7

[a]Data taken from Happich et al. (1975). Grams of amino acid residue per 100 grams of total amino acid residues.

[b]PER values corrected to that of casein at 2.5.

[c]Estimated from the manufacturers' analysis of the whey protein concentrate.

TABLE 4

PER Data on Two Beef Fatty Tissue Proteins
and Mixtures with Proteins from Other Sources[a,b]

PDBFT[c] %	Lean beef %	Whey PC[c] %	Soy PC[c] %	PER[d] #1	#3
100	--	--	--	1.1	1.7
33	67	--	--	2.4	2.5
33	--	67	--	2.6	2.7
33	--	--	67	2.0	2.0
25	25	25	25	2.5	2.6

[a]Proteins, singly or in mixture, fed as 10% of diet.
[b]Data taken from Happich et al. (1975).
[c]Product code: PDBFT, partially defatted beef fatty tissue; PC, protein concentrate.
[d]PER values corrected to that of casein at 2.5.

PER data for two of these beef fatty tissue residues and for combinations of each with lean beef, whey protein concentrate, or soy protein concentrate are given in Table 4. The PER value of one beef fatty tissue was 1.1 and the other was 1.7 (the other one analyzed and not shown here was 1.68). When either of these two, #1 (1.1) or #3 (1.7), was combined in a 33:67 protein ratio with the whey protein concentrate or the soy protein concentrate, the PER value was considerably higher than that for the beef fatty tissue alone. The PER values of the combinations with lean beef or whey concentrate proteins approach or are higher than that of casein, the standard. The essential amino acid composition and PER of the whey and the soy protein concentrates which were blended with the partially defatted beef fatty tissue and with other protein products reported in this paper, are given in Tables 3 and 9, respectively. The data indicate that the proteins of lean beef and the whey concentrate supplement the beef fatty tissue proteins to a greater degree than the proteins of the soy concentrate. This is due to the higher methionine and total sulfur amino acid content in lean beef and the whey protein concentrate.

Mixtures with 25% of the protein supplied by a beef fatty tissue and 25% supplied by each of 3 other proteins, lean beef, a whey, and a soy concentrate, had PER values of at least 2.5.

Bovine Blood

Whole bovine blood contains about 17% protein distributed in two principal fractions, a solid fraction composed of blood cells and a liquid fraction, plasma (American Meat Institute, 1950).

The solid fraction is made up of red cells, white cells, and platelets and contains 32% hemoglobin. Hemoglobin may be separated into the heme pigment and the protein globin by chemical procedures (Tybor et al., 1973).

Plasma contains 3 protein fractions: fibrinogen, albumins, and globulins. It also contains salts, fat-like bodies, and other substances such as sugar and vitamins in small quantities. Serum is the liquid fraction remaining after removal of fibrinogen from plasma.

Bovine blood is now dried and diverted to animal feed or fertilizer. It is potentially edible if handled correctly and represents an annual supply of 220 million pounds of protein available for food utilization. Freeze-dried samples of citrated whole blood and of serum were prepared. The latter was separated from freshly collected and clotted blood. Their proximate compositions are given in Table 5. PER tests are in progress at this time.

Literature data on the amino acid composition of whole beef blood and globin show them to be very low in isoleucine (Table 6). Beef blood plasma and serum contain larger amounts of isoleucine. All fractions appear to be low in methionine but contain some cystine. All fractions are high in leucine, lysine, phenylalanine, tryptophan, and valine as compared with casein or whole egg protein.

Blood fractions have not been used to any extent as food components in the United States. In 1970 Pals reported on a dried

TABLE 5

Composition of Freeze-Dried Bovine Blood[a]

Item	Percentages				
	Ash	Fat	N	Protein, N x 6.25	Other
Whole blood	3.8	0.22	14.9	93.3	2.7
Serum	9.9	0.11	13.1	82.1	7.9

[a]Results on a moisture-free basis.

free-flowing beef blood plasma named Isolated Beef Protein (IBP) that was 88-90% protein. The amino acid analysis indicated that isoleucine was low (2.9%), about 55% that of casein. Methionine was low, 1.1%, but IBP contained cystine. The tryptophan content was the same and the lysine content was higher than that of casein. The amino acid analyses indicate this protein would be useful in supplementing foods low in lysine but having adequate to high iso-leucine and sulfur amino acids.

There is little data on the PER of blood fractions in the literature. Young and co-workers (1973) determined the PER of the spray-dried globin and plasma fractions of Tybor et al. (1973). The plasma fraction had a PER of about 2.2. Although globin did not support life (rats died during the sixth week of continued feeding on the globin diet), supplementing it with isoleucine in rat feeding studies produced an apparent PER of 2.2.

Bovine blood collected and prepared for food use offers possi-bilities as protein food supplements, food emulsifying and binding agents, and other uses.

In 1973 Tybor and co-workers reported on the emulsification capacity of spray-dried globin, plasma, and serum concentrates. Satterlee, Free, and Levin (1973) reported from their investiga-tions of the use of several high protein tissue powders as binder/extenders in meat emulsions that whole beef blood had high emulsion capacity and stability. Crenwelge et al. (1974) reported on the effects of pH, protein solubility, and concentration on the

NUTRITIVE VALUE OF MEAT EXTENDERS

TABLE 6

Essential Amino Acid Composition of Bovine Blood Fractions[a]

Amino acid	Blood[b]	Globin[c]	Plasma[c]	Serum[d]	Fibrin[d]
Histidine	--	6.6	3.0	1.9	2.5
Isoleucine	0.4	0.3	3.1	3.4	5.8
Leucine	13.6	13.2	9.2	10.1	10.7
Lysine	9.4	9.8	8.9	7.9	8.7
Methionine	1.8	1.6	1.0	1.7	2.6
Cystine	--	0.1	2.2	3.6	2.0
Phenylalanine	8.0	7.6	5.1	5.0	4.5
Tyrosine	2.6	2.5	4.9	5.0	5.6
Threonine	4.7	4.1	6.0	6.3	7.3
Tryptophan	1.4	2.0	1.9	1.8	3.5
Valine	8.0	9.4	6.9	7.5	4.1
Total	49.9	57.2	52.3	54.2	57.3

[a]Analyses taken from the literature.

[b]Percentage of total protein (Olson, 1970).

[c]Grams per 100 grams protein. Rounded off to first decimal (Young et al., 1973).

[d]Grams of amino acid per 16.0 grams of nitrogen (Block and Weiss, 1956).

emulsification capacity of decolorized bovine hemoglobin (Tybor et al., 1973).

The technology for recovering beef blood proteins for food use is fairly well developed (Gordon, 1971; Halliday, 1973; Porter and Michaels, 1971; Garner et al., 1971; Tybor et al., 1973). However, we find that there is considerable need for studies concerned with obtaining optimum functionality, including uses strictly for nutritional purposes. We have such work in progress.

Soy Proteins

Recently we had the opportunity, in collaboration with USDA Food and Nutrition Service, to determine the amino acid composition of 4 commercial samples of textured vegetable protein and 3 samples of meat patties containing textured vegetable protein.

The PER value was determined for each product. Values ranged from 1.7 to 2.1 for the four samples of textured vegetable protein. Those for meat patties with textured vegetable protein ranged from 2.1 to 2.3 and do not meet USDA regulations. They were not much higher than the PERs of the textured vegetable protein samples. An amino acid analysis for each type of product is given in Table 7. These analyses indicate that the meat patties with textured vegetable protein contained higher amounts of glycine and proline than either textured vegetable protein or lean beef, and 2.6-3.2% hydroxyproline (textured vegetable protein had no hydroxyproline and lean beef contained only a slight trace of hydroxyproline, Table 9), indicating a higher collagen content than was found in lean beef. There are products on the market that contain some partially defatted beef fatty tissue with meat and soy and this may explain the composition of these products. The total sulfur amino acids were low, about 65% of those found in lean beef and lower than those in textured vegetable protein.

Recently investigators have been obtaining information on the use of soy proteins in meat and meat products. Korslund et al. (1973) and Kies and Fox (1973) studied the nutritive value of beef and soy proteins using human feeding tests. Rakosky (1974) reported on the nutritive value of soy products and of mixtures of soy and meat protein. Wilding (1974) reported on the nutritional quality of blends of textured soy and beef proteins and Wolford (1974) reported on consumer acceptance of beef/soy. The functionality and performance of soy proteins in meat blends in comminuted meat systems and in processed meat products were recently investigated by Judge et al. (1974), Schweiger (1974), and Roberts (1974).

Recently, we had PERs determined on mixtures containing 60,

70, or 80% lean beef proteins and 40, 30, or 20%, respectively, of the proteins of a soy concentrate, PER 2.2. The PER results are found in Table 8. There was no significant difference between the PER values of these three mixtures or between either one and the PER of casein at 2.5. However, mixtures containing higher concentrations of soy would be expected to have lower PERs than casein.

The essential amino acid composition of lean beef, the lean beef-soy mixtures, and the soy protein concentrate is shown in Table 9. The amino acid compositions for the beef-soy mixtures were calculated from the determined amino acid composition of lean beef and of the soy protein concentrate. All PER values were determined by rat feeding tests.

The essential amino acids which have the greatest variation throughout the five samples are histidine, lysine, methionine, and the total sulfur amino acids. Methionine sulfoxide, an oxidation product of methionine, was also found in these samples. Bennett (1939) reported that under the conditions of her experiments DL-methionine sulfoxide was able to replace DL-methionine in the diet of the albino rat. Kohler et al. (1974) touched on the nutritive value of methionine sulfoxide. Compared with lean beef, the soy protein concentrate contains about 26% methionine; 55% methionine plus methionine sulfoxide; and 71% total sulfur amino acids, methionine, methionine sulfoxide, and cystine. Methionine is the first limiting amino acid. Although the proteins of soy contain only 74% as much lysine as lean beef protein, soy proteins have about the same lysine as whole egg, a reference protein of high quality. Tryptophan varies little. There is a linear correlation between the PER values and each essential amino acid in the five samples. The correlation coefficient (r) equals ± 0.97 with one exception, r = 0.98 for isoleucine.

Combinations of Lean Beef Proteins with Four Protein Concentrates

PER values for combinations of lean beef proteins and proteins of whey, whole fish, soy, or cottonseed protein concentrates in

TABLE 7

Amino Acid Composition and PER Value of
a Textured Vegetable Protein and a Sample
of Meat Patties with Textured Vegetable Protein[a]

Amino acid	Textured vegetable protein	Meat patties with textured vegetable protein
Histidine	3.2	2.9
Isoleucine	5.3	4.5
Leucine	7.9	7.3
Lysine	6.8	6.3
Methionine	1.0	1.0
Methionine sulfoxide	0.9	0.6
1/2 cystine	1.2	1.0
Phenylalanine	5.9	4.9
Tyrosine	4.3	3.7
Threonine	4.2	3.7
Tryptophan	1.3	1.0
Valine	5.2	5.2
Alanine	4.2	5.7
Arginine	8.0	7.3
Aspartic acid	10.8	9.8
Glutamic acid	16.0	15.1
Glycine	3.8	6.4
Hydroxylysine	0.0	Trace
Hydroxyproline	0.0	3.2
Proline	5.0	6.3
Serine	4.9	4.1
Approximate % of total N accounted for	84.7	89.3
PER[b]	2.1	2.1

[a]Grams of amino acid residues per 100 grams of total amino acid residues.

[b]PER values corrected to that of casein at 2.5.

TABLE 8

PER Data on Protein Mixtures of
Lean Beef and a Soy Protein Concentrate (PC)[a]

Lean beef, %	Soy PC, %	PER[b]
100	--	2.8
--	100	2.2
80	20	2.5[c]
70	30	2.6[c]
60	40	2.5[c]

[a]Proteins, singly or in mixture, fed as 10% of diet.

[b]PER values corrected to that of casein at 2.5.

[c]These PER values were not significantly different from each other or from the PER of casein.

mixtures of 70 and 30%, respectively, are in Table 10. All mixtures met the minimum PER requirement of 2.5, complying with USDA regulations for meat products for the School Lunch Program. The whey-lean beef mixture had the highest PER, although it was not significantly better than the lean beef-soy or lean beef-fish mixtures. The animal proteins tested had higher PER values and tended to produce mixtures with higher PERs than the plant proteins tested. This suggests the possible advantages of combining lean beef and soy proteins with a third protein of good quality, such as whey, fish, or perhaps blood plasma proteins to ensure nutritious meat products with a PER similar to that of lean beef, particularly if there is mutual supplementation of the amino acids. PER tests are in progress now of 70-20-10 and 60-20-20 combinations of lean beef, soy, and a third protein, either whey, fish, or cottonseed protein concentrate, respectively. We also plan to determine PERs of cooked mixtures of lean beef and soy proteins and cooked mixtures with a third protein.

TABLE 9

Amino Acid Composition and PER Data for
Lean Beef and Soy Proteins and their Mixtures[a]

Amino acid		Lean beef	Lean beef-soy protein mixtures[b,c]			Soy protein[b]
			80-20	70-30	60-40	
Essential amino acids:						
Histidine		4.3	4.1	3.9	3.8	3.2
Isoleucine		5.2	5.2	5.2	5.1	5.0
Leucine		8.2	8.0	7.9	7.9	7.4
Lysine		9.0	8.6	8.3	8.1	6.7
Methionine		2.7	2.3	2.1	1.9	0.7
Methionine sulfoxide		0.4	0.5	0.6	0.6	1.0
1/2 cystine		0.92	0.96	0.98	1.0	1.15
Phenylalanine		4.9	5.1	5.1	5.2	5.6
Tyrosine		3.8	3.9	3.9	4.0	4.2
Threonine		4.7	4.6	4.5	4.5	4.2
Tryptophan		0.89	0.90	0.91	0.91	0.94
Valine		5.6	5.5	5.4	5.4	5.1
	Total	50.21	49.16	48.19	47.81	44.19

Nonessential amino acids:

Alanine	5.5	5.2	5.0	4.9	4.0
Arginine	6.9	7.2	7.3	7.5	8.3
Aspartic acid	9.4	9.8	10.0	10.3	11.6
Glutamic acid	14.5	15.0	15.3	15.5	17.1
Glycine	4.5	4.3	4.3	4.2	3.6
Hydroxyproline	very slight trace	--	--	--	0.0
Proline	4.5	4.6	4.7	4.8	5.3
Serine	4.0	4.2	4.3	4.4	4.9
Total	49.70	50.80	51.50	52.20	55.80
Approximate % of total N accounted for	84.13	--	--	--	88.86
PER[d]	2.8	2.54	2.57	2.46	2.2

[a] Grams of amino acid residues per 100 grams of total amino acid residues.

[b] The soy protein was soy protein concentrate.

[c] The amino acid compositions of the lean beef-soy protein mixtures were calculated from the determined amino acid composition of lean beef and soy protein.

[d] PER values corrected to that of casein at 2.5.

TABLE 10

PER Data on Protein Mixtures of
Lean Beef and Several Protein Concentrates[a]

Lean beef %	Whey %	Whole fish %	Soy %	LCP[b] cottonseed %	PER[c]
70	30	--	--	--	2.7
70	--	30	--	--	2.6
70	--	--	30	--	2.6
70	--	--	--	30	2.5

[a]Proteins in mixture fed as 10% of the diet.

[b]Liquid cyclone process.

[c]PER values corrected to that of casein at 2.5.

Cattlehide Collagen

Collagen, a high-molecular-weight, insoluble, fibrous protein, is a promising food texturizing agent. Food components such as soy flours, whey, dry milk powder, gums, or gelatine may be used in admixture with meat or in meat analogues for economical and nutritional reasons. They produce products with textures that frequently are undesirable and there is evidence that collagen in small quantities can improve the texture of such products.

Our research is mainly concerned with utilizing the fibrous collagen present in mature cattlehides and especially the lower layer of lime-unhaired hide called the flesh split (Whitmore et al., 1970). The Engineering and Development Laboratory at the Eastern Regional Research Center has developed processes for comminuting the collagen in splits into small particles and produced 5 wet products, their differences being particle size (Komanowsky et al., 1974).

Fibrous collagen has unique physical and chemical properties. It is practically odorless and tasteless, has a bland flavor and a hydrothermal shrinkage temperature of about 60-65°C. It is amphoteric and may act as a buffer. It absorbs and binds a large quantity of water. Whitmore et al. (1972) found that fibrous, insoluble, limed collagen will form a wide variety of aqueous dispersions producing characteristics from a fibrous paste to a liquid virtually free of fibers. The dispersions may be thixotropic. This technology has made it possible to prepare collagen foams, films, coatings, emulsions, gels, and pastes. Collagen offers the potential of varying the character, viscosity, consistency, mouth feel, tenderness, and juiciness (succulence) of extended meat and other food products to meet consumers' expectations.

Fibrous cattlehide collagen was about 90% digestible in rat feeding tests. It has an unusual and characteristic amino acid composition. About one-third of the amino acid residues is glycine. It contains hydroxyproline and hydroxylysine and is completely lacking in tryptophan and cystine. It is deficient in all the other essential amino acids as compared with casein or whole egg. A PER of zero was obtained when rats were fed a diet containing 10% collagen as the only source of protein. However, probing tests supplementing collagen with DL-tryptophan and DL-methionine and feeding it at 20% of the diet resulted in a positive PER value.

To establish parameters on combinations of collagen with other proteins, we have obtained the PER values listed in Table 11, on three combinations of collagen and lean beef proteins and on lean beef-collagen protein blends in combination with proteins of a whey or soy protein concentrate.

The PER of lean beef was 2.8. Adding 10% collagen to lean beef reduced the PER to about 2.5, the PER of the standard casein. A mixture of 50% collagen and lean beef proteins had a PER of 1.7.

All of the PER values of lean beef-collagen protein mixtures with whey protein were similar to the PER for casein. Those with soy protein were lower. Of the two products used, the whey protein supplemented the lean beef-collagen blend proteins to a greater degree. They have a higher methionine and total sulfur amino acid content and methionine is probably the second limiting amino acid in the lean beef-collagen blend.

TABLE 11

PER Data on Lean Beef, Whey and Soy Proteins,
and Mixtures with Lean Beef and Collagen Proteins[a]

Lean beef, %	Collagen, %	Whey[b], %	Soy[b], %	PER[c]
100	--	--	--	2.8
90	10	--	--	2.5
50	50	--	--	1.7
10	90	--	--	0
--	--	100	--	2.7
90	5	5	--	2.5
50	25	25	--	2.4
25	25	50	--	2.6
--	--	--	100	2.2
50	25	--	25	2.2
25	25	--	50	2.1

[a]Proteins, singly or in mixture, fed as 10% of diet.
[b]Protein concentrate.
[c]PER values corrected to that of casein at 2.5.

These data indicate that collagen as an added component in meat products or meat analogues in limited quantities can result in products that have a satisfactory PER.

ACKNOWLEDGMENTS

The authors thank Stauffer Chemical Company for a sample of whey protein concentrate, Enrpro 50; Central Soya for a sample of soy protein concentrate, Promosoy-100; Astra Nutrition (USA) Incorporated for a sample of whole fish protein concentrate; the Southern Regional Research Center for a sample of liquid cyclone process cottonseed flour; and National Marine Fisheries Service, USDC, for a sample of fish protein concentrate.

Reference to brand or firm names does not constitute

endorsement by the U.S. Department of Agriculture over others of a similar nature not mentioned.

REFERENCES

American Meat Institute. 1950. By-products of the Meat Packing Industry, Institute of Meat Packing, Chicago, Illinois.

AOAC. 1970. Official Methods of Analysis (11th Ed.). Association of Official Agricultural Chemists. Washington, D.C.

Bennett, M.A. 1939. Metabolism of sulphur.X. The replaceability of DL-methionine in the diet of albino rats with its partially oxidized derivative, DL-methionine sulphoxide Biochem. J. 33-1794.

Bird, K.M. 1974. Plant proteins: progress and problems. Food Technol. 28:3:31.

Block, R.J. and K.W. Weiss. 1956. Amino Acid Handbook, Methods and Results of Protein Analysis. Charles C. Thomas, Springfield, Illinois. pp. 252-253.

Crenwelge, D.D., C.W. Dill, P.T. Tybor and W.A. Landmann. 1974. A comparison of the emulsification capacities of some protein concentrates. J. Food Sci. 39:175.

Derse, P.H. 1965. Evaluation of protein quality (biological method). J. Ass. Offic. Anal. Chem. 48:847.

Edwards, R.H., R.E. Miller, D. De Fremery, B.E. Knuckles, E.M. Bickoff and G.O. Kohler. 1973. Presented at the 166th Meeting of the American Chemical Society, August 27-30, Chicago, Illinois. (Abstract).

Garner, R.G., G.J. Mountney and S.E. Zobrisky. 1971. Agricultural processing wastes: a review. Proceedings of the 68th Annual Convention of the Association of Southern Agricultural Workers, Inc. (Abstract).

Gordon, A. 1971. Animal blood as a source of protein in food products. Food Trade Rev. 41:4:29.

Halliday, D.A. 1973. Blood - a source of proteins. Process Biochem. 8:12:15.

Happich, M.L., R.A. Whitmore, S. Feairheller, M.M. Taylor, C.E. Swift, J. Naghski, A.N. Booth and R.H. Alsmeyer. 1975. Composition and protein efficiency ratio of partially defatted chopped beef and of partially defatted beef fatty tissue and combinations with selected proteins. J. Food Sci. 40:35.

Judge, M.D., C.G. Haugh, G.L. Zachariah, C.E. Parmelee and R.L. Pyle. 1974. Soya additives in beef patties. J. Food Sci. 39:137.

Kies, C. and H.M. Fox. 1971. Comparison of the protein nutritional value of TVP, methionine-enriched TVP and beef at two levels of intake for human adults. J. Food Sci. 36:841.

Knox, R., G.O. Kohler, R. Palter and H.G. Walker. 1970. Determination of tryptophan in feeds. Anal. Biochem. 36:136.

Kohler, G.O. 1974. Private communication.

Kohler, G.O., H.G. Walker Jr., D.D. Kuzmicky and S.C. Witt. 1974. Problems in analysis for sulfur amino acids in feeds and foods. Presented at the 168th Meeting of the American Chemical Society, September 9-13, Atlantic City, New Jersey. (Abstract). See also this volume, Part 1.

Komanowsky, M., H.I. Sinnamon, S. Elias, W.K. Heiland and N.C. Aceto. 1974. Production of comminuted collagen for novel applications. J. Amer. Leather Chem. Ass. 69:410.

Korslund, M., C. Kies and H.M. Fox. 1973. Comparison of the protein nutritional value of TVP, methionine-enriched TVP and beef for adolescent boys. J. Food Sci. 38:637.

Liu, T.Y. and Y.H. Chang. 1971. Hydrolysis of proteins with p-toluenesulfonic acid. J. Biol. Chem. 246:2842.

Olson, F.C. 1970. Nutritional aspects of offal proteins. Proceedings of the Meat Industry Research Conference, University of Chicago, March 26-27. p. 23.

Pals, C.H. 1970. The practical aspects of blood component procurement. Proceedings of the Meat Industry Research Conference, University of Chicago, March 26-27. p. 17.

Piez, K.A. and L. Morris. 1960. A modified procedure for the automatic analysis of amino acids. Anal. Biochem. 1:187.

Porter, M.C. and A.S. Michaels. 1971. Membrane ultrafiltration. 3. Applications in the processing of meat by-products. Chem. Technol. July, p. 440.

Rakosky, Joseph Jr. 1974. Soy grits, flour, concentrates, and isolates in meat products. J. Amer. Oil Chem. Soc. 51:1:123A.

Rama Rao, P.B., H.W. Norton and B.C. Johnson. 1961. The amino acid composition and nutritive value of proteins. J. Nutr. 73:38.

Roberts, L.H. 1974. Utilization of high levels of soy protein in comminuted processed meat products. J. Amer. Oil Chem. Soc. 51:1:195A.

Rose, W.C. and R.L. Wixom. 1955. The amino acid requirements of man. XIII. The sparing effect of cystine on the methionine requirement. J. Biol. Chem. 216:763.

Rose, W.C. and R.L. Wixom. 1955. The amino acid requirements of man. XIV. The sparing effect of tyrosine on the phenylalanine requirement. J. Biol. Chem. 217:95.

Satterlee, L.D., B. Free and E. Levin. 1973. Utilization of high protein tissue powders as a binder/extender in meat emulsions. J. Food Sci. 38:306.

Schweiger, R.G. 1974. Soy protein concentrates and isolates in comminuted meat systems. J. Amer. Oil Chem. Soc. 51:1:192A.

Sidwell, V.D., B.R. Stillings and G.M. Knobl Jr. 1970. The fish protein concentrate story. 10. U.S. Bureau of Commercial Fisheries FPCs: nutritional quality and use in foods. Food Technol. 24:8:40.

Tybor, P.T., C.W. Dill and W.A. Landmann. 1973. Effect of decolorization and lactose incorporation on the emulsification capacity of spray-dried blood protein concentrates. J. Food Sci. 38:4.

Vix, H.L.E., P.H. Eaves, H.K. Gardner Jr. and M.G. Lambou. 1971. Degossypolized cottonseed flour--the liquid process. J. Amer. Oil Chem. Soc. 48:611.

Watt, B.K. and A.L. Merrill. 1963. Composition of Foods, Agric. Handbook No. 8. USDA, Washington, D.C. p. 15, no. 352.

Whitmore, R.A., H.W. Jones, W. Windus and J. Naghski. 1970. Preparation of hide collagen for food. J. Amer. Leather Chem. Ass. 65:383.

Whitmore, R., H. Jones, W. Windus and J. Naghski. 1972. Preparation and visco-elastic properties of fibrous collagen dispersions from limed cattlehide splits. J. Food Sci. 37:302.

Wilding, M.D. 1974. Textured proteins in meats and meat-like products. J. Amer. Oil Chem. Soc. 51:1:128A.

Wolford, K.M. 1974. Beef/soy: consumer acceptance. J. Amer. Oil Chem. Soc. 51:1:131A.

Young, C.R., R.W. Lewis, W.A. Landmann and C.W. Dill. 1973. Nutritive value of globin and plasma protein fractions from bovine blood. Nutr. Rep. Int. 8:4:211.

8

NUTRITIONAL EVALUATION OF HORSEMEAT

S. J. Pintauro, K-T Yuann, and J. G. Bergan

Departments of Food and Nutritional Science and
Food and Resource Chemistry

University of Rhode Island
Kingston, Rhode Island

Commercially available ground horsemeat was subjected to proximate analysis. On a wet weight basis, the horsemeat contained 69.0, 1.0, 7.6, and 22.6 percent of moisture, ash, fat, and protein, respectively. An amino acid analysis showed that the sulfur amino acids were limiting and that the chemical score and calculated protein efficiency ratio (PER) compared favorably with ground beef. An analysis of the fatty acid composition by gas-liquid chromatography showed a relatively high concentration of linolenic acid. The cholesterol content was determined to be approximately 70 mg per 100 grams of sample. In addition, a relationship was found to exist between the intensity of the color of the rib adipose tissue and the levels of β-carotene present. Organoleptic rating showed that horsemeat frankfurters, when compared to commercial products, were slightly less acceptable, but that little difference was detected among ground meat samples.

INTRODUCTION

In recent years, with the unceasing rise in the price of meats, most notably beef, the search for a more economical source

187

of protein has resulted in an interest in horsemeat. A recent review (Root, 1974) points out that horses are among the game animals depicted in the cave paintings of France and Spain dating back as far as the Paleolithic era. They were also a significant part of the diet of the Tartars and Mongols, as well as many other populations. After 1200 A.D., consumption of horsemeat in Europe had almost ceased, except during periods when food, particularly animal protein, was not readily available. Great Britain is an excellent example: as recent as 1951, 53,000 horses were consumed primarily due to the postwar meat shortage. Coincidently, the Harvard Faculty Club still has horsemeat on its menu, since it was first served during World War II, when it was difficult to obtain beef.

Today, horsemeat is a significant part of the diet only of certain South American Indians, some North Africans, to a slight extent the Swedes, and the French, whose total consumption of horsemeat surpasses that of all other populations.

The purpose of this study is to ascertain horsemeat's nutritional value, as well as its acceptability. A proximate analysis, amino acid analysis (including chemical score and calculated PER), fatty acid analysis, β-carotene determination, and cholesterol determination were run, as well as a simple organoleptic evaluation.

EXPERIMENTAL PROCEDURE

Commercially available fresh ground horsemeat was analyzed for moisture, crude protein, crude fat, and ash content, according to the procedures outlined in the Official Methods of Analysis of the AOAC (1970).

Amino acid content was determined with the Technicon Auto-analyzer in a standard 21-hour chromatogram. Samples were prepared for analysis by heating with excess 6N HCl at 110°C, for 24 hours, in an evacuated, sealed pyrex tube. Following complete hydrolysis, the excess HCl was removed under reduced pressure. Tryptophan was separately analyzed following alkaline hydrolysis. A chemical score (FAO, 1973) was calculated according to the formula:

Chemical Score =

$$\frac{\text{mg of amino acid per gram of test protein}}{\text{mg of amino acid per gram of reference pattern}} \times 100$$

A PER was calculated according to the equations derived by Alsmeyer, Cunningham, and Happich (1974). This new method of predicting PER is a result of correlating known PER values and amino acid analyses and the relationship between PER and specific amino acids. It must be noted, as the authors are careful to point out, that the amino acids used in these equations do not necessarily have more biological significance than other amino acids, but simply a more significant mathematical relationship to PER.

Cholesterol content was determined on ground horsemeat as well as two grades of ground beef, extra lean and regular. The principle method used was that of Tu, Powrie, and Fennen (1967). Basically, this procedure involves a cold extraction of the lipid material, saponification of the extract, reextraction of the cholesterol after saponification, and finally, addition of a stable color-forming reagent, in this case ferric perchlorate dissolved in ethyl acetate and concentrated sulfuric acid as outlined by Wybenga et al. (1970). Boiling a small amount of the extracted cholesterol in combination with this reagent produces a stable color which can be measured photometrically. An analysis of the β-carotene levels of rib adipose tissue, in order to examine the possible relationship between the levels of this pigment and the yellow color of the adipose tissue, was determined according to Winsten and Dalal (1972). Determinations were conducted on three samples of rib adipose tissue with obvious differences in yellow intensity. The three samples were classified according to color as, a) very light yellow, b) slightly yellow, and c) very yellow.

The fatty acid composition of horsemeat was determined by

gas-liquid chromatography. Samples of adipose tissue were prepared according to the method of Metcalfe, Schmitz, and Pelka (1968) and chromatographed on a 10% Hi-Eff 1BP/Chromosorb WAW (80-100 mesh) column using a Varian Aerograph Series 1800 Gas Chromatograph, equipped with a hydrogen flame ionization detector. Operating conditions were: injection-port temperature 275°C, detector temperature 250°C, column temperature 180°C, and a nitrogen gas flow rate of 50 cc/min.

Finally, in order to assess the acceptability of horsemeat, we set up a simple organoleptic evaluation using a nine-point hedonic scale ranging from a score of nine for excellent to a score of one for extremely poor. The evaluation was conducted on two consecutive days.

On the first day, five brands of frankfurter were tested. They were: 1) Horse--pork, 2) Spicy--pork beef, 3) Skinless--all beef, 4) Kosher--all beef (deli purchased), and 5) Kosher--all beef (packaged). All frankfurters were boiled for approximately ten minutes and served immediately. Participants were instructed to evaluate each sample separately, according to appearance, smell, texture, and taste. Water and soda crackers, to be used between samplings, were available. Participants were not informed as to the identity of the various samples.

On the second day, six varieties of ground meat were tested. They were: 1) Regular beef, 2) Lean beef, 3) Extra lean beef, 4) Lamb, 5) Horse, and 6) Horse with beef fat. The samples were prepared by broiling until thoroughly cooked and served immediately. All data were statistically tested using a simple analysis of variance (IBM Statistical Package, Version 2, 1970).

RESULTS AND DISCUSSION

The results of the proximate analysis are given in Table 1. Literature values are included for the sake of comparison. Although it has been reported that horsemeat is richer in glycogens than

TABLE 1

Proximate Analysis

Item	Horse		Beef	
	Experimental	USDA[a]	USDA[b]	
			Regular	Lean
Moisture	69.0 ± 1.19 (S.D.)	76.0	60.2	68.3
Fat	7.6 ± 0.17	4.1	21.2	10.0
Protein	22.6 ± 0.41	18.1	17.9	20.7
Ash	1.0 ± 0.05	0.9	0.9	0.9

[a]USDA, 1973. Unpublished Data. Agric. Research Service, Hyattsville, Maryland.

[b]Watt and Merrill, 1963.

other meats (Root, 1974), the carbohydrate content in this study was assumed to be negligible.

The crude fat content of horsemeat gave an interesting comparison. The experimental value of 7.55% is the highest of all reported values for horsemeat, but it is still lower than the lowest of any value reported for beef. The protein content is slightly higher than for lean beef and the ash contents of beef and horse are comparable. Further analysis of the ash showed that the iron content of the horsemeat was approximately 5 mg per 100-gram sample (J. Spirn, Personal Communication).

The results of the amino acid analysis for horsemeat and the chemical score are shown in Table 2. The reference pattern used for the determination of the chemical score was that of the new 1973 FAO provisional pattern based on the derived estimates of amino acid requirements, rather than the earlier pattern based on egg protein. Using this reference pattern, a chemical score of 73 was calculated, with the essential, sulfur-containing amino acids, methionine and cystine, being limiting.

The equations derived by Alsmeyer et al. (1974), and given below, were used for the prediction of PER from amino acid analysis.

191

1)   PER = -0.684 + 0.456 (LEU) - 0.047 (PRO)

2)   PER = -0.468 + 0.454 (LEU) - 0.105 (TYR)

3)   PER =

     -1.816 + 0.435 (MET) + 0.780 (LEU) + 0.211 (HIS) - 0.944 (TYR)

In an attempt to predict PER, all three equations and the results of the amino acid analysis as well as the FAO amino acid values for horsemeat and ground beef were tested. The results are illustrated in Table 3. All three equations predicted accurately the PER for ground beef based on the FAO values. However, equation 3 yielded a very high PER value for horsemeat; apparently, the first two equations are more accurate predictions.

The results of the cholesterol and β-carotene determinations are given in Table 4. The cholesterol content of ground horsemeat is lower than that of the regular ground beef samples, but no significant difference is evident between the extra lean beef and horse. Although the β-carotene values showed poor reproducibility, the results do demonstrate a definite relationship between the

TABLE 2

Amino Acid Analysis of Horsemeat (MG/G Nitrogen)[a,b]

Aspartic acid	581	Methionine	134
Threonine	270	Isoleucine	272
Serine	251	Leucine	455
Glutamic acid	734	Tyrosine	134
Proline	279	Phenylalanine	261
Glycine	354	Lysine	595
Alanine	426	Histidine	205
Valine	274	Arginine	405
Cystine	26	Tryptophan	63

[a]Chemical Score = 73.

[b]Limiting Amino Acids = Methionine and Cystine.

TABLE 3

Calculated PER[a]

Test	Equation 1	Equation 2	Equation 3
Beef (FAO values)[b]	2.95	2.94	3.16
Horse (FAO values)[b]	3.65	3.64	4.18
Horse (experimental values)	2.71	2.90	3.96

[a]Amino acids expressed as grams of the individual amino acid residue per 100 grams of the total amino acid residue.

[b]FAO Nutrition Studies No. 24, 1970.

intensity of the yellow color and the levels of β-carotene present. In fact, the very yellow adipose tissue had a carotene value of more than 10 μg per gram of sample.

The fatty acid composition of the horse adipose tissue is given in Table 5. As expected, palmitic acid and oleic acid comprised the largest percentages with 29 and 35%, respectively. The experimental values generally agree with other published values (Swern, 1964; Otake et al., 1972). Although Swern (1964) reported a higher proportion of linolenic acid than does the present study (16.3 versus 10.0%), a relatively high concentration of this fatty acid is present

TABLE 4

Cholesterol and β-Carotene Concentrations

Cholesterol (mg/100 g meat sample)	
Regular ground beef	76.7 ± 1.72 (S.D.)
Extra lean ground beef	70.1 ± 1.27
Ground horsemeat	70.3 ± 1.43
β-Carotene (μg/g fat sample)	
Horse adipose tissue	
Very light yellow	1.47 ± 0.56 (S.D.)
Slightly yellow	3.54 ± 1.22
Very yellow	10.44 ± 2.84

TABLE 5

Fatty Acid Analysis of Horse Rib Adipose Tissue

Fatty acid	%
$C_{10} - C_{12}$	Trace
Myristic	4.6
$C_{14:1} - C_{15:0}$	0.9
Palmitic	28.7
Palmitoleic	8.7
Stearic	4.5
Oleic	34.2
Linoleic	6.3
Linolenic	10.0

in the horse adipose tissue.

The results of the organoleptic evaluation are shown in Table 6. There were a total of 16 judges and 5 samples in the frankfurter evaluation and 13 judges and 6 samples in the ground meat evaluation. F-values were calculated between samples and between judges and the standard F-values at $\alpha = 0.05$, with the appropriate degrees of freedom, are given in the left-hand column of the table. The figures reported for each sample and category are the mean values of all judges for that sample.

In the frankfurter evaluation, analysis of variance showed no significant difference between samples or judges in the appearance and texture category, but a difference was demonstrated between both samples and judges for smell and taste. The ground meat evaluation showed a significant difference in all categories between judges; however, no difference was detected between the six samples, except in appearance. Accordingly, the ground horsemeat proved as acceptable as ground beef or lamb.

TABLE 6

Organoleptic Evaluation

Frankfurters	Appearance	Smell	Texture	Taste
Kosher--all beef (deli purchased)	5.8	5.1	5.9	5.0
Horse--pork	4.6	4.3	4.4	3.6
Skinless--all beef	6.1	4.9	5.5	6.1
Spicy--pork beef	6.3	5.2	6.8	6.6
Kosher--all beef (packaged)	6.4	6.1	6.1	5.8
Between samples				
$F_{.05}$ (4,60) = 2.53	F=2.320	F=3.457	F=1.221	F=5.883
Between judges				
$F_{.05}$ (15,60) = 1.84	F=1.899	F=3.128	F=1.596	F=2.652
Ground meat	Appearance	Smell	Texture	Taste
Lean beef	6.9	6.2	5.6	5.8
Lamb	6.4	5.6	5.4	5.1
Extra lean beef	6.3	6.1	5.5	5.1
Horse	4.8	6.3	4.9	5.0
Regular beef	6.1	6.2	5.6	5.4
Horse with beef fat	5.4	4.8	5.1	4.1
Between samples				
$F_{.05}$ (5,60) = 2.37	F=4.195	F=2.130	F=0.658	F=1.859
Between judges				
$F_{.05}$ (12,60) = 1.92	F=5.855	F=3.173	F=12.007	F=6.195

REFERENCES

Alsmeyer, R.H., A.E. Cunningham and M.L. Happich. 1974. Equations predict PER from amino acid analysis. Food Technol. 28:7:34.

AOAC. 1970. Official Methods of Analysis (11th Ed.). Association of Official Agricultural Chemists. Washington, D.C.

FAO Nutrition Studies No. 24. 1970. Amino acid content of foods and biological data on proteins. Rome, Italy.

FAO Nutritional Meetings Report Series No. 52. WHO Technical Report Series No. 522. 1973. Energy and protein requirements. Rome, Italy.

Metcalfe, L.D., A.A. Schmitz and J.R. Pelka. 1966. Rapid preparation of fatty acid esters from lipids for gas chromatographic analysis. Anal. Chem. 38:514.

Otake, Yoshiyuki Takayuki and Nakazato. 1972. Fatty acid and triglyceride composition of horsemeat. Nippon Chikusan Gakkai-Ho. 43:11:631.

Root, Waverly. 1974. They eat horses, don't they? Esquire. 81:82.

Swern, D. 1964. Bailey's Industrial Oil and Fat Products (3rd Ed.). Interscience Publishers, New York.

Tu, C., W.D. Powrie and D. Fennen. 1967. Free and esterified cholesterol content of animal muscles and meat products. J. Food Sci. 32:30.

Watt, B.K. and A.L. Merrill. 1963. Composition of Foods, Agric. Handbook No. 8. USDA, Washington, D.C.

Winsten, S. and F. Dalal. 1972. Manual of Clinical Laboratory Procedures for Non-Routine Problems. CRC Press, Cleveland.

Wybenga, D.R., V.J. Pileggi, P.H. Dirstine and J. DiGiorgio. 1970. Direct manual determination of serum cholesterol with a single stable reagent. Clin. Chem. 16:12:980.

9

NUTRITIONAL AND CHEMICAL EVALUATION
OF THE PROTEIN OF VARIOUS FINFISH AND SHELLFISH

Virginia D. Sidwell and Mary E. Ambrose

Southeast Utilization Research Center
National Marine Fisheries Service, NOAA
U.S. Department of Commerce
College Park, Maryland

The proximate composition of the muscle of the twelve species
of finfish and shellfish agreed well with values in literature,
although surf clams contained less protein than the reported values.
With the exception of thread herring, variation in the amino acid
profile of the other four finfish was not extensive. Except for
mahogany (ocean) quahog, which was especially low in lysine and
methionine, the amino acid profile for the protein in the muscle of
shellfish was not too greatly different. The protein efficiency
ratio (PER) values, with the exception of thread herring, mahogany
(ocean) quahog, and Atlantic squid, were equal to or better than
that of casein.

INTRODUCTION

Forty billion pounds of marine finfish and shellfish are
potentially available for harvesting along the nearly 90 thousand
miles of tidal coasts of the United States. Since the availability
of traditionally caught fisheries products is decreasing and the
demand for animal protein is growing, it is becoming necessary to

look at the many species of finfish and shellfish that are not commercially harvested or are presently underutilized. Reasons for their underutilization are generally at least one of the following: 1) no efficient method for harvesting; 2) no adequate method either to process the product or to stabilize it to retain its initial quality; 3) insufficiently developed foreign or domestic market. Consequently, the monetary return from these underutilized species is at a minimum.

The American consumer is quite nutrition-conscious. To establish a market for these relatively new products, it is important for the consumer to know the quality of the protein in these species of finfish and shellfish. This investigation reports the proximate composition, amino acid profile, and nutritive quality of the protein in 12 underutilized species of finfish and shellfish.

PROCEDURE

Sources of Samples

The following finfish and shellfish were evaluated in this study:

Finfish
     American eel--*Anguilla rostrata*
     Croaker--*Micropogon undulatus*
     Mullet--*Mugilidae* spp.
     Sablefish--*Anoplopoma fimbria*
     Thread herring--*Opisthonema oglinum*

Shellfish
     Mollusca
          Mahogany (ocean) quahogs--*Mercenaria mercenaria*
          Surf clams--*Spisula solidissima*
     Crustacea
          Red crab--*Podaphehalmus vigil*
          Rock shrimp--*Silyomia brevirostris*
          Squid, Atlantic--*Loligo pealei*
          Squid, Pacific--*Illex opalescens*
          Tanner crab--*Chronoectes tanneri*

The following species of finfish and shellfish were purchased from the market: American eel, croaker, mullet, thread herring, mahogany quahog, surf clam, red crab, rock shrimp, and tanner crab.

The other species were obtained from the fisherman by the personnel of the Northeast Utilization Research Center, Gloucester, Massachusetts, or from the research vessel by the Northwest Utilization Research Center, Seattle, Washington, personnel. No effort was made to determine when the fish were caught. All samples were packed in dry ice and shipped to the Southeast Utilization Research Center, College Park, Maryland. Before the samples were prepared for analysis, they were allowed to thaw at room temperature.

Preparation of Samples. Finfish and shellfish samples were finely ground by a Hobart grinder in preparation for analysis. All fish obtained were ready to grind (skinned fillet or muscle portion) with the following exceptions: American eel, croaker, and sablefish were obtained dressed and had to be filleted and skinned; thread herring, obtained in the round, had head and tail cut off, and was gutted and scaled. The raw flesh of all the finfish and mollusks was used to prepare samples for analysis. The muscle of the red crab and tanner crab had been cooked, removed from the shell, and frozen in 5- or 10-pound blocks, respectively. The rock shrimp had been headed, cooked, split (muscle not removed from the shell), and then frozen. Before grinding, the meat was removed from the shell. The squid was obtained whole, and had to be gutted and skinned. The mantle and tentacles were used in analysis.

One half of each ground lot was spread in shallow pans and freeze-dried for animal feeding studies to determine the nutritive quality of the protein. The other half was packed in 4-ounce plastic cups, covered tightly, frozen, and stored at -40°F until analyzed.

Method of Analysis. The finfish and shellfish muscle samples were analyzed for crude protein (N x 6.25) and ether-extractable fat by the methods described in Sections 2.051 and 7.048, respectively, of the Official Methods of Analysis (AOAC, 1970). Moisture content was analyzed by drying the samples in a forced-air oven for 16 hours at 100°C. Ash was determined by burning the samples in a muffle furnace for 16 hours at 550°C. Amino acids were determined

with the automatic amino acid analyzer by the method described by
Moore et al. (1958). Each single sample was analyzed in duplicate;
three samples of each finfish and shellfish were submitted for
analysis. The average and standard error of the mean are thus based
on six determinations.

Rat feeding studies were conducted to determine the nutritive
quality of the protein in the muscle of the finfish and shellfish.
The freeze-dried product was ground in a Wiley Mill before it was
incorporated into the experimental diet. The diets were formulated
to contain 10% protein. The composition of the diet is tabulated
in Table 1, and the method used for conducting the rat feeding
studies is described by Stillings et al. (1969). All diets but one
were isocaloric. The exception, the sablefish diet, was mixed
without the addition of fat and still contained 14% fat. Consequently, two control diets were used in this evaluation. Both contained 10% protein, but one had 10% fat and the other 14% fat.

Each diet was fed to ten Charles River male albino 23-day-old
rats for four weeks. The amounts of food consumed and of weight
gained were recorded three times a week. At the end of four weeks,
the protein efficiency ratio (PER) was calculated by dividing the
weight gained by the protein consumed. PER values are used as a
measure of nutritive value or nutritional quality of the protein.

Since the feeding trials were not conducted at the same time,
the PER values were adjusted to a casein value of 3.0. By this
adjustment, it was possible to compare the results of the three
feeding trials.

RESULTS AND DISCUSSION

Proximate Composition

The proximate composition of the 12 finfish and shellfish
samples is tabulated in Table 2. With the exception of thread
herring, the values obtained in this study are within the range of
the values that Sidwell et al. (1974) reported. Thompson (1959a, b)

EVALUATION OF FINFISH AND SHELLFISH

TABLE 1

Composition of the Basic Diet Used to Evaluate
the Nutritive Quality of the Protein
in the Muscle of the Finfish and Shellfish

Item	%
Cornstarch	35[a]
Sucrose	35[a]
Protein	10
Vitamins	1
Minerals	4
Fat	10
Non-nutritive cellulose	5

[a]This amount is not always the same, depending on
the amount of test material needed to make up 10% protein. The remaining ingredients are held constant.

reported values for whole thread herring, as it is used in the pet
food industry.

In another investigation, Sidwell et al. (1973) reported that
the protein content of surf clams is 15.6 g/100 g. That figure is
nearly 4 g/100 g higher than the results of this study. The range
of values in literature for protein in squid (*Loliginidae* spp.) was
from 11.9 to 16.4 g/100 g (Valenzuela, 1928; Santos and Ascalon,
1931; Jaffe, 1956). The protein content for the squid used in this
study was within that range. Krzeczkowski and Stone (1974) reported
18.8 percent protein for cooked snow crab (*Chionoecetes biardi*), a
close relative to the tanner crab. No data are available in literature for the composition of the edible portion of the red crab or
rock shrimp.

Amino Acid Profile

Table 3 shows the amino acid content of the protein in the
muscle of 4 finfish and on the basis of protein in whole, gutted
thread herring (bones and skin included). In general, the variation

201

TABLE 2

Proximate Composition of Edible Portions of Various Finfish and Shellfish

Species	Protein (N x 6.25), %	Moisture, %	Fat (ether), %	Ash, %
Finfish				
American eel (raw)	19.5 ± 0.21[a]	68.0 ± 0.29[a]	11.6 ± 0.34[a]	1.4 ± 0.07[a]
Croaker (raw)	18.8 ± 0.10	79.9 ± 0.17	0.6 ± 0.04	1.0 ± 0.02
Mullet (raw)	20.4 ± 0.37	73.5 ± 0.66	4.8 ± 0.54	1.2 ± 0.06
Sablefish (raw)	11.3 ± 0.32	72.1 ± 0.35	15.8 ± 0.51	0.83 ± 0.04
Thread herring (raw)	21.4 ± 0.16	74.7 ± 0.12	2.4 ± 0.07	1.8 ± 0.05
Shellfish				
Mollusca				
Ocean quahog (raw)	10.7 ± 0.16	85.2 ± 0.13	0.3 ± 0.05	1.2 ± 0.01
Surf clams (raw)	11.7 ± 0.20	85.5 ± 0.21	0.3 ± 0.01	0.5 ± 0.02
Crustacea				
Red crab (cooked)	14.7 ± 0.11	81.1 ± 0.33	0.4 ± 0.03	2.5 ± 0.09
Rock shrimp (cooked)	21.6 ± 0.45	76.7 ± 0.30	0.5 ± 0.03	1.6 ± 0.05
Squid, loligo (raw)	14.5 ± 0.22	82.7 ± 0.35	0.9 ± 0.12	0.8 ± 0.05
Squid, illex (raw)	16.7 ± 0.24	80.1 ± 0.17	0.5 ± 0.06	1.1 ± 0.05
Tanner crab (cooked)	16.0 ± 0.21	81.5 ± 0.20	0.3 ± 0.02	1.8 ± 0.04

[a]Standard error of the mean.

TABLE 3

Amino Acid Profile of the Protein in the Edible Portion of Various Finfish

Amino acid	American eel (raw)	Croaker (raw)	Mullet (raw)	Sablefish (raw)	Thread herring (raw, whole)
			% of total protein		
Lysine	9.7 ± 0.44[a]	9.5 ± 0.56[a]	9.3 ± 0.82[a]	8.4 ± 0.92[a]	8.2 ± 0.80[a]
Histidine	4.5 ± 0.23	2.18 ± 0.09	3.7 ± 0.28	1.8 ± 0.15	2.9 ± 0.13
Arginine	6.6 ± 0.36	6.4 ± 0.30	6.8 ± 0.31	6.3 ± 0.22	4.9 ± 0.11
Aspartic acid	13.6 ± 0.34	13.3 ± 1.11	14.1 ± 1.17	12.8 ± 1.23	8.1 ± 0.57
Threonine	4.4 ± 0.15	4.3 ± 0.32	4.6 ± 0.27	4.0 ± 0.26	3.4 ± 0.04
Serine	3.8 ± 0.08	4.0 ± 0.23	4.1 ± 0.25	3.4 ± 0.33	3.0 ± 0.05
Glutamic acid	15.3 ± 0.33	16.4 ± 0.81	16.2 ± 1.19	15.0 ± 1.20	12.6 ± 0.43
Proline	4.20 ± 0.24	3.3 ± 0.24	3.8 ± 0.22	2.8 ± 0.83	4.2 ± 1.11
Glycine	5.8 ± 0.27	4.5 ± 0.21	5.5 ± 0.42	4.7 ± 0.41	4.5 ± 0.26
Alanine	6.5 ± 0.27	6.0 ± 0.26	6.6 ± 0.46	5.5 ± 0.39	4.9 ± 0.05
Valine	5.2 ± 0.30	4.8 ± 0.33	5.5 ± 0.33	5.0 ± 0.19	3.6 ± 0.30
Methionine	2.8 ± 0.12	3.0 ± 0.12	2.9 ± 0.11	2.8 ± 0.16	2.2 ± 0.13
Isoleucine	4.7 ± 0.20	4.5 ± 0.20	5.0 ± 0.20	4.6 ± 0.24	3.5 ± 0.07
Leucine	8.2 ± 0.25	7.8 ± 0.67	8.7 ± 0.46	7.7 ± 0.43	6.8 ± 0.35
Tyrosine	3.2 ± 0.22	3.1 ± 0.25	3.4 ± 0.05	2.8 ± 0.12	2.5 ± 0.09
Phenylalanine	3.7 ± 0.23	3.4 ± 0.29	3.9 ± 0.04	3.1 ± 0.16	2.9 ± 0.10

[a]Standard error of the mean.

in amino acid composition is not extensive. The greatest variations appear in the amounts of histidine and proline in sablefish and of arginine, valine, and isoleucine in thread herring. The histidine values for American eel and mullet are higher than the amount found in whole egg (2.40 g/100 g of protein), which is considered to be the most balanced natural protein. Fish protein is higher in lysine than whole egg protein, 8-9 g and 6 g, respectively. The amino acid profile for the protein in the flesh of the various species of finfish has not been studied extensively.

The values of lysine, histidine, and arginine in croaker and mullet flesh determined microbiologically by Pottinger and Baldwin (1946) were lower than those determined chemically by Master and Magar (1954). Master and Magar also found lower values for tyrosine, but higher ones for methionine, threonine, and leucine. Other amino acid values were comparable to those listed in Table 3. Only these papers mentioned data on amino acid in the muscle protein of finfish. Since the values presented in this paper are from single lots, variations from lot to lot cannot be ascertained.

As it may be seen in Table 4, the whole mahogany (ocean) quahog tends to be low in lysine and methionine compared to the muscle only of the surf clam. The values for the other amino acids appear to be within the same limits as those of the muscle protein of the finfish.

In several instances, the amino acid profile of the two crabs, red and tanner, does differ. The red crab is caught off the northeast coast of the U.S. and the tanner off the southeast coast of Alaska. The greatest discrepancies are in the amounts of lysine, histidine, glycine, leucine, and arginine. Rock shrimp appears to have an amino acid pattern very much like that of red crab. The squids contain the same amount of aspartic acid as the finfish, but less than the other shellfish. Krzeczkowski and Stone (1974) reported the amino acid profile for canned snow crab. The values listed in Table 4 for arginine, aspartic acid, and glycine are lower, but the other amino acids are either comparable or higher than the ones reported for canned snow crab.

TABLE 4

Amino Acid Profile of the Protein in the Edible Portion of Various Shellfish

Amino acid	Mahogany quahog (raw, whole)	Surf Clams (raw)	Red Crab (cooked)	Rock shrimp (cooked)	Squid Atlantic (raw)	Squid Pacific (raw)	Tanner crab (cooked)
	% of total protein						
Lysine	5.1 ± 0.28[a]	8.2 ± 1.31[a]	9.0 ± 0.68[a]	9.3 ± 1.68[a]	7.2 ± 0.38[a]	7.5 ± 0.72[a]	7.2 ± 0.50[a]
Histidine	1.4 ± 0.02	1.7 ± 0.05	2.4 ± 0.27	2.4 ± 0.73	1.5 ± 0.10	2.5 ± 0.54	1.7 ± 0.05
Arginine	6.4 ± 0.42	7.6 ± 0.29	8.2 ± 1.25	9.6 ± 1.43	5.7 ± 0.79	6.3 ± 0.21	11.2 ± 0.44
Aspartic acid	10.2 ± 1.18	12.7 ± 1.11	11.6 ± 2.46	13.2 ± 2.65	10.7 ± 1.23	10.9 ± 0.69	11.6 ± 0.71
Threonine	4.1 ± 0.04	4.3 ± 0.13	4.8 ± 0.32	3.7 ± 0.52	3.5 ± 0.22	3.7 ± 0.07	3.9 ± 0.15
Serine	3.6 ± 0.19	4.3 ± 0.13	4.2 ± 0.43	3.7 ± 0.53	3.3 ± 0.39	3.7 ± 0.09	3.8 ± 0.10
Glutamic acid	13.3 ± 0.32	15.9 ± 0.89	16.8 ± 1.00	16.5 ± 2.59	13.7 ± 0.51	13.2 ± 0.40	13.8 ± 0.21
Proline	3.8 ± 0.18	5.6 ± 2.6	4.3 ± 0.33	3.5 ± 0.47	4.7 ± 0.64	5.6 ± 0.11	4.0 ± 0.10
Glycine	5.3 ± 0.13	5.9 ± 0.11	4.7 ± 0.26	6.0 ± 0.76	4.4 ± 0.13	5.0 ± 0.19	7.0 ± 0.16
Alanine	6.6 ± 0.10	6.5 ± 0.32	5.8 ± 0.27	5.4 ± 0.83	5.4 ± 0.12	5.5 ± 0.17	5.3 ± 0.11
Valine	3.6 ± 0.16	3.7 ± 0.30	4.9 ± 0.16	4.0 ± 0.60	3.0 ± 0.01	3.3 ± 0.09	4.1 ± 0.22
Methionine	1.9 ± 0.12	2.4 ± 0.07	2.5 ± 0.33	2.8 ± 0.36	2.3 ± 0.05	2.2 ± 0.05	2.3 ± 0.14
Isoleucine	3.5 ± 0.07	4.1 ± 0.04	5.0 ± 0.23	4.1 ± 0.63	3.7 ± 0.10	3.7 ± 0.12	4.0 ± 0.14
Leucine	6.2 ± 0.13	7.7 ± 0.27	8.6 ± 0.46	7.7 ± 1.11	6.9 ± 0.20	6.9 ± 0.20	6.9 ± 0.20
Tyrosine	2.9 ± 0.30	3.2 ± 0.33	4.4 ± 0.18	2.9 ± 0.57	1.8 ± 0.44	2.3 ± 0.13	3.1 ± 0.28
Phenyl-alanine	2.4 ± 0.21	3.1 ± 0.33	4.4 ± 0.23	3.1 ± 0.81	2.7 ± 0.10	2.6 ± 0.13	3.5 ± 0.32

[a] Standard error of the mean.

TABLE 5

Food Consumed, Weight Gained, and Protein Efficiency Ratio (PER) of Rats
Fed a Diet Containing 10 Percent Protein from Finfish, Shellfish, and Casein

Protein source	No. of rats	Average food intake	Average weight gained	PER[a]	Adjusted PER[b]
Finfish					
American eel (raw)	8	17.3 ± 0.40[c]	6.5 ± 0.24[c]	3.7 ± 0.08[c]	3.28
Croaker (raw)	10	16.6 ± 0.40	6.5 ± 0.21	3.8 ± 0.05	3.34
Sablefish (raw)	10	16.5 ± 0.51	6.4 ± 0.23	3.8 ± 0.04	3.46
Thread herring (raw, whole)	9	16.6 ± 0.41	6.0 ± 0.26	3.5 ± 0.09	2.94
Shellfish					
Mollusca					
Ocean quahogs (raw)	10	14.6 ± 0.39	4.8 ± 0.17	3.1 ± 0.08	2.73
Surf clams (raw)	9	14.2 ± 0.43	4.6 ± 0.20	3.5 ± 0.07	3.07
Crustacea					
Red crab (cooked)	9	17.2 ± 0.61	6.7 ± 0.29	3.8 ± 0.06	3.32
Rock shrimp (cooked)	10	16.6 ± 0.47	6.1 ± 0.24	3.7 ± 0.07	3.25
Squid, Atlantic (raw)	9	13.8 ± 0.46	4.6 ± 0.21	3.3 ± 0.06	2.99
Squid, Pacific (raw)	9	15.5 ± 0.61	5.3 ± 0.29	3.4 ± 0.07	3.00
Tanner crab (cooked)	10	18.2 ± 0.60	6.8 ± 0.33	3.6 ± 0.07	3.04

Controls

Casein 10% fat	9[d]	15.1 ± 0.52	5.2 ± 0.22	3.4 ± 0.06	3.00
Casein 10% fat	9[e]	15.5 ± 0.17	5.3 ± 0.12	3.6 ± 0.06	3.00
Casein 10% fat	9[f]	15.2 ± 0.65	5.3 ± 0.32	3.4 ± 0.08	3.00
Casein 14% fat	10[g]	14.9 ± 0.40	4.9 ± 0.19	3.3 ± 0.06	3.00

[a] $PER = \dfrac{\text{weight gained}}{\text{protein consumed}}$

[b] Adjusted the PER value of the control diet containing casein to 3.00.

[c] Standard error of the mean.

[d] Control diet for rock shrimp and the two squids.

[e] Control diet for thread herring and tanner crab.

[f] Control diet for croaker, surf clam, red crab, quahog, and American eel.

[g] Control diet for sablefish.

Nutritional Quality of the Protein

Table 5 shows the results of the feeding studies when the protein from the muscle of the various fishery products was incorporated into the diets at the 10% level. Except for thread herring, the nutritive quality of the finfish muscle protein was better than that of casein. The results for the other finfish were surprisingly alike. The presence of collagen from skin and bones in the muscle of the thread herring is reflected in its lower PER value.

The PER value for the mahogany (ocean) quahog is a little lower than for the surf clam. This may be due to the use of the whole animal, as opposed to the muscle of the surf clam, or to the lower content of lysine, histidine, and methionine in the quahog.

The nutritive quality of the flesh of the crustacea was equal to or better than that of casein. The PERs for red crab and rock shrimp were comparable to those of the muscle of finfish.

In conclusion, it appears that the nutritive quality of these underutilized finfish and shellfish is quite acceptable, and that the development of this important resource should not be delayed on the grounds of inadequacy as a food.

ACKNOWLEDGMENTS

The authors appreciate the work done by Audrey Smith, who assembled the data; by Herta Lagally and Donald Briscoe, who conducted the animal feeding trials; and by Dee Cosgrove and James Bonnet, who conducted some of the chemical analyses.

Reference to trade names does not imply endorsement by the National Marine Fisheries Service.

REFERENCES

AOAC. 1970. Official Methods of Analysis (11th Ed.). Association of Official Agricultural Chemists, Washington, D.C.

Clark, E.D. and L.H. Almy. 1918. A chemical study of food fish. The analysis of twenty common food fishes with especial reference to a seasonal variation in composition. J. Biol. Chem. 33:483.

Jaffe, W.G. 1956. Composition of Venezuelan fishes. Arch. Venezuelan Nutr. 7:163.

Krzeczkowski, R.A. and F.E. Stone. 1974. Amino acid, fatty acid and proximate composition of snow crab (*Chionoecetes biardi*). J. Food Sci. 39:386.

Laver, B.H., M.C. Murray, W.E. Anderson and E.B. Guptill. 1974. Atlantic queen crab (*Chionoecetes opilio*), Jonah crab (*Cancer borealis*) and red crab (*Geryon quinquedens*). Proximate composition of crabmeat from edible tissues and concentrations of some major mineral constituents in the ash. J. Food Sci. 39:383.

Master, F. and N.G. Magar. 1954. Studies in the nutritive value of Bombay Duck. II. Amino acid composition. Indian J. Med. Res. 42:509.

Moore, S., D.H. Spackman and W.H. Stein. 1958. Chromatography of amino acids on sulfonated polystyrene resins. Anal. Chem. 30:1185.

Ousterhout, L.E. 1960. Technical Note No. 56--Chemical composition and laboratory fillet yield of 13 species of middle and south Atlantic fish. Commercial Fisheries Rev. 22:15.

Pottinger, S.R. and W.H. Baldwin. 1946. The content of certain amino acids in seafoods. Commercial Fisheries Rev. 8:5.

Santos, F.O. and S.J. Ascalon. 1931. Amount of nutrients in Philippine food materials. Philippine Agr. Rev. 20:402.

Sidwell, V.D., J.C. Bonnet and E.G. Zook. 1973. Chemical and nutritive values of several fresh and canned finfish, crustaceans and mollusks. I. Proximate composition, calcium and phosphorus. Marine Fisheries Rev. 35:16.

Sidwell, V.D., P.R. Foncannon, N.S. Moore and J.C. Bonnet. 1974. Composition of the edible portion of raw (fresh or frozen) crustaceans, finfish and mollusks. I. Protein, fat, moisture, ash, carbohydrate energy value, and cholesterol. Marine Fisheries Rev. 36:21.

Stillings, B.R., O.A. Hammerle and D.G. Snyder. 1969. Sequence of limiting amino acids in fish protein concentrate produced by isopropyl alcohol extraction of red hake (*Urophycis chuss*). J. Nutr. 97:70.

Thompson, M.H. 1959a.Proximate composition of Gulf of Mexico industrial fish. I. Winter and spring of 1958 studies. Commercial Fisheries Rev. 21:17.

Thompson, M.H. 1959b.Proximate composition of Gulf of Mexico industrial fish. II. Summer of 1958 studies. Commercial Fisheries Rev. 21:22.

Valenzuela, A. 1928. Composition and nutritive value of Philippine food fish. Philippine J. Sci. 36:235.

10

FACTORS AFFECTING RUMINANT RESPONSES TO PROTECTED AMINO ACIDS AND PROTEINS

G. A. Broderick

Department of Animal Science
Texas A & M University
Texas Agricultural Experiment Station
College Station

The general aspects of ruminal protein degradation and resynthesis are reviewed, including quantitative estimates of protein
from both microbial synthesis and normal dietary by-pass which is
available to the host for intestinal digestion and absorption.
Evidence from reviewed reports indicates that protein supplied from
both sources may be qualitatively or quantitatively inadequate in
some circumstances. Considerable data indicate that sheep will
generally respond with increased wool growth and body-weight gains
when supplementated post-ruminally with methionine alone or with
good-quality proteins. Abomasal infusion studies indicate that
performance of growing beef and lactating dairy cattle will sometimes be improved with post-ruminal protein supplementation, but
there appears to be little potential for post-ruminal supplementation with a single essential amino acid (EAA). The most promising
techniques for protecting dietary EAA from ruminal degradation
include lipid encapsulation, chemical derivatization, and use of
inhibitors of microbial amino acid deamination. This review dis-
cusses the major processing techniques used to protect dietary proteins from ruminal breakdown. These include treatment with heat,
tannins and aldehydes, with formaldehyde-treatment being the most
thoroughly studied and reviewed of these processes. If properly

applied, all three treatments will reduce ruminal protein losses and increase the amounts of protein intestinally digested and absorbed. However, animal production responses with these various treatments have been inconsistent. Possible explanations for this inconsistency, such as over-protection with heat or formaldehyde-treatments, are also discussed.

INTRODUCTION

Ruminants are well adapted to the utilization of low quality, high fiber diets. The microorganisms of the forestomach ferment fibrous feeds which are of little or no direct value to the animal, and the host in turn utilizes the products of this fermentation. But ruminal intervention also has effects which may be deleterious. For example, the fats in meat and milk from ruminants are highly saturated, partly because of ruminal hydrogenation of polyunsaturated fatty acids (PUFA) normally present in the diet. Techniques are now available which can be used to protect dietary PUFA supplements from ruminal hydrogenation, and allow direct incorporation of the PUFA into the fats of ruminant products (Scott, Cook and Mills, 1971). Use of protected PUFA to increase the unsaturation of ruminant fats has been the subject of recent reviews (Bitman et al., 1974; Dinius, 1974), and will not be considered further here.

Although the tissue requirements for essential amino acids (EAA) are qualitatively the same in ruminants as in monogastrics (Black et al., 1952; Downes, 1961), the action of the microorganisms in the forestomach makes ruminant protein nutrition markedly different from that of monogastrics. The EAA needs of ruminants are met primarily from microbial protein synthesis in the rumen, and the synthetic ability of the ruminal microbes allows utilization of non-protein nitrogen (NPN) compounds, such as urea, as dietary protein sources. However, ruminal intervention may result in losses of preformed dietary proteins that could be directly

212

RUMINANT RESPONSES TO PROTECTED AMINO ACIDS AND PROTEINS

digested and absorbed in the small intestine (Black and Tribe, 1973). The action of the ruminal microbes also prevents normal oral supplementation of amino acids. The possibility that reducing ruminal degradation could improve the efficiency of utilization of both preformed proteins and NPN compounds has stimulated considerable interest in the use of various techniques for ruminally protecting dietary proteins and amino acids.

RUMINAL PROTEIN METABOLISM

Ruminant protein metabolism has been the topic of several recent and excellent reviews. Allison (1970) thoroughly reviewed the nitrogen (N) metabolism of ruminal microorganisms. A series of excellent papers appeared in 1973 in the Proceedings of the Nutrition Society (Proc. Nutr. Soc., 32:79-122) which covered most areas of ruminant protein nutrition. Hogan (1975) has reviewed thoroughly the quantitative aspects of N-utilization in ruminants. The most complete coverage of all areas of ruminant nutrition and metabolism is of course Hungate's text (1966).

Ruminal Protein Degradation

The process of ruminal protein degradation consists of proteolysis and deamination by enzymes of microbial rather than animal origin. Most of the microbial proteolytic enzymes are not free in the rumen, but are closely associated with the bacterial and protozoal cells (Blackburn and Hobson, 1960). Work with a pure strain of ruminal bacteria indicates that these enzymes are bound to the outer surface of the bacterial cell wall (Blackburn and Hullah, 1974). Proteolysis in the rumen is always an active process, and appears to be more a function of microbial cell numbers (Blackburn, 1968) than of content of protein or other constituents in the diet (Annison, 1956; Warner, 1956). The free amino acids released by proteolysis of dietary proteins are rapidly deaminated to ammonia and carbon-chains. Unlike proteolytic activity, deamination activity is directly related to dietary protein content (Lewis, 1955; Annison, 1956; Warner, 1956). That the capacity for amino acid deamination generally exceeds the rate of amino acid release by proteolysis is indicated by the fact that amino acids accumulate only transiently, if at all, even when large amounts of very digestible proteins are introduced into the rumen (Annison et al., 1959; Lewis, 1962). Therefore, proteolysis is thought to be the step limiting ruminal degradation of proteins.

The susceptibility of different feed proteins to degradation is considered mainly a function of the protein's solubility in ruminal liquor (Henderickx and Martin, 1963; Hungate, 1966; Sniffen, 1974). However, work by Mangan (1972) showed that the protein ovalbumin, although quite soluble in ruminal liquor, was very resistant to degradation. This worker, noting that oval- bumin's polypeptide chain is cyclic, suggested that the proteoly- tic activity of ruminal microbes may be relatively more exopepti- dase than endopeptidase in nature. Therefore, proteins such as ovalbumin, without C- or N-terminal amino acid residues available for exopeptidase attack may be poor substrates for ruminal proteo- lysis.

Many studies show that dietary proteins vary greatly as to degree of ruminal degradation, and observed values range from less than 30% (Ely et al., 1967) to as high as 90% (McDonald and Hall, 1957) of the protein consumed. In spite of considerable study, little is known concerning the amounts of protein from common feedstuffs which escape ruminal degradation and are directly available for digestion in the intestine. Two new feeding systems (Burroughs et al., 1974; Satter and Roffler, 1975) which require this information are now gaining acceptance, and this has added increased impetus to study in this area. Use of processing techniques and chemical treatments of feed proteins to reduce ruminal breakdown, and hopefully to increase intestinal digestion, will be considered later in considerable detail.

RUMINANT RESPONSES TO PROTECTED AMINO ACIDS AND PROTEINS

Microbial Protein Synthesis

Bacteria account for 80% or more of ruminally synthesized protein (Hogan and Weston, 1970). Most bacterial species can utilize or require ammonia as their only N-source (Bryant and Robinson, 1962). There is little direct use made of amino acids by growing bacteria (Borchers, 1967), probably due to lack of specific systems to transport amino acids into the bacterial cells (Allison, 1969). This suggests that NPN sources can serve satisfactorily as the major N-source for most ruminal bacteria, with little benefit to be gained from amino acid supplementation at the ruminal level.

There is however, some evidence that proteins and NPN are not nearly equal as N-sources for ruminal microbes. Direct incorporation of peptides by bacteria occurs to some degree (Wright, 1967), and a few important strains of ruminal bacteria require certain fatty acids which serve as carbon backbones for specific amino acids (Allison, 1969). Moreover, supplementation of all-NPN diets with specific amino acid carbon-chains has increased N-retention in growing sheep (Cline et al., 1966), and ruminal microbial protein synthesis (Hume, 1970a). Also, Hume (1970b) has shown substantial improvements in yields of ruminal microbial protein when proteins were added to all-NPN diets already supplemented with the required amino acid carbon-chains. Other workers have obtained significant improvements in N-utilization by ruminants fed high-urea diets with oral amino acid supplementation (Loosli and Harris, 1945; Lofgreen et al., 1947; Williams and Moir, 1951; McLaren et al., 1965; Bunn et al., 1968). It is possible that degradation of ruminally synthesized proteins could supply some if not all of these required amino acid carbon-chains (Hungate, 1966; Virtanen, 1971). Although ruminal protozoa appear to obtain most of their protein requirements by engulfment of bacteria (Hungate, 1966), their amino acid requirements are similar to those of higher animals. Therefore, intact proteins or amino acids may have an effect through stimulation of protozoal growth. Such a possibility is suggested by the results of feeding studies in which supplements of methionine and its hydroxy analog significantly increased ruminal protozoal numbers (Patton et al., 1970).

The above considerations imply that it may not be safe to assume that urea and other NPN compounds are N-sources equivalent to preformed proteins at the ruminal level. Protection of dietary proteins from ruminal degradation may result in deleterious effects on ruminal function due to reduced supply of essential non-ammonia factors normally derived from protein fermentation. This possibility deserves further study before the general application of the technique of ruminal protection of dietary proteins.

Quantitative Amino Acid Supply in Ruminants

Both the quantity and quality of ruminally synthesized microbial protein may be inadequate for optimal performance. The amount of microbial crude protein (CP) formed is limited energetically by the amount of substrate fermented in the rumen (Hungate, 1966). Evidence now indicates that the ruminal microbes are much more efficient converters of fermented material into cellular protoplasm than was previously thought. A wide range of microbial CP yields have been reported, but recent in vivo experiments with sheep fed diets with optimal protein levels indicate that the yield of microbial CP may average as high as 23 gm/100 g ruminally digested organic matter (DOM_r) (Hume, 1970b; Hogan and Weston, 1970). Although even higher yields have been obtained (Hogan and Weston, 1971), under practical conditions a yield of about 18 to 20 g microbial CP/100 g DOM_r (Hogan, 1973) would be expected. About 70% of the total digestion of feed dry matter occurs in the rumen (Topps et al., 1968), and consumption of 1 kg of a ration of 70% overall digestibility will give about 0.5 kg DOM_r. Thus, consumption of 1 kg of a 70% digestible ration should yield about 90-100 g microbial CP.

The usefulness of ruminally synthesized microbial CP is also limited because a considerable proportion of the N is present as nucleic acids and because of relatively low digestibility. Nucleic

acids apparently account for nearly 20% of the N in ruminal
bacteria (Smith and McAllan, 1970), and only about 70% of the
total microbial -N is present in the normal protein amino acids
(Hogan and Weston, 1971). The low digestibility of microbial
CP equivalent is apparently due to the presence of much of the N
as indigestible bacterial cell wall components (Allison, 1970).
Mason and Palmer (1971) found that about 20% of bacterial -N,
mainly present in the cell wall, is not digested by the rat.
Assuming 20% indigestibility and 20% nucleic acid -N, it can be
estimated that bacterial CP, which comprises most of the ruminally
synthesized microbial protein, would yield only about 60% digestible protein amino acids. The EAA composition of both bacterial
and protozoal proteins of ruminal origin is very constant, and
unaffected by diet composition (Weller, 1957; Purser and Buechler,
1966). Both protein sources have biological values of about 80
(McNaught et al., 1954), indicating good, if not ideal, EAA
patterns.

Applying the values derived above, one could expect about 54
to 60 g absorbable protein amino acid residues (metabolizable
protein) to be contributed from ruminal microbial synthesis with
consumption of one kg of a ration of 70% digestibility. Burroughs
et al. (1974) estimated a microbial yield of 84 g metabolizable
protein/kg total digestible nutrients (TDN) consumed. This
corresponds to a value of 59 g of absorbable protein amino acid
residues/kg of 70% TDN ration consumed. Applying values of 40%
by-pass (Satter and Roffler, 1975) and 90% true intestinal digestibility (Burroughs et al., 1974) to dietary protein, it can be
estimated that one kg of a diet containing 13% natural protein
would yield 47 g amino acid residues for intestinal absorption
due to by-pass of dietary protein. If ruminal synthesis supplied
between 50 and 60 g, ruminal synthesis plus by-pass would contribute about 100 g of metabolizable protein with consumption of one
kg of this ration. Differences in ration digestibility or replacement of preformed protein with NPN would of course alter these

values. For ruminants to respond to protection of dietary amino acids or proteins, the pattern or quantity of EAA supplied from both ruminal synthesis and by-pass must be inadequate. The next section presents evidence that, in certain circumstances, this is true.

EVIDENCE OF AMINO ACID AND PROTEIN
INSUFFICIENCY IN RUMINANTS

Intervention of ruminal microorganisms and the difficulties involved in measuring the quantities of amino acids absorbed from the small intestine complicate the matter of determining EAA requirements of the various ruminant classes. It is therefore necessary to use indirect procedures to determine limiting EAA (Nimrick et al., 1970; Schwab, 1974) and to estimate EAA requirements (Armstrong, 1973; Williams and Smith, 1974).

Early reports from sheep feeding experiments showed that dietary protein quality was important in ruminants as well as monogastrics. Lofgreen et al. (1947); Williams and Moir (1951), and Ellis et al. (1956) all observed that the quality of dietary protein had a marked effect on N-retention and on estimated "biological value" in growing lambs. Although the clear differences in N-utilization normally observed in monogastrics for these proteins were not seen here, preformed proteins were found to be considerably better N-sources than urea or urea supplemented with methionine. Part of the difference could be explained on the basis of improved microbial protein synthesis with the protein-containing diets (Williams and Moir, 1951), but the importance of feed protein by-passing the rumen is clearly implied from these results. There is now a large body of literature showing production responses to amino acid and protein supplements given post-ruminally (i.e., supplements given in such a way as to avoid the action of the rumen, making the amino acids and proteins available for intestinal digestion and absorption).

RUMINANT RESPONSES TO PROTECTED AMINO ACIDS AND PROTEINS

Wool Growth in Sheep

Beginning in the early 1960's, Australian reports began to
appear which indicated that large increases in wool growth could
be obtained with small abomasal supplements of sulfur-amino acids
or protein. A typical experiment was that of Reis and Schinckel
(1964) in which 70 to 100% increases in wool growth, due to
increases in both fiber length and diameter, were obtained with
abomasal infusion of about 1 g/day of either methionine or cystine.
Similar results were also obtained with intravenous and intraperitoneal infusions of methionine or cystine (Downes et al., 1970a),
and with abomasal casein supplements (Reis and Schinckel, 1964).
These dramatic wool growth responses with post-ruminal methionine
and cystine supplementation are due to the fact that, while wool
proteins are very high in sulfur-amino acids, particularly cystine,
microbial and by-passed feed proteins are relatively low. Abomasal
infusion studies with various proteins (Reis and Colebrook, 1972)
showed the importance of overall EAA patterns as well as sulfur-
amino acid content, and that proteins of highest biological value
yielded the largest wool growth responses.

Growing Sheep

Abmosally infused methionine has also improved N-balance in
growing lambs fed diets containing all-NPN (Schelling and Hatfield,
1968) or all natural protein (Schelling et al., 1973). Mowat and
Deelstra (1972) observed improved feed efficiency in growing lambs
fed some natural diets supplemented with encapsulated methionine
(a lipid-coated methionine product which allows post-ruminal
absorption of the amino acid). It must be pointed out, however,
that a considerable proportion of the retained N, even in growing
lambs, will be deposited in the form of high-sulfur wool proteins
(Reis and Tunks, 1969). Wright (1971) intravenously injected
graded supplements of methionine into growing lambs and obtained
results suggesting that wool and muscle protein synthesis respond

separately to nutritional factors. In Wright's work, the lowest methionine supplement resulted in substantial increases in both wool growth and body weight gain. However, further increases in methionine injection had the toxic effect of decreasing feed intake and weight gain, but wool growth continued at the same high level obtained with the initial methionine level. The fact the wool growth responds separately from muscle and has much higher levels of sulfur-amino acids must be borne in mind when results obtained with sheep are extrapolated to growing or lactating cattle. Using abomasal infusions, Nimrick et al. (1970) identified the first 3 limiting EAA to be methionine, lysine and threonine for growing lambs fed all-NPN diets.

That sheep will respond to post-ruminal supplementation of preformed proteins has been shown in several experiments. Enhanced N-retentions have been obtained with abomasal infusion versus oral feeding of casein (Cuthbertson and Chalmers, 1950; Little and Mitchell, 1967) and casein hydrolysate (Schelling and Hatfield, 1968). Ørskov and co-workers used the novel technique of esophageal groove closure in young lambs to get ruminal by-pass of dietary proteins (Ørskov and Benzie, 1969). Using this method of post-ruminal protein supplementation, increased weight gains, feed efficiencies and substantially improved N-retentions were obtained (Ørskov and Fraser, 1969; Ørskov et al., 1970). Other work by Ørskov's group indicated that oral feeding of fish meal, a feed protein naturally resistant to ruminal degradation, lowered ruminal protein losses and increased the amount of total protein (ruminally synthesized plus dietary by-pass protein) that passed to the small intestine (Ørskov et al., 1971), and was digested in the small intestine (Ørskov et al., 1974). This corroborated an earlier report of improved N-utilization in lambs with the feeding of herring meal (Chalmers and Synge, 1954).

Growing Cattle

The most definitive and basic work on post-ruminal amino acid and protein supplementation in growing cattle has been that of Chalupa and colleagues of SmithKline Corporation. These workers obtained marked improvement in N-retention in 200 kg growing steers when abomasally supplementing feed-lot type rations with casein, casein hydrolysate or all 10 EAA (Chalupa, Chandler and Brown, 1972). Chalupa and co-workers have not observed consistent increase in N-balance with abomasally infused methionine alone (1972), or with other EAA infused individually (1973). Similarly, Steinacker et al. (1970) were unable to detect a consistent growth response to feeding of encapsulated methionine to growing Holstein steers. These results indicate that several EAA may be nearly co-limiting, and that the situation occuring in sheep of methionine being clearly first limiting, does not occur in growing cattle. It should also be noted that, under feed-lot conditions, growing cattle derive no additional benefit from preformed protein, compared to urea, after reaching a body weight of about 300 kg (Preston, 1972). This implies that ruminal protein foundation may be adequate to meet tissue amino acid needs in heavier growing cattle, and that post-ruminal protein supplements would no longer improve performance.

Lactating Cattle

That lactating cows will respond to post-ruminal protein was shown in several experiments in which abomasal casein infusions resulted in increases of 11 to 13% in milk protein production (Broderick et al., 1970; Vik-Mo et al., 1974; Derrig et al., 1974). Although Fisher (1972) obtained improved milk protein secretion with intravenous methionine infusion, other studies with feeding of encapsulated methionine gave no change in production of milk or milk components (Broderick et al., 1970; Williams et al., 1970). Broderick et al. (1974) obtained plasma free amino acid patterns which suggested that lysine, methionine and valine may be nearly equally limiting for lactating dairy cows consuming a diet based on corn silage and corn grain. Schwab (1974) used abomasal

221

infusions of EAA to lactating cows fed a similar diet, and determined lysine, methionine, and possibly threonine to be first,
second and third limiting, respectively. Although an order of
limitation was definable, these 3 EAA appeared to be closely co-
limiting. These results tend to discourage hope that one would
obtain a clear-cut lactation response to post-ruminal supplementation of a single EAA.

In summary, because of ruminal degradation of dietary proteins
and limited synthesis of microbial protein, ruminants will sometimes respond to post-ruminal supplements of amino acids or proteins. Sheep are the most promising candidates for post-ruminal
supplementation of a single EAA, methionine, for growth and
especially wool production. Substantial weight gain and wool
growth responses are possible with post-ruminal supplement of
proteins of good quality. There appears to be no outstanding first
or second limiting EAA for growing beef and lactating dairy cattle,
but both will sometimes give improved performance with post-ruminal
feeding of preformed proteins.

PROTECTION OF AMINO ACIDS FROM RUMINAL DEGRADATION

That the rapid deaminative activity of ruminal microorganisms
would prevent intestinal absorption by the ruminant of orally fed
amino acids has been shown by several workers. Lewis (1955),
Annison et al., (1959), Lewis (1962), and Lewis and Emery (1962)
have all observed rapid rates of deamination of free amino acids
in the rumen, especially when added as mixtures of the protein
amino acids. Chalupa (1975) estimated in vivo half-lives $(t_{1/2})$ of
about 2 hours or less for 8 EAA from ruminal in vitro incubations.
It is possible to use Chalupa's data to calculate the proportion
of free amino acids escaping ruminal degradation. From Hungate's
(1966) application of continuous flow theory to the rumen, the proportion of a compound which passes out of the rumen without being
fermented equals $k_r/(k_r + k_d)$, where k_r and k_d are respectively,

the rate constants for turnover of ruminal contents and for degradation of the compound in the rumen (J. H. Matis, personal communication). Assuming a turnover constant, k_r, of .04 hr^{-1} for ruminal contents, and calculating the degradation rate constants from the data of Chalupa (1975) using the equation $k_d = .693/t_{1/2}$ the estimated proportions of EAA directly available for intestinal absorption are very low, ranging from 3 to 11%. The proprotions of by-pass estimated by this procedure for 8 EAA are given in Table 1.

TABLE 1

Estimated Proportions of Unprotected Essential Amino Acids
Escaping Ruminal Degradation

Essential Amino Acid	$t_{1/2}^a$	k_d^b	Proportion[c] Escaping
	hr	hr^{-1}	%
Arginine	0.79	0.88	4.3
Isoleucine	1.75	0.40	9.1
Leucine	2.16	0.32	11.1
Lysine	1.31	0.51	7.0
Methionine	0.53	1.31	3.0
Phenylalanine	1.25	0.55	6.8
Threonine	1.12	0.62	6.1
Valine	2.12	0.33	10.8

[a]*In vivo* half-life values, $t_{1/2}$, reported by Chalupa (1975).

[b]Degradation rate constants, k_d, calculated from data of Chalupa (1975) by equation: $k_d = 0.693/t_{1/2}$.

[c]Estimated proportion of essential amino acids escaping ruminal degradation, calculated from equation: Proportion Escaping, % = $[k_r/(k_r + k_d)]$ x 100, where k_r, the turnover constant for ruminal contents, is set equal to 0.04 hr^{-1}, and k_d values are the calculated degradation rate constants.

Techniques of Amino Acid Protection

Although feeding protected methionine to sheep is the only situation in which feeding of a single protected EAA now shows promise, several methods of post-ruminal amino acid supplementation have received considerable study. These methods, which deal mainly with the protection of methionine, are the subject of an excellent review by Chalupa (1975).

Oral feeding to ruminants of the calcium salt of methionine hydroxy analog (MHA) received considerable attention several years ago. It was originally thought that MHA was stable in the rumen, and served as a source of methionine to the ruminant's tissues (Belasco, 1972). However, others have observed extensive ruminal degradation (Salsbury et al., 1971), and failure of oral MHA to give the same wool growth response (Reis, 1970) and plasma methionine concentrations (Papas et al., 1974) obtained with abomasal MHA, thus indicating that oral MHA is not a satisfactory post-ruminal methionine supplement. Moreover, it appears that the possible beneficial effects reported with MHA feeding to lactating cows may be mediated through some action in the rumen (see Broderick, 1973, for a more detailed discussion).

Delmar Chemicals of Canada worked out a procedure for encapsulating methionine with a coating of lipid. The product these workers developed consisted of a core of DL-methionine, kaolin and tristearin, which was physically covered with kaolin and tristearin, and contained 20% methionine by weight (Sibbald et al., 1968). This product gave increased plasma methionine:valine ratios (Broderick et al., 1970), and the methionine appeared to the 65% available for intestinal absorption (Neudoerffer et al., 1971). Other lipid-protected methionine products have been prepared and patented (Grass and Unangst, 1972; J. P. Hogan, personal communication), but none is commercially available at this time. The lipid-protected product of Grass and Unangst (1972) incorporated some polyunsaturated fat into the lipid coat. According to these workers, the amino acid was protected in the rumen just as well as with a coat of all saturated fat, but was more available for absorption in the intestine. The technique of lipid encapsulation is potentially applicable to EAA other than methionine.

A comparatively new technique for imparting ruminal protection to amino acids is the use of chemical blocking groups to structurally modify the amino acid to prevent action of microbial enzymes. The most recent and thorough work in this area is that of Kentucky scientists (Digenis et al., 1974a,b; Amos et al., 1974b) in which various derivatives of methionine were tested as potential oral methionine sources to ruminants. Two of the tested compounds, N-acetyl-DL-methionine and particularly DL-homocysteine thiolactone appear to be quite stable with respect to the ruminal microbial activity in vitro (Digenis et al., 1974a), and both are biologically active methionine sources in the rat (Amos et al., 1974b). Although there was some evidence with DL-homocysteine thiolactone of preintestinal absorption and conversion to methionine, most of the in vivo data was unfavorable and suggested that both derivatives may not be effective oral methionine sources in sheep (Amos et al., 1974b).

Australian workers had little success with N-formyl-DL-methionine and polymethionine as sources of protected methionine (Downes et al., 1970b). However, N-steroyl-DL-methionine appears stable in the rumen and will serve as a methionine source in the rat (Langer et al., 1973). Also, Ku and Simon (1973) have prepared amino acid imides that appear stable at prevailing ruminal pH's, degrade to the amino acid at abomasal pH's, and will elevate the circulating levels of the amino acid in ruminants. These results show that tools for oral supplementation of protected amino acids in ruminants may soon be available.

A new and exciting technique now receiving considerable study is the use of inhibitors to reduce amino acid degradation in the rumen. So long as general ruminal functions (such as cellulose digestion and protein synthesis) are not interfered with, this method could potentially prevent considerable wastage of preformed

225

protein amino acids from the diet, and perhaps decrease the necessity of feeding expensive protein supplements. Presumably, amino
acids would be released by normal ruminal proteolysis, but not
degraded further, which would increase the supply of all amino
acids to the lower gut. Hogan and Weston (1969) studied the use
of 6 antibiotics as possible agents for reducing amino acid degradation in the rumen. In initial studies, chloramphenicol gave
a 50% reduction in ruminal ammonia levels, and appeared quite
promising. However, in later experiments, 1 g/day of chloramphenicol gave only slight reduction in ruminal ammonia, and may have
reduced feed intake.

Kentucky workers have conducted extensive trials using oxytetracycline as a model compound for inhibition of ruminal amino
acid deamination. Feeding 1 g/day of oxytetracycline, along with
unprotected methionine or lysine, gave elevated levels of these
2 EAA in the plasma of lambs (Schelling et al., 1973). Performance
was slightly depressed with methionine plus oxytetracycline, possibly due to overfeeding in this study of the methionine. The
Kentucky group is continuing study of these techniques (Schelling
et al., 1974). Scientists at SmithKline Corporation are also
pursuing this line of research, and have tested over 2000 compounds
for inhibitory action on ruminal amino acid degradation (W. Chalupa,
personal communication. SmithKline workers have identified a group
of aryl-iodonium salts, of which diphenyliodonium chloride is the
parent compound, which are effective inhibitors of amino acid
deamination at very low ruminal concentrations (Chalupa et al.,
1975 U. S. Patent 3,862,333).

PROTECTION OF DIETARY PROTEINS FROM
RUMINAL DEGRADATION

The idea of protecting dietary proteins from ruminal breakdown originated from research begun in Great Britain about 25
years ago. Cuthbertson and Chalmers (1950) found that sheep fed a
protein deficient diet had improved N-retention, due to much lower

urinary N excretion, when supplemental casein was infused into the duodenum rather than into the rumen. The explanation of these results was that ruminal administration resulted in considerable breakdown of the casein to ammonia, without corresponding resynthesis into microbial protein. The excess ammonia was absorbed from the rumen, converted to urea by the liver, and excreted in the urine. Duodenally infused casein was of course directly available to the sheep for digestion and absorption as amino acids. In subsequent and more thorough studies by this same group, heat-treated casein gave reduced ammonia production and improved N-retention, when fed to sheep (Chalmers et al., 1954). Herring meal, which is subjected to considerable amounts of heat in normal processing, was also found to a better utilized protein source than untreated casein (Chalmers and Synge, 1954). These workers also report trying formaldehyde-treatment of casein (Chalmers et al., 1954) and herring meal (Chalmers and Synge, 1954), but little improvement in utilization of either protein was obtained in these early studies.

Out of this classic British work came several important concepts regarding utilization of proteins by ruminants.

1. The amino acid composition of a feed protein may be less important in determining its utilization than its susceptibility to ruminal degradation (Synge, 1952).

2. Simple digestibility figures for a protein may be of little value in ruminant nutrition because these tell nothing about the relative amounts digested to ammonia in the rumen and digested to amino acids in the intestine (Chalmers et al., 1954).

3. Processing steps, such as heat treatments, which decrease the value of proteins for monogastric species may actually improve their value to ruminants (Chalmers et al., 1954).

4. Any treatment of a feed protein for ruminants which decreases its ruminal degradation, without sacrificing too much intestinal digestibility, will result in greater

amino acid absorption in the lower gut, so long as the factors normally released from protein degradation in the rumen are not limiting for microbial growth.

The mechanism of ruminal protein degradation was discussed in detail earlier. The major property which is thought to influence ruminal breakdown of proteins is their solubility in ruminal contents (Hungate, 1966). Indeed, the terms ruminal solubility and ruminal breakdown are frequently used interchangeably. There is, however, some evidence that other properties of proteins, such as availability of peptide bonds or N- or C-terminal amino acids to enzymatic attack, will influence their rate of ruminal breakdown (Mangan, 1972). Nevertheless, in practice it may be permissible to assume that protein solubility and susceptibility to ruminal breakdown are synonymous, because processes which reduce protein solubility also reduce ruminal degradation.

In their excellent review, Goering and Waldo (1974a) presented the theoretical relationship between protein solubility and utilization shown in Figure 1. Processing effects that reduce protein

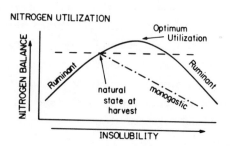

FIG. 1. Theoretical relationships between dietary N-utilization (e.g., N-balance) and insolubility of the dietary-N. Figure illustrates how processing treatments that reduce protein solubility decrease monogastric protein-utilization, but may actually improve protein-utilization in ruminants. Figure taken from Goering and Waldo (1974a) by permission of the authors.

solubility, while reducing utilization by monogastrics, may actually improve utilization by ruminants. Although processing may have reduced intestinal digestibility, ruminal degradation may be reduced even more. This is possible because ruminal proteolysis, the limiting step in ruminal protein breakdown, is probably less efficient than proteolysis in the small intestine. The net result will be that reducing protein solubility will yield a greater net absorption of amino acids at the intestine. Beyond the point of optimal utilization, processing which results in too great a decrease in protein solubility will reduce overall protein utilization. Overprocessing, while greatly reducing ruminal degradation, will also sacrifice too much intestinal digestibility; the over-protected protein will be excreted in the feces.

Natural feed proteins differ greatly in their ruminal solubility (Henderickx and Martin, 1963; Wohlt et al., 1973), and probably susceptibility to ruminal degradation. Therefore, one would expect different responses in protein utilization to treatments which reduce ruminal digestibility, depending on the properties of feed proteins prior to treatment. For example, some feed proteins may already have optimal or nearly optional ruminal solubilities, and further treatment with heat or formaldehyde may actually impair protein utilization. It must be further noted that most feed proteins are really mixtures of many different proteins which also possess different solubility properties and presumably have different susceptibilities to ruminal degradation. Sniffen (1974) states that processes which are thought to improve ruminant protein utilization, apparently shift the proportion of total protein in a feed from the more soluble albumin and globulin fractions to the less soluble prolamin and glutelin fractions. Sniffen (1974) also notes that the feed proteins of best EAA pattern are generally the most in need of ruminal protection.

Heat Treatment

One of the first processes used to give improved dietary

protein utilization in ruminants was heat treatment. Heating will
result in crosslinking within and between protein molecules mainly
because of reactions between free amino groups (largely the ε-amino
group of lysine residues) and other reactive groups on amino acid
residues (Finley and Friedman, 1973). Most feed proteins, particularly those in grains and oilseed meals, are present in the diet
with large amounts of carbohydrate. Heating of proteins in the
presence of carbohydrate results in the well known Schiff's base
formation between free amino and aldehyde groups, as well as many
other reactions. The chemistry of this process is very complex and
not completely understood. Heating decreases a protein's susceptibility to ruminal proteolytic attack by physically reducing contact
of the protein with microbial enzymes through reducing the proteins
solubility, and by blocking, through chemical modification, the
sites of enzymatic attack.

Heating has not only improved utilization of casein by sheep
(Chalmers et al., 1954), but also has substantially improved N-
retention and milk protein production in goats fed heat-treated
groundnut meal (Chalmers et al., 1964) and herring meal, a protein
normally heated extensively in its preparation (Chalmers and
Marshall, 1964). Tagari et al. (1962) conducted an excellent
study on the effects of heat-treatment of soybean meal for ruminants.
From experiments in which sheep were feed soybean meal preparations
subjected to three levels of heating, soybean meal steamed at 120°C
for 15 minutes was found to have the lowest solubility and ruminal
ammonia release rate,and to give the best N-retention.

Workers at the Rowett Research Institute in Scotland studied
the effects of heating on the utilization of various protein
supplements by ruminant calves. Whitelaw (1961), compared the
value of commercial decorticated groundnut meal with heat-treated
groundnut meal and a Peruvian fish meal of "high quality." N-
retention and weight gain in 11-week old calves were highest on
the fish meal diet, next highest on the heat-treated groundnut meal
diet, and lowest on the diet containing unheated groundnut meal.

In a later experiment (Whitelaw and Preston, 1963), although no advantage was seen for heat-treatment of groundnut meal, the heat-treatment of herring meal improved its utilization in young calves. In still another experiment (Whitelaw et al., 1964), four fish meal preparations were compared, again as protein sources for early-weaned calves. There were strong positive relationships among the amounts of heat used in processing, protein insolubility, and effectiveness of the fish meals to support higher N-retention and weight gain. All three reports by Whitelaw and coworkers indicated that improved N-retention with the effective heat-treatments was due to improved utilization of absorbed N.

Use of heat-treatment of oilseed meals to reduce ruminal degradation and to increase protein utilization has been studied extensively in America. Sherrod and Tillman (1962) conducted growth and metabolism trials with wether lambs fed soybean or cottonseed meals autoclaved at 120°C for varying lengths of time. Heat-treatment of both oilseed meals, although decreasing overall protein digestibility, reduced ruminal ammonia concentration and urinary-N losses, and increased N-retention and rate of gain. In subsequent experiments with growing sheep, Sherrod and Tillman (1964) studied the effects of six graded levels of heat-treatment (by autoclaving for different lengths of time) of cottonseed meal alone. With increased heat-treatment, there was a linear decrease in urinary-N excretion and a linear increase in fecal-N excretion. The responses of N-retention, weight gain and feed efficiency to increased heat-treatment were curvilinear--increasing to maxima before falling as heat-treatment was increased beyond the point of optimal effect. These relationships between degree of heat-treatment and N-utilization are shown in Figure 2, and illustrate clearly the possibility of overprotection as well as beneficial effects from heat-treatment of dietary proteins for ruminants. Similar findings were reported in a later paper by this same group (Danke et al., 1966).

The improved efficiency of utilization of heat-treated soybean meal protein was shown by reports from the Kentucky Station. Dry-

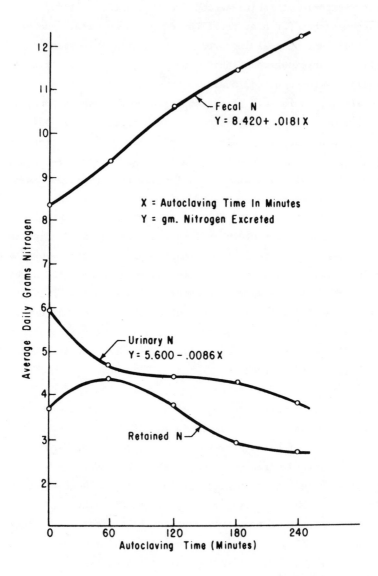

FIG. 2. Effects of autoclaving CSM at 120°C for various lengths of time on N-excretion and N-retention in growing lambs. Figure taken from Sherrod and Tillman (1964) by permission of the American Society of Animal Science.

heating soybean meal at 149°C for 4 hours decreased protein solubility (Glimp et al., 1967), increased the amount of protein bypassing the rumen (Hudson et al., 1970), and resulted in the N-
retention on a 12% CP diet, containing heated soybean meal, being
comparable to that with 17% CP diet containing unheated soybean
meal (Glimp et al., 1967). Later studies at the Kentucky Station
with feeding heat-treated soybean meal to lambs showed improved
N-retention (Nishimuta et al., 1973), and increased amounts of
protein amino acids reaching the abomasum (Nishimuta et al., 1974).
The data in Table 2, taken from a review by Goering and Waldo
(1974b), summarizes well the effects of heat-treatments on utilization of proteins by ruminants.

Tannin Treatments

A procedure which has received considerable recent attention
is use of tannins (polyphenolic compounds of plant origin) to
prevent ruminal degradation of dietary protein. Leroy et al.,
(1965) reported that addition of aqueous tannin solutions to groundnut and soybean meals, when incubated with ruminal contents in
vitro, significantly reduced ammonia release without affecting
cellulose digestibility. Work by the same group indicated that
treatment of groundnut meal with 13% tannin almost completely
inhibited ammonia production in vivo, and gave improved efficiency
of utilization of dietary protein for growth and milk production
(Delort-Laval and Zelter, 1968). Driedger and Hatfield (1972)
report on the effects of treating soybean meal with graded levels
of tannic acid. From ammonia release rates, treatment with 10%
tannic acid (1 g tannic acid/10 g soybean meal) gave complete protection for 8 hours, and protection was almost comparable to that

TABLE 2

Effects of Heating on Protein Utilization by Ruminants
(Data from Goering and Waldo (1974b) by Permission of the Authors)

Protein Source	Digestibility[a] %	N-Retention[b] g/day
Alfalfa		
Field-Dried Hay	69.3	-0.9
Artificially-Dried Hay	61.7	0.1
Grass		
Fresh Material	68.0	1.0
Dried at 40°C	70.3	2.3
Dried at 90°C	66.3	2.5
Dried at 90°C-2x as long	65.0	3.0
Dried at 120°C	65.7	3.6
Dried at 120°C-2x as long	60.6	2.3
Soybean Meal		
Solvent Removed-Room Temp	46.1	0.6
Solvent Removed-80°C (10 min)	48.5	1.7
Solvent Removed-120°C (15 min)	50.4	2.3

[a]Apparent N-digestibility in growing lambs.

[b]N-retention in growing lambs.

with 25% tannic acid after 24 hours of in vitro ruminal incubation. In vitro pepsin-pancreatin digestions suggested that tannic acid treatment would not interfere with intestinal protein digestion. In lamb feeding studies, Driedger and Hatfield (1972) found that pelleting of soybean meal treated with 10% tannic acid gave significantly improved N-retention, weight gain, and feed efficiencies, compared to pelleted diets supplemented with untreated soybean meal or urea.

The evidence that tannin-treatment will improve protein utilization by ruminants is not uniformly favorable. Nishimuta et al. (1973), although finding substantial reductions in ruminal ammonia concentration and urinary-N excretion, found that fecal-N excretion increased, resulting in no net improvement in N-retention in lambs fed soybean treated with 9% tannic acid. In a later study (Nishimuta et al., 1974), tannic acid treatment of soybean meal was observed to have no effect on the amount of protein by-passing the rumen in lambs. In ruminal in vitro studies, Tagari et al. (1965) found that the tannins extraction from carob pods, although having no effect on cellulose digestion and inhibiting ruminal proteolytic activity (which would favor by-pass of dietary protein), appeared not to change ammonia production and strongly inhibited microbial protein synthesis. It should be noted however, that in the Tagari et al. (1965) study, carob tannins were added directly to the ruminal in vitro medium. In the other tannin-treatment work cited here, tannins were allowed to react with the proteins prior to feeding or in vitro incubation. Also, Tagari et al. (1965) observed that the inhibitory effect of tannins on microbial protein synthesis was substantially reversed by addition of readily fermentable carbohydrate to the incubation medium.

The mechanism by which tannins reduce ruminal protein degradation is unclear. It has been suggested that tannins form hydrogen bonds with proteins (Haslam, 1966) which interfere with proteolytic attack by ruminal microbes, and the tannin-protein complex may be dissociated at the acid pH's found in the abomasum and upper small

235

intestine (Van Buren and Robinson, 1969; Driedger and Hatfield, 1972). It is also possible that, where the pH of small intestine has returned to neutrality, the tannin-protein complex may recombine (Driedger and Hatfield, 1972), or that tannins may inhibit proteolytic enzymes directly (Feeney, 1969), rendering the proteins less digestible than without the presence of tannins. The technique of tannin-treatment to protect dietary proteins is covered by a patent licensed to Kent Feeds, Incorporated.

Miscellaneous Treatments

Two miscellaneous procedures used to reduce ruminal protein degradation deserve mention. Jayasinghe (1961) observed substantial reductions in ruminal ammonia concentrations when he added fats (either groundnut or coconut oil) to groundnut or coconut meal fed to sheep. Atwal et al. (1974) studied the effects of pelleting protein concentrates with a mixture of volatile fatty acids (VFA) which contained 83% propionic acid. It was found that addition of 5, 10, 15 and 20 g VFA/100g of a mixture of soybean meal plus promine proteins, inhibited ruminal ammonia release rates in vivo to, respectively, 43, 28, 20 and 16% of control. It was suggested that the presence of propionic acid in close proximity to the proteins had a bacteriostatic effect on the ruminal microbes. When followed for 24 hours after a protein-VFA preparation was added to the rumen, ammonia levels rose somewhat at 18 hours, suggesting that the protective effect may be removed with time. However, with normal ruminal turnover times, this protective effect should have been sufficient to allow by-pass of a substantial portion of the protein-VFA supplement, and this technique deserves further study.

Treatment with Formaldehyde and Other Aldehydes

The procedure for increasing ruminal by-pass of proteins which has received by far the most attention is aldehyde-treatment, principly formaldehyde-treatment of dietary proteins. The first

prominent use of formaldehyde for this purpose was reported by
Chalmers and coworkers, for the protection of casein (Chalmers et
al., 1954) and herring meal (Chalmers and Synge, 1954) from ruminal
degradation in sheep. Although these initial trials were unsuccess-
full, the procedure was resurrected by Australian scientists of the
Commonwealth Scientific and Industrial Research Organization (CSIRO).
In their paper (Ferguson et al., 1967), formaldehyde-treatment of
casein was reported to give significant reductions in ruminal ammonia release in vitro, and when fed to sheep, to increase wool growth
70% (compared to a 15% increase in wool growth with untreated casein). In subsequent experiments, feeding of formaldehyde-treated
casein was shown to increase not only wool growth, but also rate of
gain and N-retention in lambs (Faichney, 1971), and the amount of
protein digested in the intestines of lambs (Faichney and Weston,
1971). These successful results led to the patenting of this process (Ferguson and Solomon, 1971). In the United States, this
patent is now licensed to Dow Chemical Corporation.

The chemistry of formaldehyde-protein reactions is well defined,
but several aspects regarding the mechanism by which formaldehyde-
treatment increases intestinal digestion of dietary proteins in
ruminants remain uncertain. Walker (1964) has thoroughly reviewed
the chemistry of formaldehyde interaction with proteins. Under the
mild conditions generally used to feed proteins, formaldehyde probably reacts principally with the free amino groups of lysine and N-
terminal amino acid residues, forming Schiff's bases and methylene
cross-links between peptide chains. In addition to that of lysine,
the residues of arginine, histidine, methionine, tryptophan and
tyrosine will react with formaldehyde, as will the amide groups of
asparagine, glutamine and the peptide bond. Aldehydes other than
formaldehyde would presumably react in a similar way. The effect
of reducing ruminal degradation is thought to be due to reduced
solubility of the formaldehyde-treated protein (Ferguson et al.,
1967), and increased resistance of the treated proteins to enzymatic attack (Walker, 1964).

One of the supposed advantages of formaledhyde-treatment of protein fed to ruminants is that the reaction may be reversed in the acid medium of the abomasum and upper small intestine (Ferguson et al., 1967). Most of the products of formaldehyde-protein reaction are reversed by acid treatment (Walker, 1964), and the pH of the ruminant small intestine remains lower for a greater length of the tract than occurs in the monogastric (Kay, 1969; Ben-Ghedalia et al., 1974). This would give the technique of formaldehyde-treatment of proteins an advantage over such procedures as heat-treatment, which are probably not reversed in the lower gut.

Reversal of the formaldehyde-protein reaction in the lower gut was one of the principles upon which the formaldehyde-treatment technique was patented (Ferguson and Solomon, 1971). Evidence favoring this hypothesis was obtained by Mills et al. (1972), who recovered, as expired carbon dioxide and methane, 60-80% of the label from a ^{14}C-formaldehyde-treated casein-oil complex that was fed to sheep. Fecal and urinary excretion accounted for 11-27% and 5-6% of the ingested label, respectively. Assuming all of the ^{14}C-formaldehyde had reacted with protein before feeding,these results suggest that about 70% of the protein-bound formaldehyde was re- moved due to the low pH of the lower gut. It is interesting to note that recovery of label in expired air tended to be lower, and fecal recovery higher, as time after treatment increased, indicating a change to more irreversible binding with time. Another important finding of these workers was that very little radioactivity was recovered in carcass tissues of sheep or in milk secreted by lactating goats, and feeding of the dietary formaldehyde did not increase the levels of unlabeled formaldehyde found in tissues or milk.

There is some information indicating that the formaldehyde- treatment of protein may not be reversed in the abomasum and upper small intestine. It is recognized by the author that monogastrics may be less effective in removing protein-bound formaldehyde, but rat feeding studies show continuing decreases in protein digestibi-

lity with increasing levels of formaldehyde-treatment. Schmidt
et al., (1973a) found that treatment of soybean meal protein with
0,0.4,0.8,1.2 and 1.6% w/w formaldehyde (g formaldehyde/100g protein) gave apparent protein digestibilities in the rat of 86.4,
85.6, 77.4, 66.4 and 54.5%. Similar trends were observed by
Broderick (1972) who found that increasing the level of formaldehyde-treatment of casein gave a linear drop in both the rates of
rat growth and release of amino acids during in vitro pepsin-
pancreatin digestions. The results of several digestion trials
indicate that protein digestibility falls in ruminants as well,
when the protein is treated with formaldehyde. Feeding sheep diets
in which 40% of the protein came from casein, Faichney (1971) found
the apparent digestibility of a diet containing formaldehyde-treated
casein was 5 percentage units lower than that of the same diet
containing untreated casein. Although MacRae et al. (1972) observed
only slightly lowered protein digestibility in sheep fed diets containing formaldehyde-treated casein, Faichney and Davies found
protein digestibilities decreased about 7 percentage units when
calves were fed diets containing formaldehyde-treated peanut meal
(1972), or when the whole diet was treated (1973).

Reis and Tunks (1970) observed, with feeding of formaldehyde-
treated casein to sheep, a six-fold increase in plasma concentration of a compound identified as ε-N-methyl lysine, which was
thought to be formed from ε-N-methylol lysine released during digestion of treated casein. Although not quantitative, these data imply
that the groups which form when protein reacts with formaldehyde are
incompletely removed by the action of lower gut. The overall evidence is strongly suggestive that the reaction between dietary protein and formaldehyde is only partially reversed in the acid
environment of the abomasum and upper small intestine. Some intestinal digestibility is sacrificed when protein is treated with
formaldehyde to protect it from ruminal degradation. Therefore,
it is very important to determine the minimum level of formaldehyde-treatment necessary to achieve maximal or nearly maximal

ruminal protection, without reducing intestinal protein digestion too greatly.

Hemsley et al., (1973) reported on experiments using casein treated with various levels of formaldehyde. Figure 3 shows the

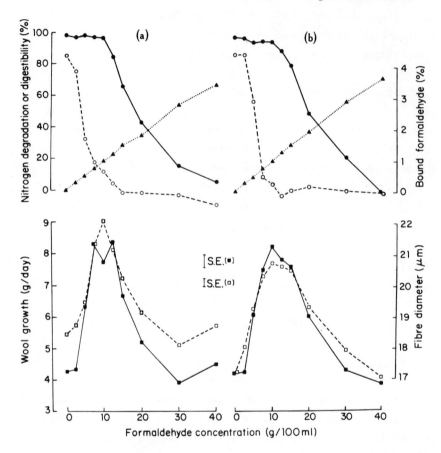

FIG. 3. Effect of treating casein with 100 ml formaldehyde solution per kg casein on bound formaldehyde content (g/100 g casein dry matter, ▲), on degradation of casein-N to ammonia-N by ruminal microbes *in vitro* (o), on *in vivo* casein-N digestibility (●), on wool growth rate (g/day clean dry wool, ■), and on adjusted fiber diameter (□). Experiment (a), products of formaldehyde-treatment unheated; experiment (b), products of formaldehyde-treatment heated for 24 hr at 70°C. Figure taken from Hemsley et al. (1973) by permission of the Commonwealth Scientific and Industrial Research Organization.

effect of level of formaldehyde-treatment of casein on in vitro degradation to ammonia, in vivo digestibility, amount of formaldehyde bound to the protein, wool growth and wool fiber diameter. It appears that application of about 1.0% w/w formaldehyde gives the maximal wool growth response and nearly maximal protection from ruminal degradation, without adversely affecting overall digestibility of casein protein. These results indicate that optimal level of treatment lies within a very narrow range between about 0.8 and 1.2% formaldehyde which may make this procedure difficult to apply in a practical feeding situations. Other protein supplements have not been studied as extensively as casein, and their optimal level of formaldehyde-treatment has not been as precisely determined. However, CSIRO workers feel that approximately 2% w/w formaldehyde is probably near to the optimal treatment level for most oilseed meal proteins (J. P. Hogan, personal communication).

There is now a very large body of literature dealing with the effects on animal performance of treating part of all of the dietary protein with formaldehyde or other aldehydes. This topic has been the subject of recent reviews of greater (McGilliard, 1972; Hatfield, 1973; Goering and Waldo, 1974a,b) and lesser quality (Broderick, 1973; See also J. H. Clark, this volume). Casein is the protein which has been the most studied in formaldehyde-treatment experiments. Formaldehyde-treatment of casein has been shown to substantially reduce ruminal solubility and degradation to ammonia (Ferguson et al., 1967; Hemsley et al., 1973). Compared to untreated casein, feeding formaldehyde-treated casein to sheep resulted in significant increases in plasma free amino acid concentrations (Reis and Tunks, 1970), in protein digested in the small intestine (Faichney and Weston, 1971; MacRae et al., 1972), in wool growth (Ferguson et al., 1967; Reis and Tunks, 1969; Langlands, 1971a; Wright, 1971; Hemsley et al., 1973), in N-retention (Reis and Tunks, 1969; Faichney, 1971, MacRae et al., 1972), and in weight gain and feed efficiency (Reis and Tunks, 1969; Faichney, 1971; Wright, 1971). Canadian workers also found improved N-retention

(Sharma and Ingalls, 1974) and flow of protein and EAA to the lower gut (Sharma, Ingalls, and Parker, 1974) with formaldehyde-treatment of casein fed to steers. Not all of the experiments have shown increased production when casein was formaldehyde-treated. Several workers found no advantage over untreated casein with formaldehyde-treatment of casein for wool growth (Carrico et al., 1970; Henderson et al., 1970) or for milk production in dairy cattle (Wilson, 1970; Broderick and Lane, 1974).

The results from experiments using treatment with formaldehyde or other aldehydes of proteins commonly fed in ruminant nutrition are much less definitive than results obtained with casein. The effect of aldehyde-treatment of soybean meal protein has been the subject of several reports. Illinois workers (Peter et al., 1971; Hatfield, 1973) obtained reduced ruminal degradation, and improved N-retention, weight gains and feed efficiencies when lambs were fed soybean meal treated with formaldehyde, glutaraldehyde or glyoxal (another aldehyde). Nishimuta et al. (1974) observed significant increases in the amounts of protein and amino acids passing to the abomasum when they treated soybean meal with formaldehyde. Preston and Smith (1974) found that steers supplemented with 0.23 kg/day of formaldehyde-treated soybean meal had weight gains and feed efficiencies almost comparable to steers given 0.45 kg/day of untreated soybean meal. However, others have found no improvements, with formaldehyde-treatment of soybean meal, in weight gains and feed efficiencies in lambs (Schmidt et al., 1974; Wachira et al., 1974) and steers (Schmidt et al., 1974), or in production of milk or milk components in dairy cows (Clark et al., 1974; Wachira et al., 1974). Moreover, some workers have been found reduced N-retention in lambs (Nishimuta et al., 1973; Amos et al., 1974a), decreased weight gains in steers (Schmidt et al., 1973b), and reduced N-digestibilities in cattle (Clark et al., 1974) and lambs (Schmidt et al., 1974; Amos et al., 1974a) when dietary soybean meal was treated with formaldehyde.

Contradictory results were also obtained in feeding studies

with other formaldehyde-treated protein supplements. Saville et al. (1971) and Langlands (1971b) found no improvement in wool growth when cottonseed meal was treated with formaldehyde, even though ruminal degradation was decreased. Rattray and Joyce (1970) observed increased N-retention with formaldehyde-treatment of linseed meal but reduced N-retention with treatment of meat meal fed to young lambs. Sharkey et al. (1974) obtained improved feed intakes and growth rates, but no improvement in feed efficiency, when barley and linseed meal diets were treated with formaldehyde. Entwistle (1973) found in one experiment that formaldehyde-treatment of a grain plus meat meal diet improved weight gains in lambs, but had no effect in another study. Formaldehyde-treatment of rapeseed meal reduced ruminal ammonia concentrations, but also reduced overall protein digestibility (Sharma et al., 1972; Sharma and Ingalls, 1974), and had no effect on growth rates of calves (Sharma et al., 1972). Formaldehyde-treatment of wheat fed to sheep tended to increase N-retention, N-digestion in the intestines (Langlands, 1973a), and wool growth (Langlands, 1973b), while formaldehyde-treatment of barley fed to steers decreased feed intakes, weight gain, feed efficiency and overall protein digestion (Davies and Faichney, 1973).

Groundnut meal appears to respond well to formaldehyde-treatments. Although their initial studies showed little improvement in performance of calves with formaldehyde-treatment of groundnut meal, Faichney and Davies (1972) found that complete treatment of a groundnut meal diet with 12% CP gave a 9% increase in weight gains of calves. Other studies have also shown that formaldehyde protection of groundnut meal fed to sheep substantially increased intestinal digestion of dietary protein (Miller, 1972) and wool growth (Hughes and Williams, 1971).

The majority of the protein consumed by ruminants generally comes from forages in the diet. Forage protein quality, especially that of leaf proteins, is usually very good. Therefore, in a time when grains and protein concentrates are being increasingly diverted

to human nutrition, a practical approach to the problem of increasing the amount of protein reaching the ruminant small intestine
may be to use formaldehyde-treatment of the forage proteins normally
present in the diet. Hemsley et al. (1970) reported that formaldehyde-treatment of clover hay increased wool growth 15%, while
Sharkey et al. (1972) found that treatment of clover-grass hay had
no effect on wool growth, and actually reduced weight gain and N-
retention in sheep. Barry treated ryegrass-clover herbage with
various levels of formaldehyde and found marked reduction of ruminal ammonia concentrations (1973a), but little change in wool growth
in sheep fed at or slightly below maintenance (1973b). Although
observing no wool responses under the conditions of his experiment,
Barry (1973a) felt that formaldehyde-treatment had increased the
amount of dietary protein digested in the lower gut.

An application where formaldehyde-treatment of herbage, particularly legumes and other high-protein forages, may be practical and
convenient is during herbage ensiling. With high protein forages,
the silage making process frequently results in reduced feeding value
(e.g., degradation of forage protein after ensiling), and in
objectionable characteristics which reduce silage consumption by
animals. Brown and Valentine (1972) used formaldehyde-treatment to
reduce the detrimental effects due to ensiling lucerne, but also
found marked reduction in N-digestibility (probably due to over-
treatment with formaldehyde--17g/100g CP was the lowest formaldehyde level applied). In a subsequent study (Valentine and Brown,
1973), formaldehyde was added alone, or together with formic acid,
to lucerne silage. Formaldehyde-treatment alone, but especially in
combination with formic acid, produced significant increases in dry
matter intake and wool growth, compared to untreated silage and
silage treated with formic acid alone. Treatment of grass-legume
silages with formaldehyde-formic acid mixtures was found by others
to improve N-retention in steers (Waldo et al., 1973) and to slightly
improve milk production in dairy cows (Barker et al., 1973). Barry
and coworkers also found that treatment of a mixed grass-clover
silage with slightly less than 3g formaldehyde/100g CP, decreased

protein breakdown during ensiling (Barry and Fennessy, 1972) and in the rumen (Barry and Fennessy, 1973), and increased silage intake, weight gain and wool growth in sheep (Barry, Fennessy and Duncan, 1973). Goering and Waldo (1974b) have reviewed the use of formaldehyde-treatment of silages.

There are several possible explanations for the great diversity of responses to protein treatment in ruminants, most of which have been touched on previously. For improved protein utilization due to formaldehyde or other treatments to be clearly shown experimentally, it is probable that, prior to treatment, the protein must be relatively susceptible to ruminal degradation. This may be why treatment responses of casein, groundnut meal and forages (especially the very soluble leaf proteins), which are all readily degraded in the rumen, are more easily detected experimentally. Because most other feed proteins are of lower ruminal solubility and breakdown, the degree of improvement in intestinal availability due to treatment of these proteins, while still real and important, would be smaller and therefore harder to detect.

The importance of the amino acid pattern of the protected protein, and how well it complements the amino acid pattern of the mixture of microbial protein and feed protein which normally by-passes the rumen, was discussed earlier. That not all feed proteins are equal as post-ruminal supplements was shown in the esophagel groove experiments of Ørskov et al. (1970).

In many experiments, it is probable that the proteins were not properly protected. Some of the heat-treatment and formaldehyde-treatment studies referred to earlier showed substantial over-protection of proteins. Australian workers (Hemsley et al., 1973) found a very narrow range of 0.8-1.2% w/w within which formaldehyde-treatment of casein was effective for giving optimal wool growth responses. Other results suggested that formaldehyde-treatment levels of about 2% for oilseed meal proteins (J. P. Hogan, personal communication) and 3% for legume-grass silage proteins (Barry et al., 1973) may give optimal utilization. Considerable loss of the applied protecting agent, as probably would occur with formaldehyde-application during hay-making, must also be considered when deciding on the appropriate level of treatment.

ACKNOWLEDGMENT

The author wishes to thank Dr. W. C. Ellis for his helpful advice during preparation of this manuscript.

REFERENCES

Allison, M. J. 1969. Biosynthesis of amino acids by ruminal micro-organisms. J. Anim. Sci. 29:797.

Allison, M. J. 1970. Nitrogen metabolism of ruminal micro-organisms. In A. T. Phillipson (Ed.) Physiology of Digestion and Metabolism in the Ruminant. Oriel Press, Newcastle-upon-Tyne, England.

Amos, H. E., D. Burdick and T. L. Huber. 1974a. Effects of formaldehyde treatment of sunflower and soybean meal on nitrogen balance in lambs. J. Anim. Sci. 38:702.

Amos, H. E., C. O. Little, G. A. Digenis, G. T. Schelling, R. E. Tucker and G. E. Mitchell, Jr. 1974b. Methionine, DL-homocysteine thiolactone and N-acetyl-DL-methionine for ruminants. J. Anim. Sci. 39:612.

Annison, E. F. 1956. Nitrogen metabolism in the sheep. Protein digestion in the rumen. Biochem. J. 64:705.

Annison, E. F., D. Lewis and D. B. Lindsay. 1959. The metabolic changes which occur in sheep transferred to lush spring grass. I. Changes in blood and rumen constituents. J. Agr. Sci. 53:34.

Armstrong, D. G. 1973. Amino acid requirements and amino acid supply in the sheep. Proc. Nutr. Soc. 32:107.

Atwal, A. S., L. P. Milligan and B. A. Young. 1974. Effects of volatile fatty acid treatment on the protection of protein in the rumen. Can. J. Anim. Sci. 54:393.

Barker, R. A., D. N. Mowat, J. B. Stone, K. R. Stevenson and M. G. Freeman. 1973. Formic acid or formic acid-formalin as a silage additive. Can. J. Anim. Sci. 53:465.

Barry, T. N. 1973a. Effect of Treatment with formaldehyde and intraperitoneal supplementation with D-L methionine on the digestion and utilization of a hay diet by sheep. I. The digestion of energy and nitrogen. New Zealand J. Agr. Res. 16:185.

Barry, T. N. 1973b. Effect of treatment with formaldehyde and intraperitoneal supplementation with D-L methionine on the digestion and utilization of a hay diet by sheep. II. Live-weight change and wool growth. New Zealand J. Agr. Res. 16: 191.

Barry, T. N. and P. F. Fennessy. 1972. The effect of formaldehyde treatment on the chemical composition and nutritive value of silage. I. Chemical composition. New Zealand J. Agr. Res. 15:712.

Barry, T. N. and P. F. Fennessy. 1973. Effect of formaldehyde treatment on the chemical composition and nutritive value of silage. II. Digestibility of the silages and the chemical composition of rumen fluid in sheep supplemented or not supplemented with D-L methionine. New Zealand J. Agr. Res. 16:59.

Barry, T. N., P. F. Fennessy and S. J. Duncan. 1973. Effect of formaldehyde treatment on the chemical composition and nutritive value of silage. III. Voluntary intake, live-weight gain, and wool growth in sheep fed the silages with or without intraperitoneal supplementation with D-L methionine. New Zealand J. Agr. Res. 16:64.

Belasco, I. J. 1972. Stability of methionine hydroxy analog in rumen fluid and its conversion in vitro to methionine by calf liver and kidney. J. Dairy Sci. 55:353.

Ben-Ghedalia, D., H. Tagari, A. Bondi and A. Tadmor. 1974. Protein digestion in the intestine of sheep. Brit. J. Nutr. 31:125.

Bitman, J., T. R. Wrenn, L. P. Dryden, L. F. Edmonson and R. A. Yoncoskie. 1974. Encapsulated vegetable fats in cattle feeds. In J. E. Vandager (Ed.) Microencapsulation: Processes and Applications. Plenum Publishing Corp., New York.

Black, A. L., M. Kleiber and A. H. Smith. 1952. Carbonate and fatty acids as precursors of amino acids in casein. J. Biol. Chem. 197:365.

Black, J. L. and D. E. Tribe. 1973. Comparison of ruminal and abomasal administration of feed on the growth and body composition of lambs. Australian J. Agr. Res. 24:763.

Blackburn, T. H. 1968. Protease production by *Bacteroides amylophilus* strain H18. J. Gen. Microbial. 53:27.

Blackburn, T. H. and P. N. Hobson. 1960. Proteolysis in the sheep rumen by whole and fractionated rumen contents. J. Gen. Microbiol. 22:272.

Blackburn, T. H. and W. A. Hullah. 1974. The cell-bound protease of *Bacteroides amylophilus* H18. Can. J. Microbial. 20:435.

Borchers, R. 1967. Incorporation of radioactive carbon from glucose or amino acids by rumen microorganisms. J. Dairy Sci. 50:242.

Broderick, G. A. 1972. Protein and amino acid studies. 1. Effects of post-ruminal casein supplementation on lactating cows. 2. Gas-liquid chromatography of amino acids. Ph.D. Thesis, University of Wisconsin, Madison.

Broderick, G. A. 1973. Potential for "protected" proteins and amino acids in ruminant feeding. Proc. 28th Ann. Tex. Nutr. Conf. p. 111.

Broderick, G. A., T. Kowalczyk and L. D. Satter. 1970. Milk production response to supplementation with encapsulated methionine per os or casein per abomasum. J. Dairy Sci. 53:1714.

Broderick, G. A. and G. T. Lane. 1974. Response of lactating cows to supplemental feeding of formaldehyde-treated casein. Rep. Conf. Rumen Function p. 6.

Broderick, G. A., L. D. Satter and A. E. Harper. 1974. Use of plasma amino acid concentration to identify limiting amino acids for milk production. J. Dairy Sci. 57:1015.

Brown, D. C. and S. C. Valentine. 1972. Formaldehyde as a silage additive. I. The chemical composition and nutritive value of frozen lucerne, lucerne silage, and formaldehyde-treated lucerne silage. Australian J. Agr. Res. 23:1093.

Bryant, M. P., and I. M. Robinson. 1962. Some nutritional characteristics of predominant culturable ruminal bacteria. J. Bact. 84:605.

Bunn, C. L., J. J. McNeill and G. Matrone. 1968. Comparison of amino acid and alfalfa supplementation of purified diets for ruminants. J. Nutr. 94:47.

Burroughs, W., A. H. Trenkle and R. L. Vetter. 1974. A system of protein evaluation for cattle and sheep involving metabolizable protein (amino acids) and urea fermentation potential of feedstuffs. Vet. Med. Small Anim. Clin. 69:713.

Carrico, R. G., F. R. M. Cockrem, D. D. Haden and G. A. Wickham. 1970. Wool growth and plasma amino acid responses of N. Z. Romney sheep to formalin-treated casein and methionine supplements. New Zealand J. Agr. Res. 13:631.

Chalmers, M. I., D. P. Cuthbertson and R. L. M. Synge. 1954. Ruminal ammonia formation in relation to the protein requirement of sheep. I. Duodenal administration and heat processing as factors influencing fate of casein supplements. J. Agr. Sci. 44:254.

Chalmers, M. I., J. B. Jasasingke and S. B. M. Marshall. 1964. The effect of heat treatment in the processing of groundnut meal on the value of the protein for ruminants with some additional experiments on copra. J. Agr. Sci. 63:283.

Chalmers, M. I., and S. B. M. Marshall. 1964. Ruminal ammonia formation in relation to the utilization of groundnut meal and herring meal as protein sources for milk production. J. Agr. Sci. 63:277.

Chalmers, M. I. and R. L. M. Synge. 1954. Ruminal ammonia formation in relation to the protein requirement of sheep. II. Comparison of casein and herring meal supplements. J. Agr. Sci. 44:263.

Chalupa, W. 1975. Rumen bypass and protection of proteins and amino acids. J. Dairy Sci. 58:1198.

Chalupa, W., J. E. Chandler and R. E. Brown. 1972. Amino acid nutrition of growing cattle. Fed. Proc. 31:681 (Abstr.).

Chalupa, W., J. E. Chandler and R. E. Brown. 1973. Abomasal infusion of mixtures of amino acids to growing cattle. J. Anim. Sci. 37:339 (Abstr.).

Clark, J. H., C. L. Davis and E. E. Hatfield. 1974. Effects of formaldehyde treated soybean meal on nutrient use, milk yield and composition, and free amino acids in the lactating bovine. J. Dairy Sci. 57:1031.

Cline, T. R., U. S. Garrigus and E. E. Hatfield. 1966. Addition of branched- and straight-chain volatile fatty acids to purified lamb diets and effects on utilization of certain dietary components. J. Anim. Sci. 25:734.

Cuthbertson, D. P. and M. I. Chalmers. 1950. Utilization of a casein supplement administered to ewes by ruminal and duodenal fistulae. Biochem. J. 46:xvii (Abstr.).

Danke, R. J., L. B. Sherrod, E. C. Nelson and A. D. Tillman. 1966. Effects of autoclaving and steaming of cottonseed meal for different lengths of time on nitrogen solubility and retention in sheep. J. Anim. Sci. 25:181.

Davies, H. L. and G. J. Faichney. 1973. The effect of formaldehyde treatment of barley on productive performance of Friesian steers. Australian J. Exp. Agr. Anim. Husb. 13:142.

Delort-Laval, J., and S. Z. Zelter. 1968. Improving the nutritive value of proteins by tanning process. Second World Conf. Anim. Nutr. (Abstr.).

Derrig, R. G., J. H. Clark and C. L. Davis. 1974. Effect of abomasal infusion of sodium caseinate on milk yield, nitrogen utilization and amino acid nutrition of the dairy cow. J. Nutr. 104:151.

Digenis, G. A., H. E. Amos, K. Yang, G. E. Mitchell, C. O. Little, J. V. Swintosky, R. C. Parish, G. T. Schelling, E. M. Dietz and R. E. Tucker. 1974a. Methionine substitutes in ruminant nutrition. 1. Stability of nitrogenous compounds related to methionine during in vitro incubation with rumen microorganisms. J. Pharm. Sci. 63:745.

Digenis, G. A., H. E. Amos, G. E. Mitchell, J. V. Swintosky, K. Yang, G. T. Schelling and R. C. Parish. 1974b. Methionine substitutes in ruminant nutrition. 2. Stability of non-nitrogenous compounds related to methionine during in vitro incubation with rumen microorganisms. J. Pharm. Sci. 63:751.

Dinius, D. A. 1974. Potential for protected fat in ruminant rations. Proc. 29th Ann. Tex. Nutr. Conf. p. 112.

Downes, A. M. 1961. The amino acids essential for the tissues of the sheep. Australian J. Biol. Sci. 14:254.

Downes, A. M., P. J. Reis, L. F. Sharry and D. A. Tunks. 1970a. Metabolic fate of parenterally administered sulphur-containing amino acids in sheep and effects on growth and composition of wool. Australian J. Biol. Sci. 23:1077.

Downes, A. M., P. J. Reis, L. F. Sharry and D. A. Tunks. 1970b. Evaluation of modified [^{35}S] methionine and [^{35}S] casein preparations as supplements for sheep. Brit. J. Nutr. 24:1083.

Driedger, A. and E. E. Hatfield. 1972. Influence of tannins on the nutritive value of soybean meal for ruminants. J. Anim. Sci. 34:465.

Ellis, W. C., G. B. Garner, M. E. Muhrer and W. H. Pfander. 1956. Nitrogen utilization by lambs fed purified rations containing urea, gelatin, casein, blood fibrin, and soybean protein. J. Nutr. 60:413.

Ely, D. G., C. O. Little, P. G. Woolfolk and G. E. Mitchell, Jr. 1967. Estimation of the extent of conversion of dietary zein to microbial protein in the rumen of lambs. J. Nutr. 91:314.

Entwistle, K. W. 1973. Formaldehyde treated diets for drought feeding of sheep. Australian J. Exp. Agr. Anim. Husb. 13:630.

Faichney, G. J. 1971. The effect of formaldehyde-treated casein on the growth of ruminant lambs. Australian J. Agr. Res. 22:453.

Faichney, G. J. and H. L. Davies. 1972. The effect of formaldehyde treatment of peanut meal in concentrate diets on the performance of calves. Australian J. Agr. Res. 23:167.

Faichney, G. J. and H. L. Davies. 1973. The performance of calves given concentrate diets treated with formaldehyde. Australian J. Agr. Res. 24:613.

Faichney, G. J. and R. H. Weston. 1971. Digestion by ruminant lambs of a diet containing formaldehyde-treated casein. Australian J. Agr. Res. 22:461.

Feeney, P. P. 1969. Inhibitory effect of oak leaf tannins on the hydrolysis of proteins by trypsin. Phytochem. 8:2119.

Ferguson, K. A., J. A. Hemsley and P. J. Reis. 1967. The effect of protecting dietary protein from microbial degradation in the rumen. Australian J. Sci. 30:215.

Ferguson, K. A. and D. H. Solomon. 1971. Method and food composition for feeding ruminants. U.S. Patent 3,619,200.

Finley, J. W. and M. Friedman. 1973. Chemical methods for available lysine. Cereal Chem. 50:101.

Fisher, L. J. 1972. Response of lactating cows to the intravenous infusion of amino acids. Can. J. Anim. Sci. 52:377.

Glimp, H. A., M. R. Karr, C. O. Little, P. G. Woolfolk, G. E. Mitchell, Jr. and L. W. Hudson. 1967. Effect of reducing soybean protein solubility by dry heat on the protein utilization of young lambs. J. Anim. Sci. 26:858.

Goering, H. K. and D. R. Waldo. 1974a. Processing effects on protein utilization by ruminants. Proc. Cornell Nutr. Conf. p. 25.

Goering, H. K. and D. R. Waldo. 1974b. Protein value of heat- and formaldehyde-treated ruminant feeds. Proc. Maryland Nutr. Conf. p. 52.

Grass, G. M. and R. R. Unangst. 1972. Glycerol tristearate and higher fatty acid mixtures for improving digestive absorption. U.S. Patent 3,655,864.

Hatfield, E. E. 1973. Treating dietary proteins with tannins or aldehydes *In* Effect of Processing on the Nutritional Value of Feeds. National Academy of Sciences, Washington, D.C.

Haslam, E. 1966. Chemistry of Vegetable Tannins. Academic Press, New York.

Hemsley, J. A., J. P. Hogan and R. H. Weston. 1970. Protection of forage protein from ruminal degradation. Proc. XI Int. Grassland Cong. p. 703.

Hemsley, J. A., P. J. Reis and A. M. Downes. 1973. Influence of various formaldehyde treatments on the nutritional value of casein for wool growth. Australian J. Biol. Sci. 26:961.

Henderickx, H. and J. Martin. 1963. In vitro study of the nitrogen metabolism in the rumen. Compt. Rend. Rech., Inst. Rech. Sci. Ind. Agr., Bruxelles 31:7.

Henderson, A. E., J. McG. Bryden, F. E. Mazzitelli and K. E. Milligan. 1970. Protein supplementation and wool growth. Proc. New Zealand Soc. Anim. Prod. 30:186.

Hogan, J. P. 1973. Intestinal digestion of subterranean clover by sheep. Australian J. Agr. Res. 24:587.

Hogan, J. P. 1975. Quantitive aspects of nitrogen utilization in ruminants. J. Dairy Sci. 58: 1164.

Hogan, J. P. and R. H. Weston. 1969. The effect of antibiotics on ammonia accumulation and protein digestion in the rumen.

Australian J. Agr. Res. 20:339.

Hogan, J. P. and R. H. Weston. 1970. Quantitative aspects of microbial protein synthesis in the rumen. *In* A. T. Phillipson (Ed.) Physiology of Digestion and Metabolism in the Ruminant. Oriel Press, Newcastle-upon-Tyne, England.

Hogan, J. P. and R. H. Weston. 1971. The utilization of alkali-treated straw by sheep. Australian J. Agr. Res. 22:951.

Hudson, L. W., H. A. Glimp, C. O. Little and P. G. Woolfolk. 1970. Ruminal and postruminal nitrogen utilization by lambs fed heated soybean meal. J. Anim. Sci. 30:609.

Hughes, J. G. and G. L. Williams. 1971. The utilization of for-maldehyde-treated groundnut meal by sheep. Anim. Prod. 13: 396 (Abstr.).

Hume, I. D. 1970a. Synthesis of microbial protein in the rumen. II. A response to higher volatile fatty acids. Australian J. Agr. Res. 21:297.

Hume, I. D. 1970b. Synthesis of microbial protein in the rumen. III. The effect of dietary protein. Australian J. Agr. Res. 21:305.

Hungate, R. E. 1966. The Rumen and Its Microbes. Academic Press, New York.

Jayasinghe, J. B. 1961. The effect of addition of fat on the breakdown of protein and the subsequent production of ammonia in the rumen. Ceylon Vet. J. 9:135.

Kay, R. N. B. 1969. Digestion of protein in the intestines of adult ruminants. Proc. Nutr. Soc. 28:140.

Ku, Y. and P. W. Simon. 1973. Ruminant feed supplement. U.S. Patent 3,751,262.

Langer, P. N., P. J. Buttery and D. Lewis. 1973. N-steroyl-DL-methionine. A new form of protected methionine for ruminant feeds. Proc. Nutr. Soc. 32:86A (Abstr.).

Langlands, J. P. 1971a. The wool production of grazing sheep supplented with casein and formaldehyde-treated casein. Australian J. Exp. Agr. Anim. Husb. 11:9.

Langlands, J. P. 1971b. The wool production of sheep supplemented with cottonseed meal and formaldehyde-treated cottonseed meal. Australian J. Exp. Agr. Anim. Husb. 11:493.

Langlands, J. P. 1973a. Wheat as a survival ration for sheep. 1. The digestion of wheat and formaldehyde treated wheat. Australian J. Exp. Agr. Anim. Husb. 13:341.

Langlands, J. P. 1973b. Wheat as a survival ration for sheep. 2. The effect of frequency of feeding and formaldehyde treat-ment on wool production and liveweight change. Australian J. Exp. Agr. Anim. Husb. 13:347.

Leroy, F., S. Z. Zelter and A. C. Francois. 1965. Protection of proteins in feeds against deamination by bacteria in the rumen. Studies with the artificial rumen. Nutr. Abstr. and Rev. 35: 444 (Abstr.).

Lewis, D. 1955. Amino acid metabolism in the rumen of the sheep. Brit. J. Nutr. 9:215.

Lewis, D. 1962. The inter-relationships of individual proteins and carbohydrates during fermentation in the rumen of the sheep. II. The fermentation of starch in the presence of proteins and other substances containing nitrogen. J. Agr. Sci. 58:73.

Lewis, T. R. and R. S. Emery. 1962. Relative deamination rates of amino acids by rumen microorganisms. J. Dairy Sci. 45:765.

Little, C. O. and G. E. Mitchell, Jr. 1967. Abomasal vs. oral administration of proteins to wethers. J. Anim. Sci. 26:411.

Lofgreen, G. P., J. K. Loosli and L. A. Maynard. 1947. The influence of protein source upon nitrogen retention by sheep. J. Anim. Sci. 6:343.

Loosli, J. K., and L. E. Harris. 1945. Methionine increases the value of urea for lambs. J. Anim. Sci. 4:435.

MacRae, J. C., M. J. Ulyatt, P. D. Pearce and J. Hendtlass. 1972. Quantitative intestinal digestion of nitrogen in sheep given formaldehyde-treated and untreated supplements. Brit. J. Nutr. 27:39.

Mangan, J. L. 1972. Quantitative studies on nitrogen metabolism in the bovine rumen. The rate of proteolysis of casein and ovalbumin and the release and metabolism of free amino acids. Brit. J. Nutr. 27:261.

Mason, V. C. and R. Palmer. 1971. Studies on the digestibility and utilization of the nitrogen of irradiated rumen bacteria by rats. J. Agr. Sci. 76:567.

McDonald, I. W. and R. J. Hall. 1957. The conversion of casein into microbial proteins in the rumen. Biochem. J. 67:400.

McGilliard, A. D. 1972. Modifying proteins for maximum utilization in the ruminant. J. Amer. Oil. Chem. Soc. 49:57.

McLaren, G. A., G. L. Anderson and K. M. Barth. 1965. Influence of methionine and tryptophan on nitrogen utilization by lambs fed high levels of non-protein nitrogen. J. Anim. Sci. 24: 231.

McNaught, M. L., E. C. Owen, K. M. Henry and S. K. Kon. 1954. The utilization of non-protein nitrogen in the bovine rumen. 8. Nutritive value of the proteins of dried rumen bacteria, rumen protozoa and brewer's yeast. Biochem. J. 56:151.

Miller, E. L. 1972. The digestion of formaldehyde-treated groundnut meal before and after the abomasum of lambs. Proc. Nutr. Soc. 31:27A (Abstr.).

Mills, S. C., L. F. Sharry, L. J. Cook and T. W. Scott. 1972. Metabolism of [^{14}C] formaldehyde when fed to ruminants as an aldehyde-casein-oil complex. Australian J. Biol. Sci. 25: 807.

Mowat, D. N. and K. Deelstra. 1972. Encapsulated methionine supplement for growing-finishing lambs. J. Anim. Sci. 34: 332.

Neudoerffer, T. S., D. B. Duncan and F. D. Horney. 1971. The extent of release of encapsulated methione in the intestine of cattle. Brit. J. Nutr. 25:333.

Nimrick, K., E. E. Hatfield, J. Kaminski and F. N. Owens. 1970. Qualitative assessment of supplemental amino acid needs for growing lambs feed urea as the sole nitrogen source. J. Nutr. 100:1293.

Nishimuta, J. F., D. G. Ely and J. A. Boling. 1973. Nitrogen metabolism in lambs fed soybean meal treated with heat, formalin and tannic acid. J. Nutr. 103:49.

Nishimuta, J. F., D. G. Ely and J. A. Boling. 1974. Ruminal by-pass of dietary soybean protein treated with heat, formalin and tannic acid. J. Anim. Sci. 39:952.

Ørskov, E. R. and D. Benzie. 1969. Using the oesophageal groove reflex in ruminants as a means of bypassing rumen fermenta-tion with high quality protein or nutrients. Brit. J. Nutr. 23:415.

Ørskov, E. R. and C. Fraser. 1969. The effect on nitrogen reten-tion in lambs of feeding protein supplements direct to the abomasum. Comparison of liquid and dry feeding and of various sources of protein. J. Agr. Sci. 73:469.

Ørskov, E. R., C. Fraser and E. L. Corse. 1970. The effect on protein utilization of feeding different protein supplements via the rumen or via the abomasum in young growing sheep. Brit. J. Nutr. 24:803.

Ørskov, E. R., C. Fraser and I. McDonald. 1971. Digestion of concentrates in sheep. 2. The effect of urea or fish-meal supplementation of barley diets on the apparent digestion of protein, fat, starch and ash in the rumen, the small intestine and the large intestine, and calculation of volatile fatty acid production. Brit. J. Nutr. 25:243.

Ørskov, E. R., C. Fraser, I. McDonald and R. I. Smart. 1974. Di-gestion of concentrates in sheep. 5. The effect of adding fish meal and urea together to cereal diets on protein diges-tion and utilization by young sheep. Brit. J. Nutr. 31:89.

Papas, A., G. A. B. Hall, E. E. Hatfield and F. N. Owens. 1974.

Responses of lambs to oral or abomasal supplementation of methionine hydroxyl analog or methionine. J. Nutr. 104:653.

Patton, R. A., R. D. McCarthy, L. G. Keske, L. C. Griel, Jr. and B.R. Baumgardt. 1970. Effect of feeding methionine hydroxy analog on the concentration of protozoa in the rumen of sheep. J. Dairy Sci. 53:933.

Peter, A. P., E. E. Hatfield, F. N. Owens and U. S. Garrigus. 1971. Effects of aldehyde treatments of soybean meal on in vitro ammonia release, solubility and lamb performance. J. Nutr. 101:605.

Preston, R. L. 1972. Source of supplemental protein and time of supplementation for growing-finishing steer calves. Proc. 27th Ann. Tex. Nutr. Conf. p. 127.

Preston, R. L. and C. K. Smith. 1974. Role of protein level, protected soybean protein, and roughage on the performance of new feeder calves. Ohio Agr. Res. Dev. Center Res. Sum. 77 p. 47.

Purser, D. B., and S. M. Buechler. 1966. Amino acid composition of rumen organisms. J. Dairy Sci. 49:81.

Rattray, P. V. and J. P. Joyce. 1970. Nitrogen retention and growth studies with young sheep using two sources of formalin-treated protein. New Zealand J. Agr. Res. 13:623.

Reis, P. J. 1970. The influence of abomasal supplements of some amino acids and sulphur-containing compounds on wool growth rate. Australian J. Biol. Sci. 23:441.

Reis, P. J. and W. F. Colebrook. 1972. The utilization of abomasal supplements of proteins and amino acids by sheep with special reference to wool growth. Australian J. Biol. Sci. 25:1057.

Reis, P. J. and P. G. Schinckel. 1964. The growth and composition of wool. II. The effect of casein, gelatin and sulphur-containing amino acids given per abomasum. Australian J. Biol. Sci. 17:532.

Reis, P. J. and D. A. Tunks. 1969. Evaluation of formaldehyde-treated casein for wool growth and nitrogen retention. Australian J. Agr. Res. 20:775.

Reis, P. J. and D. A. Tunks. 1970. Changes in plasma amino acid patterns in sheep associated with supplements of casein and formaldehyde-treated casein. Australian J. Biol. Sci. 23: 673.

Salsbury, R. L., D. K. Marvil, C. W. Woodmansee and G. F. W. Haenlein. 1971. Utilization of methionine and methionine hydroxy analog by rumen microorganisms in vitro. J. Dairy Sci. 54:390.

Satter, L. D. and R. E. Roffler. 1975. Nitrogen requirement and utilization in dairy cattle. J. Dairy Sci. 58: 1219.

Saville, D. G., A. C. Gleeson and W. R. McManus. 1971. Drought feeding of sheep. 2. Wool growth and body weight of three types of Merinos on oat based diets supplemented with formaldehyde treated cottonseed meal. Australian J. Exp. Agr. Anim. Husb. 11:488.

Schelling, G. T., J. E. Chandler and G. C. Scott. 1973. Post-ruminal supplemental methionine infusion to sheep fed high quality diets. J. Anim. Sci. 37:1034.

Schelling, G. T. and E. E. Hatfield. 1968. Effect of abomasally infused nitrogen sources on nitrogen retention of growing lambs. J. Nutr. 96:319.

Schelling, G. T., C. R. Richardson, R. E. Tucker and G. E. Mitchell, Jr. 1973. Lamb responses to dietary methionine and oxytetracycline. J. Anim. Sci. 37:356 (Abstr.).

Schelling, G. T., R. L. Stuart, R. E. Tucker and G. E. Mitchell, Jr. 1974. Addition of OTC to purified diets for lambs. J. Anim. Sci. 39:252 (Abstr.).

Schmidt, S. P., N. J. Benevenga and N. A. Jorgensen. 1973a. Effects of formaldehyde, glyoxal, or hexamethylenetetramine treatment of soybean meal on nitrogen utilization and growth in rats and in vitro rumen ammonia release. J. Anim. Sci. 37:1238.

Schmidt, S. P., N. A. Jorgensen, N. J. Benevenga and V. H. Brungardt. 1973b. Comparison of soybean meal, formaldehyde treated soybean meal, urea and starea for steers. J. Anim. Sci. 37:1233.

Schmidt, S. P., N. J. Benevenga and N. A. Jorgensen. 1974. Effect of formaldehyde treatment of soybean meal on the performance of growing steers and lambs. J. Anim. Sci. 38:646.

Schwab, C. G. 1974. Response of lactating cows to abomasal infusion of amino acids. Ph.D. Thesis. University of Wisconsin, Madison.

Scott, T. W., L. J. Cook and S. C. Mills. 1971. Protection of dietary polyunsaturated fatty acids against microbial hydrogenation in ruminants. J. Amer. Oil Chem. Soc. 48:358.

Sharkey, M. J., C. Kat and R. S. Jeffery. 1974. Some effects of formaldehyde treatment of barley/linseed meal diets on feed intake and growth rate of Friesian calves. Proc. Australian Soc. Anim. Prod. 10:82.

Sharkey, M. J., G. R. Pearce, E. K. Simmons, R. S. Jeffery and J. Clark. 1972. Some effects of formaldehyde treatment of hay on the production of Corriedale weaners fed in pens. Australian J. Exp. Agr. Anim. Husb. 12:596.

Sharma, H. R., J. R. Ingalls and J. A. McKirdy. 1972. Nutritive value of formaldehyde-treated rapeseed meal for dairy calves. Can. J. Anim. Sci. 52:363.

Sharma, H. R. and J. R. Ingalls. 1974. Effects of treating rapeseed meal and casein with formaldehyde on apparent digestibility and amino acid composition of rumen digesta and bacteria. Can. J. Anim. Sci. 54:157.

Sharma, H. R., J. R. Ingalls and R. J. Parker. 1974. Effects of treating rapeseed meal and casein with formaldehyde on the flow of nutrients through the gastrointestinal tract of fistulated Holstein steers. Can. J. Anim. Sci. 54:305.

Sherrod, L. B. and A. D. Tillman. 1962. Effects of varying the processing temperatures upon the nutritive values for sheep of solvent-extracted soybean and cottonseed meals. J. Anim. Sci. 21:901.

Sherrod, L. B. and A. D. Tillman. 1964. Further studies on the effects of different processing temperatures on the utilization of solvent-extracted cottonseed protein by sheep. J. Anim. Sci. 23:510.

Sibbald, I. R., T. C. Loughheed and J. H. Linton. 1968. A methionine supplement for ruminants. Proc. 2nd. World Conf. Anim. Prod. p. 453.

Smith, R. H. and A. B. McAllan. 1970. Nucleic acid metabolism in the ruminant. 2. Formation of microbial nucleic acids in the rumen in relation to the digestion of food nitrogen, and the fate of dietary nucleic acids. Brit. J. Nutr. 24:545.

Sniffen, C. J. 1974. Nitrogen utilization as related to solubility of NPN and protein in feeds. Proc. Cornell Nutr. Conf. p. 12.

Steinacker, G., T. J. Devlin and J. R. Ingalls. 1970. Effect of methionine supplementation posterior to the rumen on nitrogen utilization and sulfur balance of steers on a high roughage ration. Can. J. Anim. Sci. 50:319.

Synge, R. L. M. 1952. The utilization of herbage protein by animals. Brit. J. Nutr. 6:100.

Tagari, H., I. Ascarelli and A. Bondi. 1962. The influence of heating on the nutritive value of soya-bean meal for ruminants. Brit. J. Nutr. 16:237.

Tagari, H., Y. Henis, M. Tamir and R. Volcani. 1965. Effect of carob pod extract on cellulolysis, proteolysis, deamination, and protein biosynthesis in an artificial rumen. Appl. Microbiol. 13:437.

Topps, J. H., R. N. B. Kay, E. D. Goodall, F. G. Whitelaw and R. S. Reid. 1968. Digestion of concentrate and of hay diets in the stomach and intestines of ruminants. 2. Young steers. Brit. J. Nutr. 22:281.

Valentine, S. C. and D. C. Brown. 1973. Formaldehyde as a silage additive. II. The chemical composition and nutritive value of lucerne hay, lucerne silage, and formaldehyde and formic acid-treated lucerne silages. Australian J. Agr. Res. 24:939.

Van Buren, J. P. and W. B. Robinson. 1969. Formation of complexes between protein and tannic acid. J. Agr. Food Chem. 17:772.

Vik-Mo, L., R. S. Emery and J. T. Huber. 1974. Milk protein production in cows abomasally infused with casein or glucose. J. Dairy Sci. 57:869.

Virtanen, A. I. 1971. Protein requirements of dairy cattle--Artificial nitrogen sources and milk-production. Milchwissenschaft 26:129.

Wachira, J. D., L. D. Satter, G. P. Brooke and A. L. Pope. 1974. Evaluation of formaldehyde-treated protein for growing lambs and lactating cows. J. Anim. Sci. 39:796.

Waldo, D. R., J. E. Keys, Jr. and C. H. Gordon. 1973. Formaldehyde and formic acid as a silage additive. J. Dairy Sci. 56: 229.

Walker, J. F. 1964. Formaldehyde (3rd Ed.). Reinhold Publishing Co., New York.

Warner, A. C. I. 1956. Proteolysis by rumen micro-organisms. J. Gen. Microbiol. 14:749.

Weller, R. A. 1957. The amino acid composition of hydrolysates of microbial preparations from the rumen of sheep. Australian J. Biol. Sci. 10:384.

Whitelaw, F. G. and T. R. Preston. 1963. The nutrition of the early-weaned calf. III. Protein solubility and amino acid composition as factors affecting protein utilization. Anim. Prod. 5:131.

Whitelaw, F. G., T. R. Preston and G. S. Dawson. 1961. The nutrition of the early-weaned calf. II. A comparison of commercial groundnut meal, heat-treated groundnut meal and fish meal as the major protein source in the diet. Anim. Prod. 3:127.

Whitelaw, F. G., T. R. Preston and N. A. MacLeod. 1964. The nutrition of the early-weaned calf. VII. The relative value of different fish meal products as the major protein source in the diet. Anim. Prod. 6:25.

Williams, A. P. and R. H. Smith. 1974. Concentrations of amino acids and urea in the plasma of the ruminating calf and estimation of the amino acid requirements. Brit. J. Nutr. 32:421.

Williams, L. R., F. A. Martz and E. S. Hilderbrand. 1970. Feeding encapsulated methionine supplement to lactating cows. J. Dairy Sci. 53:1709.

Williams, V. J. and R. J. Moir. 1951. Ruminal flora studies in the sheep. III. The influence of different sources of nitrogen upon nitrogen retention and upon the total number of free microorganisms in the rumen. Australian J. Sci. Res., Ser. B, Biol. Sci. 4:377.

Wilson, G. F. 1970. The influence of protein supplements on milk yield and composition. Proc. New Zealand Soc. Anim. Prod. 30: 123.

Wohlt, J. E., C. J. Sniffen and W. H. Hoover. 1973. Measurements of protein solubility in common feedstuffs. J. Dairy Sci. 56: 1052.

Wright, D. E. 1967. Metabolism of peptides by rumen microorganisms. Appl. Microbiol. 15:547.

Wright, P. L. 1971. Body weight gain and wool growth response to formaldehyde treated casein and sulfur amino acids. J. Anim. Sci. 33:137.

11

NITROGEN METABOLISM IN RUMINANTS:
PROTEIN SOLUBILITY AND RUMEN BYPASS OF PROTEIN AND AMINO ACIDS

Jimmy H. Clark

Department of Dairy Science
University of Illinois
Urbana, Illinois

INTRODUCTION

Efficient feed utilization and maximum production of milk, meat, and wool by ruminant animals are obtained by feeding large quantities of properly balanced nutrients. Maximum performance of ruminant animals may be limited by a shortage of key nutrients rather than by genetic potential. The supply of a key nutrient may be limited by the appetite of the animal, by the physical capacity of the animal to consume feedstuffs, or by the inability of the rumen microbial system and/or tissues of the animal to generate sufficient quantities of precursors to form key nutrients. If ruminants are to be fed for maximum production, nutrients that may be limiting production must be identified and methods developed to supply these nutrients in times of greatest need.

Essential amino acids are key nutrients that are required by body tissue in adequate quantities and in balanced ratios if maximum animal performance and efficient feed utilization are to be achieved. In the past, it was assumed that when ruminants were fed protein to meet their stated requirements, all essential amino acids were provided in adequate quantities to support maximum production. This assumption was based on the fact that adding protein to the diet in excess of stated requirements did not generally improve ruminant animal performance.

Protein synthesis and gluconeogenesis place a great demand on the amino acid supply of ruminant animals, especially during stressful conditions such as high production. Therefore, even though diets containing the recommended quantity of protein are being fed, it is now recognized that the supply and pattern of amino acids reaching the absorption sites may be limiting production of milk, meat, and wool (Clark, 1975; Chalupa, 1975; Hogan, 1975).

The major source of amino acids passing to the absorption sites in the small intestine of ruminants is supplied by microbial protein synthesized in the rumen and dietary protein that escapes fermentation in the rumen. Approximately 20-60% of the dietary protein escapes fermentation in the rumen and passes intact to the lower gut (Hogan, 1975; Chalupa, 1975; Satter and Roffler, 1975). The amount and composition of dietary protein eaten, the quantity and composition of microbial protein synthesized in the rumen, the rate at which microbes pass from the rumen, and the amount and composition of dietary protein escaping microbial fermentation in the rumen determine the quantity and pattern of amino acids reaching the small intestine of ruminants. Great strides have been made in the past few years toward understanding microbial metabolism in the rumen and establishing nutrient requirements of high producing ruminant animals. Numerous reviews have been written regarding the regulation of microbial protein synthesis in the rumen (Hungate, 1966; Hogan and Weston, 1970; Thomas, 1973). The discussion to follow will center on factors affecting degradation of dietary protein in the rumen and rumen bypass of protein and amino acids.

FACTORS AFFECTING DEGRADATION OF PROTEIN IN THE RUMEN

The degradation of dietary protein in the rumen varies considerably (McDonald, 1954; McDonald and Hall, 1957; Ely et al., 1967; Little et al., 1968; Hume, 1970) and is largely dependent on the solubility of the protein in rumen fluid (Henderickx and Martin, 1963; Blackburn, 1965; Smith, 1969; McGilliard, 1972; Wohlt et al., 1973; Goering and Waldo, 1974a, b; Sniffen, 1974; Chalupa, in 1975), protein intake (Orskov et al., 1971), and rate of passage of digesta through the rumen. Animal performance may be greatly influenced by the quantity of protein degraded by microorganisms in the rumen.

Protein Solubility

Solubility of protein in a nontreated feedstuff is largely determined by the composition of protein classes present in the feedstuff. Albumins and globulins are the most soluble protein fractions of feedstuffs and prolamins and glutelins are the more insoluble protein fractions of feedstuffs (Sniffen, 1974). Feedstuffs composed largely of albumins and globulins are normally more soluble and of higher quality than feedstuffs composed primarily of prolamins and glutelins (Wohlt et al., 1973). The maturity of plants at harvest affects the type of protein present in the total plant and this influences solubility of the plant protein (Waldo, 1968). As forages increase in maturity, the protein fractions, albumin, globulin, prolamin, and glutelin decrease and the nonprotein nitrogen (NPN) content increases. Therefore, the soluble nitrogen content of forage is greatest at maturity. The opposite is true for the cereal grains. Immature high moisture corn contains more soluble nitrogen than the corresponding mature dry corn (Jones, 1973). This is largely due to the conversion of NPN to protein during the maturation process in corn. The variation in protein solubility can range from 2.8 to 93.2% (Table 1) because of the ratio of protein fractions composing the total protein in the feedstuff. Casein, the major milk protein, is very soluble and is almost completely degraded when incubated in rumen contents (Pearson and Smith, 1943; Chalmers et al., 1954; Wohlt et al., 1973). Furthermore, it has been demonstrated that casein has only a 5.6-21.5 minute half-life in the rumen (Mangan, 1972). However, zein, a corn protein, is very insoluble and 40-60% of this

263

TABLE 1

Soluble Nitrogen Content of Feedstuffs[a]

Energy feeds	Soluble nitrogen %	Protein supplements	Soluble nitrogen %
Rye	41.3	Dried milk	93.2
Wheat bran	34.3	Linseed meal	50.8
Wheat	29.7	Dried whey	41.4
Oats	25.8	Alfalfa meal	22.9
Citrus pulp	25.7	Meat & bone meal	16.4
Barley	16.8	Soybean meal	13.0
Corn meal	12.0	Cottonseed meal	7.2
Beet pulp	3.9	Milo gluten	2.8

[a]Adapted from Wohlt et al. (1973).

protein escapes breakdown in the rumen (McDonald, 1954; Ely et al., 1967).

Feeding ruminants high quality protein that is highly soluble in the rumen may not be advantageous. Nonprotected feedstuffs have been blended together to provide diets varying in protein solubility. As the solubility of the protein in the diet decreased, protein degradation in the rumen and urinary nitrogen excretion decreased, and nitrogen retention increased in sheep and growing cattle (Wohlt, 1973; Sniffen, 1974). Nitrogen retention of ewes fed a low plane of nutrition was not improved by feeding a casein supplement (Cuthbertson and Chalmers, 1950), but supplying the casein postruminally improved nitrogen utilization (Chalmers et al., 1954). The amino acid composition of the soluble protein may be altered greatly during rumen fermentation and may be of no more value to the animal than NPN or a lower quality protein. In fact, a somewhat poorer quality protein with a lower solubility may be of more benefit to ruminants, if the microbial requirement for nitrogen is adequate, because of the complementary amino acids the dietary protein supplies to microbial protein in the small intestine (Hatfield, 1970). Feeding high quality protein to ruminants is beneficial only if it improves the pattern and quantity of amino acids reaching the absorption sites.

Many feed processing methods either require or generate heat which affects protein solubility. Heat treatment has been shown to substantially decrease solubility of proteins (Chalmers et al., 1954; Danke et al., 1966; Tagari et al., 1962; Little et al., 1963; Glimp et al., 1967; Hudson et al., 1970). Reducing solubility of the dietary protein has decreased degradation of protein in the rumen resulting in increased weight gain, nitrogen retention, and feed efficiency (Chalmers et al., 1954; Whitelaw et al., 1961; Tagari et al., 1962; Sherrod and Tillman, 1962, 1964; Danke et al., 1966; Glimp et al., 1967; Nishimuta et al., 1973; Goering and Waldo, 1974a, b). Because more dietary protein escapes rumen fermentation after heat treatment (Hudson et al., 1970), nitrogen retention can be increased even though nitrogen digestibility is slightly depressed (Goering and Waldo, 1974b). However, protein can be overheated resulting in a lower digestibility of the protein and poorer animal performance (Goering and Waldo, 1974a, b).

Harvesting procedures and storage conditions can greatly affect the solubility of protein in hay-crop-silage. Wilting hay-crop-silage before ensiling reduces the protein solubility of the forage and animal performance is directly related to the insoluble protein content of the forage if the forage is not overwilted (Goering and Waldo, 1974a; Waldo et al., 1973a, b). The protein in forages can be overheated resulting in poorer animal performance. This is due to the Maillard reaction between the aldehyde groups of sugars and the free amino groups of proteins. Through this reaction, the protein may be bound to the indigestible carbohydrate fraction of the plant, making it extremely insoluble and nondigestible. Temperature, length of heat treatment, and moisture content of the forage are closely related to overheating of protein in forages (Goering et al., 1973), but the protein is seldom damaged if moisture is evaporating when heat is applied. Storing wilted hay crops under conditions in which they overheat has caused a decrease in protein solubility and digestibility, which resulted in less efficient nitrogen utilization (Hill and Noller, 1963; Mohanty et al., 1969; Roffler et al., 1967; Pierson et al., 1971; Goering et al., 1972).

Altering rumen pH may decrease degradation of protein in the rumen and increase the quantity of dietary protein bypassing rumen fermentation resulting in a more efficient utilization of nitrogen. Proteins are least soluble at their isoelectric pH because at this pH the protein molecule has no net charge and, thus, no electrostatic repulsions exist between neighboring protein molecules. Since the pH of the rumen is normally 6.0-7.0, proteins with isoelectric pH's in this range may be very insoluble in rumen fluid. Determining the isoelectric pH of most feed proteins is difficult because feeds contain a mixture of proteins. However, it has indeed been demonstrated that pH alters the solubility of various proteins in in vitro rumen fluid incubations (Isaacs and Owens, 1972; Wohlt et al., 1973), and this suggests that pH of the rumen may affect the quantity of dietary protein that bypasses rumen fermentation.

Rate of Passage Through the Rumen

The quantity of protein that bypasses fermentation is somewhat dependent on factors that regulate the rate of flow of feed ingredients through the rumen since a shorter retention time in the rumen allows less time for microbial fermentation. Reducing particle size of the diet or increasing dietary feed intake, frequency of feeding, and rate of ruminal degradation will increase the rate of passage of digesta through the rumen (Balch and Campling, 1965). Frequent feeding (Beever et al., 1972) and increased protein intake (Orskov et al., 1971) have increased the quantity of nitrogen reaching the lower gut of ruminants. Feeding diets containing large quantities of salt resulted in increased water intake, which increased the rate of passage of digesta through the rumen in the study conducted by Hemsley (1967). Feeding a diet containing 20% salt resulted in a two-fold increase in wool growth of sheep (Ferguson, 1971, as cited by Chalupa, 1975).

Numerous processing procedures which alter the physical form of the diet and site of starch digestibility also affect nitrogen utilization by regulating microbial protein synthesis in the rumen (Waldo, 1973). Microbial protein synthesis in the rumen was decreased 8-23 g for each 100 g of starch that escaped ruminal degradation. Reconstitution and steam flaking of sorghum grain increases microbial degradation of protein in the rumen and increases the biological value of the protein, but micronizing has the opposite effect (Potter et al., 1971).

The amino acid composition of the protein determines to a great extent the beneficial effects of protecting protein from ruminal degradation. Destruction of high quality protein in the rumen is a wasteful process for the ruminant animal because the ammonia released in the rumen is in excess of the quantity that can be efficiently incorporated into microbial protein. Degradation of low quality protein in the rumen may or may not be beneficial to the host animal. It is beneficial only if it improves the quality of protein in postruminal digesta without altering significantly the supply of protein to the lower gut.

BENEFICIAL EFFECTS OF RUMEN BYPASS
WITH HIGH QUALITY PROTEIN OR AMINO ACIDS

Supplementing diets fed to meet stated protein requirements with additional nonprotected protein or amino acids has not consistently improved animal performance (Nelson, 1970) because the additional protein and amino acids are rapidly degraded by the microorganisms in the rumen. Therefore, postruminal infusion of proteins and/or amino acids has become the method most often used for evaluating the amino acid nutrition of ruminants. Numerous studies indicate that casein or amino acids infused into the abomasum improves performance of high producing ruminant animals fed a variety of diets. This suggests that one or more amino acids may be limiting production of milk, meat, and wool in the high producing ruminant animal (Clark, 1975; Chalupa, 1975).

Milk Yield

The milk yield of dairy cows has been increased 1-4 kg per day when casein was infused into the abomasum and compared to control cows receiving solutions of water, saline, or isonitrogenous, isocaloric mixtures of urea, monosodium glutamate, and glucose, or an equal quantity of casein in the rumen (Table 2) even though the cows were fed to meet their stated requirements for protein and energy (NRC, 1971). These studies show that cows producing the largest quantities of milk were those that responded with the greatest increase in milk yield when casein was administered postruminally. Only two studies with lactating dairy cows have failed to show a positive response in milk yield when casein was infused to bypass rumen fermentation. The lack of response in these studies was probably due to low production (Hale and Jacobson, 1972) and fluctuations in feed intake (Vik-Mo et al., 1974).

Although milk production has been increased when supplemental casein was given per abomasum, the response obtained when one or more essential amino acids was infused into the absomasum has not always given positive responses (Clark, 1975; Nelson, 1970). The infusion of one or more essential amino acids into the abomasum of lactating cows increased the milk yield of some cows, but the results were not significant (Schwab and Satter, 1973, 1974) (Table 3). Methionine, histidine, or lysine infused intravenously did not increase milk production in the cow (Fisher, 1969, 1972; Teichman et al., 1969). When lactating goats were used as experimental animals and histidine, arginine, and a mixture of nonessential amino acids were infused into the carotid artery milk production did not increase (Mepham and Linzell, 1974). In a second study, the milk yield of only one of three experimental goats increased when tyrosine, glutamic acid, and a mixture of essential amino acids were infused into the carotid artery (Linzell and Mepham, 1974). Thus, casein but not amino acids has consistently improved the milk yield of lactating ruminant animals.

268

RUMEN BYPASS OF PROTEIN AND AMINO ACIDS

Milk Protein Production

In addition to increasing the yield of milk, postruminal infusion of casein also has increased the crude protein content of
the milk. The yield of milk protein was increased by 10-15% (Table
2). As was observed for milk production the largest increase in
milk protein yield was obtained in the high producing cow. Vik-Mo
et al. (1974) indicated that the additional milk protein (N x 6.38),
produced as a result of the abomasal infusion of casein, contained
both true protein and NPN. However, it has recently been shown
that the largest increase in the additional milk protein (N x 6.38)
produced as a result of postruminal infusion is the casein fraction
(Vik-Mo et al., 1974; Blaisdell and Clark, unpublished data). Data
from these trials suggest that the true protein production of cows
fed normal diets can be increased 10-15%, depending on the level
of production. The yield of other milk components has not been
significantly influenced by abomasal supplementation of casein or
crystalline amino acids (Clark, 1975).

Infusing crystalline essential amino acids into the abomasum
also has increased both the protein content of milk and the yield
of milk protein (Schwab and Satter, 1974; Blaisdell and Clark, unpublished data) (Table 3), but these parameters are normally increased more when casein is administered postruminally. Results
of infusion trials suggest that lysine and methionine were the
amino acids in shortest supply for milk protein synthesis (Schwab
and Satter, 1974). Intravenous infusion of 11 g per day of methionine increased milk protein yield, but the infusion of histidine or
larger quantities of methionine slightly depressed milk protein
synthesis while lysine infusion did not significantly affect milk
protein yield (Fisher, 1972). Milk protein production was increased
in only one of three lactating goats by infusing essential amino
acids into the carotid artery (Linzell and Mepham, 1974). An additional supply of arginine, histidine, and nonessential amino acids
given by arterial infusion did not increase milk protein yield in
goats (Mepham and Linzell, 1974).

TABLE 2

Daily Milk and Milk Protein Yield
of Cows Infused Postruminally with Casein

Diet	Crude protein in diet (%)	Infusate	Quantity infused (g/day)	Total nitrogen supplied by infusate (%)
Concentrate, alfalfa-grass hay	16.5	Na-caseinate	440	12.6
Concentrate, alfalfa-grass hay	15.0	Na-caseinate	400	12.0
Concentrate, alfalfa-grass hay	17.0 17.0	Na-caseinate Na-caseinate + glucose	422 422 422	10.0 10.1
Concentrate, corn silage (urea added), legume-grass hay	16.0	Na-caseinate + met	770-880	16.1
Concentrate, corn silage, hay	16.4	Casein	300	12.8
Concentrate, corn silage, hay	15.0 15.0	Casein + met Casein + met + glucose	450-525 300 300	19.6 12.5
Concentrate, corn silage (urea added), hay	16.1	Na-caseinate + met	350-450	22.0
----------------	--	Casein	860	--
Concentrate, corn silage (urea added)	--	Casein Casein	-- --	-- --
Concentrate (urea added), straw	17.0 17.0 17.0	Na-caseinate Na-caseinate Na-caseinate	170 540 910	8.2 18.8 26.6

[a] $P < 0.10$.
[b] $P < 0.05$.
[c] $P < 0.01$.

TABLE 2 (continued)

Milk yield		Milk protein (N x 6.38) yield		Reference
Control	Treatment	Control	Treatment	
(kg/day)		(g/day)		
23.3	24.6[c]	719	797[c]	Derrig et al. (1974)
32.5	34.1[b]	929	1061[b]	Spires et al. (1973)
28.8	31.0[a]	963	1072[b]	Clark et al. (1973)
28.8	31.6[a]	963	1104[b]	
30.4	32.0	950	1060[b]	Broderick et al. (1970)
15.2	16.2[b]	549	597[b]	Vik-Mo et al. (1974)
24.3	26.0[a]	697	788[b]	Vik-Mo et al. (1974)
24.5	25.6[a]	669	773[b]	
12.9	13.3	413	463[b]	Vik-Mo et al. (1974)
24.0	27.0	--	--	Tyrrell et al. (1972)
14.0	14.4	357	386[c]	Hale et al. (1972)
13.8	15.6[c]	361	418	
19.5	23.7	450	590	Spechter (1972)
24.8	28.7	785	910	
29.6	32.5	810	990	

TABLE 3

Daily Milk and Milk Protein Yield
of Cows Infused Postruminally with Amino Acids

Diet	Crude protein in diet (%)	Infusate
Concentrate, corn silage (urea added)	--	DL-Met
	--	DL-Met
	--	L-His
	--	L-His
	--	L-Lys
	--	L-Lys
Concentrate, mixed grass hay	11-12	Met, Lys, Val, Ile, Leu, His, Thr, Phe, Arg, Trp
	11-12	Met, Lys, Val, Ile, Leu, His, Thr, Phe
	11-12	Met, Lys, Val, Ile, Leu, His
	11-12	Met, Lys, Val, Ile
	11-12	Met, Lys, Val
	11-12	Met, Lys
	11-12	Met
Concentrate, hay	10.8	Na-caseinate
	10.8	Met, Val, Lys, Ile, Leu Phe, Thr, His
	10.8	Met, Val, Lys, Ile, Leu
Concentrate, hay	10.8	Na-caseinate
	10.8	Met, Lys, Val, Ile, Phe
	10.8	Met, Lys, Val
	10.8	Met, Lys

TABLE 3 (continued)

Milk yield		Milk protein (N x 6.38) yield		Reference
Control	Treatment	Control	Treatment	
(kg/day)		(g/day)		
16.1	16.6	490	520	Fisher (1972)
16.1	14.8	490	486	
15.8	15.9	505	484	
15.8	16.2	505	493	
15.3	16.2	481	519	
15.3	15.8	481	507	
23.0	24.8	--	--	Schwab and Satter (1973)
23.0	25.2	--	--	
23.0	24.3	--	--	
23.0	23.3	--	--	
23.0	24.0	--	--	
23.0	23.0	--	--	
23.0	23.0	--	--	
29.1	30.8	793	892	Schwab and Satter (1974)
29.1	29.4	793	876	
29.1	29.8	793	853	
27.2	27.7	761	835	Schwab and Satter (1974)
27.2	27.0	761	807	
27.2	26.4	761	794	
27.2	27.1	761	803	

Data collected using numerous methods have been interpreted
to suggest that one of five amino acids may be first limiting for
milk protein synthesis (Clark, 1975). Most data suggest phenylalanine, methionine, lysine, threonine, and histidine as being in
most critical supply, but the order of limitation has not been
established. Tryptophan also is an essential amino acid that could
be in short supply and the availability of this amino acid has not
been extensively studied. Additional studies are needed to determine if rumen bypass of crystalline amino acids will increase the
milk and milk protein yield of lactating ruminants.

Nitrogen Retention, Body Weight Gain, and Wool Growth

Postruminal infusion of casein, casein hydrolysate, or a mixture of essential amino acids has consistently increased the nitrogen retention of growing steers (Chalupa et al., 1972, 1973; Chalupa
and Chandler, 1972; Chalupa, 1974) (Table 4). Similar observations
were made for lactating cows (Clark et al., 1973; Derrig et al.,
1974). The increased nitrogen balance has been associated with an
increase in nitrogen absorption and a decrease in urinary nitrogen
excretion when expressed as a percentage of nitrogen intake or
nitrogen absorbed. Therefore, the casein supplementation per
abomasum must improve both the supply and the pattern of amino
acids available for protein synthesis resulting in improved efficiency of utilization of absorbed nitrogen.

The response to postruminal supplementation of amino acids
either singly or in mixtures has been variable and has not specifically identified the most limiting amino acid for rapidly growing
cattle. The fact that the most limiting amino acid for growing
cattle and lactating cows has not been established may be due to
each amino acid giving a small response and this small response in
the animal system is not detectable until the total response from
several amino acids is added together. The continuous abomasal infusion of branched-chain amino acids plus phenylalanine into the
abomasum of urea-fed steers increased nitrogen retention similar

274

TABLE 4

Nitrogen Utilization by Growing Cattle Infused Abomasally With Essential Amino Acids[a]

Trial No.	Infusate	N-intake		Nitrogen utilization (g/day)			
		Fed	Infused	Absorbed	Fecal	Urine	Retained
1	Control (water infusion)	70.8	0	40.4[b]	30.4	21.2[b]	19.2[b]
	Thr, Val, Met, Ile, Leu, Phe, Lys, His, Arg	71.6	7.2	49.0[b,c]	29.8	24.1[b]	24.8[b,c]
	Thr, Val, Met, Ile, Leu, Phe, Lys, His, Arg	71.2	14.4	55.4[c,d]	30.2	26.4[b]	28.9[c,d]
	Thr, Val, Met, Ile, Leu, Phe, Lys, His, Arg	70.7	28.7	68.4[d]	31.0	32.6[c]	35.6[d]
2	Control[e]	75.3	0	50.4	24.9	41.7[b]	8.7[b]
	Thr, Val, Met, Ile, Leu, Phe, Trp, Lys, His, Arg, and 13.0 g glucose	58.6	13.4	45.6	26.4	30.0[c]	15.6[c]
3	Control (water)	102.3	0	58.2[b]	44.1	41.0[b]	17.2[b]
	Glucose	102.3	0	58.0[b]	44.3	38.1[b]	19.8[b,c]
	Thr, Val, Met, Ile, Leu, Phe, Trp, Lys, His, Arg	102.3	14.6	73.6[c]	43.5	48.7[c]	24.9[c]
	Thr, Val, Met, Ile, Leu, Phe, Trp, Lys, His, Arg, and 100 g glucose	101.6	14.1	70.9[c]	44.8	49.3[c]	21.5[b,c]

[a]Adapted from Chalupa (1974).

[b,c,d]Means within a given trial bearing common superscripts are not significantly different (P < 0.05).

[e]Fed same quantity of amino acids and glucose as was infused.

to the nitrogen retention of soy-fed control animals (Oltjen et al., 1970). Threonine, histidine, and lysine were suggested to be responsible for the largest increases in nitrogen balance when a mixture of essential amino acids was infused into the abomasum of growing steers fed a 10.5% crude protein diet (Chalupa et al., 1973) and positive but not always significant increases in nitrogen balance have been obtained when a combination of methionine and lysine were postruminally supplemented (W. Chalupa, personal communication). Beneficial responses have been obtained by infusing lysine into the abomasum of steers (Devlin and Woods, 1964; Burris et al., 1974), but the responses have not always been consistent (Devlin and Woods, 1965 ; Boila and Devlin, 1972).

Nitrogen and energy retention and body weight gain of growing lambs were increased about two-fold by infusing a complete liquid diet into the abomasum versus into the rumen (Table 5). This resulted in significantly more of the retained nitrogen and energy being stored in the marketable carcass (Black and Tribe, 1973). Other studies have demonstrated that casein administered into the abomasum or duodenum will increase the retention of nitrogen by sheep (Cuthbertson and Chalmers, 1950; Chalmers et al., 1954; Reis and Schinckel, 1961; Schelling and Hatfield, 1968; Egan, 1970; Johnson, 1972b; Papas et al., 1974b). Little and Mitchell (1967) also indicated that the retention of nitrogen in sheep was increased when casein or soybean meal was administered into the abomasum, but nitrogen balance was not increased when zein or gelatin were given, indicating the importance of the amino acid composition of the protein infused.

Black et al. (1973) demonstrated by infusing the whole diet, containing graded levels of protein and energy, into the abomasum of lambs that the rate of wool growth can be influenced by the quantities of protein and energy supplied to the lower gut. These data suggest there is an optimum ratio of protein to energy required for maximum nitrogen retention, wool growth, and body weight gain. Wool growth (Reis and Schinckel, 1961; Reis, 1969; Egan, 1970;

TABLE 5

Weight Gain, Wool Growth, Nitrogen Retention, and Energy Retention of Lambs Receiving a Liquid Diet in the Rumen versus the Abomasum[a]

Parameter	Site of infusion	
	Rumen	Abomasum
Nitrogen intake (g/day)	14.41	14.87
Nitrogen retained (g/day)	1.68	3.50[d]
Energy intake (MJ/day)	10.02	10.34
Energy retained (MJ/day)	1.39	3.21[d]
Weight gain (g/day)		
Bodyweight	72	126[d]
Empty bodyweight	45	131[d]
Wool growth (g/day)	3.68	5.34[d]
Nitrogen distribution in body tissue (%)		
Carcass	29	45[d]
Viscera	2.6	7.6[c]
Blood, head and hooves, skin	26	28
Wool	37	24[b]
Energy distribution in body tissue (%)		
Carcass	65	73[d]
Viscera	16	14
Blood, head and hooves, skin	9	8
Wool	10	5[c]

[a]Adapted from Black and Tribe (1973).
[b]$p < 0.05$.
[c]$p < 0.01$.
[d]$p < 0.001$.

Reis and Downes, 1971) and body weight gain (Reis, 1969; Papas et al., 1974b) have increased consistently when casein was infused per abomasum, indicating a deficiency of amino acids at the absorption sites of sheep. All proteins do not stimulate wool growth as effectively as does casein (Reis and Schinckel, 1964; Colebrook and Reis, 1969; Reis and Colebrook, 1972) and casein produces a larger response than amino acids. However, wool growth is stimulated by postruminally infusing sulfur-containing amino acids (Reis and Schinckel, 1963; Reis, 1970; Williams et al., 1972; Bird and Moir, 1972; Reis et al., 1973). Methionine has been indicated as the most limiting essential amino acid for sheep fed natural diets (Schelling et al., 1973a) or purified diets containing urea as the only source of nitrogen (Nimrick et al., 1970a, b). Data of Nimrick et al. (1970a, b) suggested lysine and threonine may be the second and third most limiting amino acids when lambs are fed a urea purified diet.

MODE OF RESPONSE FROM THE INFUSION OF HIGH QUALITY PROTEIN

The improved performance of ruminant animals resulting from postruminal infusion of high quality protein may be elicited by supplying limiting amino acids, by supplying carbon for gluconeogenesis, by altering the endocrine status of the animal, or by a combination of these factors (Clark, 1975). Earlier discussion in this review has suggested that the quantity or pattern of amino acids reaching the absorption sites was directly responsible for the improved animal production. The increased wool growth obtained when sheep were postruminally infused with sulfur-containing amino acids is the best example of a response obtained from limiting amino acids for ruminants.

The energy of casein was used more efficiently when given in the abomasum compared to administration into the rumen (Blaxter and Martin, 1962; Hedde et al., 1974). Energy losses resulting from microbial fermentation in the rumen and nitrogen losses associated with the conversion of dietary protein to microbial protein are eliminated when nutrients are digested postruminally (Black, 1971).

RUMEN BYPASS OF PROTEIN AND AMINO ACIDS

This may be the reason for the increased efficiency of energy and nitrogen utilization which results in greater animal production. Lactating ruminants require large quantities of glucose for lactose synthesis and glucose also is used for other functions by ruminant animals. Little glucose is absorbed from the digestive tract because of microbial fermentation of carbohydrates to volatile fatty acids in the rumen. Thus, the ruminant must synthesize large quantities of glucose from propionate and amino acids. Infusing casein into the abomasum increases the supply of amino acids absorbed and it has been demonstrated that the glucose entry rate of ruminants was increased when casein was administered postruminally (Lindsay and Williams, 1971; Judson and Leng, 1973; Lindsay and Dyke, 1974; Clark et al., unpublished data). Therefore, the increased availability of glucose may be the cause of the improved animal performance (Clark, 1975).

Administration of bovine growth hormone has increased milk production (Hutton, 1957; Machlin, 1973) and plasma insulin concentrations are closely related to the amount of protein digested in the lower gut of ruminants (Bassett et al., 1971). Arginine or casein hydrolysate administered into ruminants has increased the plasma concentrations of growth hormone and insulin in cattle, sheep, and goats (Hertelendy et al., 1969, 1970; McAtee and Trenkle, 1971; Stern et al., 1971). Therefore, the responses obtained from abomasal supplementation of high quality protein may be elicited through an altered endocrine status.

Protein administered into the abomasum has increased feed intake in animals fed diets thought to be adequate in protein content (Orskov et al., 1973; Papas et al., 1974b) and this may contribute to the beneficial response obtained in some studies. The increase in feed intake as a result of administering additional protein to the lower gut may be attributed to an improved amino acid status of the animal because recycling of nitrogen across the rumen wall and in saliva to the rumen as a result of abomasal infusion of urea did not give a similar response (Orskov et al., 1973). The causal mechanisms for reported increased feed intake are not fully understood.

279

METHODS USED TO PROTECT PROTEINS AND/OR
AMINO ACIDS FROM DEGRADATION IN THE RUMEN

Because of the beneficial responses that have been obtained when protein and amino acids were infused into the abomasum of ruminants, methods of protecting these nutrients from microbial degradation in the rumen are being investigated. The effects of heating on protection of protein has been discussed earlier in this chapter. Other procedures being studied include: chemical treatment, amino acid analogs, encapsulation of amino acids, alteration of rumen metabolism, and esophageal groove closure. For these techniques to be successful, they must protect the protein or amino acid from destruction in the rumen and allow enzymatic digestion and absorption in the abomasum and small intestine.

Chemical Treatment

Chemical treatment of protein decreases solubility and microbial degradation in the rumen by cross-linking peptide chains and tightly binding the protein under alkaline and neutral conditions. However, as the pH changes from about 5.5-7.0 in the rumen to 3.0 or less in the abomasum, these bonds are weakened and the protein can be degraded by enzymatic digestion. Numerous chemicals including aldehydes, tannins (Hatfield, 1973), phosphonitrilic halides, polymerized unsaturated carboxylic acids, halo-triazines, sulfonyl halides, acrolein acetals, hexamethylenetetramine, and acetylenic esters (Chalupa, 1975). have been used as protective agents, but more work has been conducted with formaldehyde than with the other chemicals (Table 6).

Feeding formaldehyde-treated casein has increased wool growth, nitrogen retention, and body weight gain in sheep (Ferguson et al., 1967; Reis and Tunks, 1969; Faichney, 1971; Wright, 1971; Hughes and Williams, 1971; MacRae et al., 1972; Barry, 1970, 1972; Hemsley et al., 1973). Feeding formaldehyde-treated casein or soybean meal has not improved milk or milk protein yield compared to feeding a nontreated protein (Wilson, 1970; Clark et al., 1974; Wachira et al., 1974; Kellaway et al., 1974).

RUMEN BYPASS OF PROTEIN AND AMINO ACIDS

Formaldehyde has been used to protect supplemental dietary proteins that were fed to ruminants (Rattray and Joyce, 1970; Nimrick et al., 1972; Peter et al., 1971; Schmidt et al., 1973b, 1974; Amos et al., 1974; Faichney and Davies, 1972, 1973; Faichney, 1972; Sharma et al., 1972, 1974; Sharma and Ingalls, 1973, 1974; Dinius et al., 1974; Clark et al., 1974; Wachira et al., 1974) and, although results have been inconsistent, positive responses have been obtained (Rattray and Joyce, 1970; Nimrick et al., 1972; Peter et al., 1971). Treating forages with formaldehyde and/or formic acid at the time of ensiling sometimes has increased dry matter intake (Waldo et al., 1969, 1973b; Valentine and Brown, 1973), animal weight gain (Waldo et al., 1971, 1973a, b), and wool growth (Valentine and Brown, 1973) but not always (Brown and Valentine, 1972; Barker et al., 1973). Differences in performance are probably associated with type of forage and level of chemical treatment. When increased animal performance is obtained, it is probably related to reduced microbial breakdown of the dietary protein in the rumen. However, formaldehyde, because of its bacteriostatic properties, reduces proteolysis during storage (Waldo et al., 1973b) and may increase the protein value of the silage.

Apparent digestibility of formaldehyde-treated protein by ruminants is reduced if excessive quantitities of formaldehyde are applied to the protein (Faichney, 1971; Faichney and Davies, 1972; Miller, 1972; Nishimuta et al., 1973; Clark et al., 1974) and the digestibility of plant protein is generally reduced more than casein (Chalupa, 1975). Other studies (Faichney and Weston, 1971; MacRae et al., 1972) have shown that formaldehyde treatment of casein decreased total nitrogen digestibility, but significantly increased the amount of nonammonia nitrogen entering the intestine and the quantity of nitrogen apparently absorbed. A comparison of digestibility of formaldehyde-treated casein fed in the diet and untreated casein infused into the abomasum indicated the infused casein was 6-8% more digestible (Reis and Tunks, 1969). In other studies (Faichney, 1971, 1974; MacRae et al., 1972), urinary nitrogen excretion was reduced and nitrogen retention was increased, even though nitrogen digestibility was somewhat reduced when formaldehyde-treated casein was fed to sheep.

TABLE 6

Effect of Feeding Chemically Treated Protein on Nitrogen Utilization and Animal Performance

Protein treated	Chemical applied	Quantity applied (g/100g)	Animal	Nitrogen utilization			Weight gain (kg/day)	Wool growth (% of un- treated)	Milk yield (kg/day)	Reference
				Feces	Urine	Retained				
				(% of nitrogen intake)						
Casein										
Untreated	--	0	Sheep	16	82	2[a]	--	100[a]	--	Reis & Tunks (1969)
Treated	Formaldehyde	40	Sheep	19	71	10[b]	--	162[b]	--	
Untreated in abomasum	--	0	Sheep	15	76	9[b]	--	162[b]	--	
Casein										
Untreated	--	0	Sheep	24	61	15	0.154[a]	100	--	Faichney (1971)
Treated	Formaldehyde	1.5	Sheep	29	53	18	0.166[b]	97	--	
Linseed meal										
Untreated	--	0	Sheep	31	60	9[a]	--	100	--	Rattray & Joyce (1970)
Treated	Formaldehyde	1.3-2.0	Sheep	33	48	19[b]	--	92	--	

Meat meal										
Untreated	--	0	Sheep	24ᵃ	56ᵃ	20ᵃ	--	100	--	Rattray & Joyce (1970)
Treated	Formaldehyde	1.3-2.0	Sheep	44ᵇ	45ᵇ	11ᵇ	--	96	--	
Sunflower meal										
Untreated	--	0	Sheep	35	31ᵃ	34	--	--	--	Amos et al. (1974)
Treated	Formaldehyde	1.33	Sheep	40	23ᵇ	37	--	--	--	
Treated	Formaldehyde	2.66	Sheep	44	25ᵇ	32	--	--	--	
Treated	Formaldehyde	3.99	Sheep	42	24ᵇ	34	--	--	--	
Alfalfa silage										
Untreated	--	0	Sheep	30ᵃ	--	--	--	100ᵃ	--	Valentine & Brown (1973)
Treated	Formaldehyde	1.0	Sheep	38ᵇ	--	--	--	139ᵇ	--	
Fish meal										
Untreated	--	0	Sheep	34ᵃ	44ᵃ	22ᵃ	--	--	--	Nimrick et al. (1972)
Treated	Glyoxal	3.75	Sheep	40ᵇ	32ᵇ	27ᵇ	--	--	--	

TABLE 6 (continued)

Protein treated	Chemical applied	Quantity applied (g/100g)	Animal	Nitrogen utilization Feces (% of nitrogen intake)	Urine	Retained	Weight gain (kg/day)	Wool growth (% of un-treated)	Milk yield (kg/day)	Reference
Soybean meal										
Untreated	--	0	Sheep	25	55	21	--	--	--	Nishimuta et al. (1973)
Treated	Formalin	1.0	Sheep	54	29	17	--	--	--	
Treated	Tannic acid	9.0	Sheep	32	44	24	--	--	--	
Soybean meal										
Untreated	--	0	Sheep	29	38	34[a]	0.177[a]	--	--	Driedger & Hatfield (1972)
Treated	Tannic acid	10.0	Sheep	28	33	38[b]	0.217[b]	--	--	
Soybean meal										
Untreated	--	0	Sheep	--	--	--	0.246[a]	100	--	Peter et al. (1971)
Treated	Formaldehyde	0.6	Sheep	--	--	--	0.290[b]	117	--	
Treated	Glyoxal	1.5	Sheep	--	--	--	0.280[b]	97	--	

Soybean meal										
Untreated	--	0	Cattle	36	29	35	1.31^a	--	--	Schmidt et al. (1974)
Treated	Formaldehyde	1.5	Cattle	38	29	33	$1.27^{a,b}$	--	--	
Treated	Formaldehyde	3.0	Cattle	38	28	33	1.20^b	--	--	
Peanut meal										
Untreated	--	0	Cattle	20	--	--	0.734	--	--	Faichney & Davies (1972)
Treated	Formaldehyde	0.5	Cattle	27	--	--	0.737	--	--	
Soybean meal										
Untreated	--	0	Cattle	36^a	27^a	37^a	--	--	17.2	Clark et al. (1974)
Treated	Formaldehyde	0.9	Cattle	43^b	22^b	35^b	--	--	17.1	
Soybean meal										
Untreated	--	0	Cattle	--	--	--	--	--	21.3	Wachira et al. (1974)
Treated	Formaldehyde	3.2	Cattle	--	--	--	--	--	20.5	
Total concentrate										
Untreated	--	0	Cattle	--	--	--	--	--	21.0	Wachira et al. (1974)
Treated	Formaldehyde	0.5	Cattle	--	--	--	--	--	21.0	

[a,b] Means within a given trial bearing common superscripts are not significantly different (P < 0.05).

Although casein has been successfully protected resulting in improved animal performance, protecting plant proteins by formaldehyde treatment may be difficult to achieve without altering microbial protein synthesis or intestinal digestion and absorption. Numerous investigations conducted to determine the optimum level of formaldehyde treatment of soybean meal for improving animal performance have shown only limited success (Schmidt et al., 1973a, b, 1974; Wachira et al., 1974). However, additional studies using more refined treatment techniques may improve the utilization of treated plant proteins resulting in improved animal performance.

Proteins are rendered less soluble when treated with tannins because of the formation of hydrogen bonds between the hydroxyl groups of the tannin and the carboxyl groups of the peptide chains of the protein. The reduced solubility of the protein increases the quantity of dietary protein bypassing rumen fermentation and improves animal performance if the protein is properly treated (Driedger and Hatfield, 1972; McGilliard, 1972; Hatfield, 1973).

It appears that the quantity of either formaldehyde or tannin that is required for optimum protection is related to the initial solubility of the protein before treatment and to the strength of the chemical bonds which develop between the peptide cross-linkages as a result of the treatment. Since optimum conditions for treating protein to achieve rumen bypass without reducing digestibility are not well defined, additional studies will be required to establish proper treatment procedures.

Analogs of Amino Acids

Amino acids have been structurally altered to form analogs. For these analogs to be beneficial for feeding ruminant animals, they must escape degradation in the rumen, be absorbed from the small intestine, and be biologically active. A synthetic analog of methionine, α-hydroxy-γ-methylmercaptobutyric acid (MHA) has been extensively studied and is both absorbed (Papas et al., 1974a) and biologically active (Belasco, 1972; Reis, 1970). MHA is less soluble

in rumen fluid than methionine (Belasco, 1972) but does not completely escape destruction in the rumen (Emery, 1971; Gil et al.,
1973; Papas et al., 1974a, Salsbury et al., 1971). MHA supplementation in dairy cattle diets has been reported to increase nitrogen
retention (Polan et al., 1970b) and milk production (Griel et al.,
1968; Polan et al., 1970a). However, other studies have shown no
improvement in milk yield from feeding dairy cows MHA (Polan et al.,
1970b; Holter et al., 1972; Burgos and Olson, 1970; Whiting et al.,
1972). Performance of feedlot animals has been improved by feeding
MHA (Burroughs et al., 1970), but in other studies steers did not
respond to MHA supplementation when fed a diet containing urea
(Gossett et al., 1962). Feeding MHA to ruminant animals has produced variable responses and a beneficial mode of action for increasing animal performance has not been demonstrated. Other synthetic analogs also have been investigated but to date have demonstrated only limited potential for use in feeding ruminants (Chalupa,
1975).

Encapsulation of Amino Acids

Numerous materials including a mixture of kaolin and tristearin
(Sibbald et al., 1968), basic polymers of amino acrylates or meth-
acrylates, cellulose propionate-3-morpholino butyrate, and imidamine
polymers (Chalupa, 1975)   have been investigated as vehicles
for bypassing rumen fermentation with amino acids. The product that
has been investigated most thoroughly is the kaolin and tristearin
mixture designed by Sibbald et al. (1968). This product contained
20% DL-methionine, 20% kaolin, and 60% tristearin and physically
consisted of a core of methionine, colloidal kaolin, and tristearin
covered with a continuous film of tristearin. The particles were
small, ranging from about 300 to 1,000 microns in diameter.

Plasma methionine:valine ratios were increased when the encapsulated protected methionine was fed to lactating cows (Broderick
et al., 1970) and growing steers (Linton et al., 1968) suggesting an
increase in methionine absorption. However, Neudoerffer el al. (1971)

indicated that destruction of 30% of the material in the rumen and incomplete breakdown of 60-65% of the material which reached the lower gut resulted in only a small amount of the total methionine being absorbed. Adding a liquid unsaturated fatty acid or oil, such as oleic acid, has been used to overcome the low methionine release in the lower digestive tract (Grass and Unangst, 1972, as cited by Chalupa, 1975). Feeding this preparation to sheep increased nitrogen retention. However, feeding other forms of encapsulated methionine has not been completely successful in improving feed efficiency and weight gain of sheep (Chalupa, 1975). Mowat and Deelstra (1972) fed encapsulated methionine (Sibbald et al., 1968) to sheep and improved weight gains and feed efficiency; however, no effect on milk production or composition has been observed using this protective material (Broderick et al., 1970; Williams et al., 1970).

The lack of response from feeding encapsulated methionine in various studies may be attributed to destruction of the material in the rumen, poor release in the lower gut, or to postruminal digesta containing an adequate supply of methionine. The quantity of an amino acid in the encapsulated product that is absorbed from the small intestine and the cost of the encapsulation material are the major factors in determining the feasibility of this procedure for bypassing amino acids to the lower gut.

Alteration of Rumen Metabolism

Altering the metabolic pathways of rumen metabolism has been reported to influence both the quantity and rate of formation of the end products of fermentation in the rumen which in turn affect animal performance. Feeding antibiotics to alter breakdown of protein and amino acids has not improved animal performance but has lowered rumen ammonia concentrations. Hogan and Weston (1969) fed penicillin and erythromycin to sheep and reduced feed intake. Rumen ammonia concentrations also were lowered by 35%. Rumen ammonia concentrations were depressed by 15% when chloramphenicol was added to the diet of sheep, but efficiency of nitrogen utilization was not improved. It was postulated that feed intake would have been reduced if the animals had been fed ad libitum. Feeding neomycin, oxytetracycline, and streptomycin also lowered rumen ammonia concentrations, but results were not consistent and animal performance was not improved. Rumen metabolism appeared unaltered and the concentration of methionine and lysine in the abomasum and plasma was increased when a combination of oxytetracycline, methionine, and lysine was fed to sheep (Schelling et al., 1972). Supplementing the diet with a mixture of methionine and oxytetracycline also increased plasma concentrations of methionine but decreased feed intake and caused temporary digestive disturbances (Schelling et al., 1973b). Feeding the above antibiotics to alter rumen metabolism does not appear to improve animal performance largely because of a depression in feed intake.

Proteolytic activity of rumen microbes is probably not affected by type of diet (Chalupa, 1975) but the deamination of amino acids may be influenced by diet since microbes from animals fed low-protein molasses-urea diets have depressed deamination activity (Ramirez, 1972, as cited by Chalupa, 1975). Several compounds have decreased urease activity in the rumen and have lowered the concentration of ammonia in rumen fluid (Chalupa, 1972; Tillman and Sidhu, 1969). These alterations in rumen metabolism should improve urea utilization since ammonia is normally liberated much faster than it can be incorporated into microbial protein. Feeding aceto-hydroxyamic acid, an inhibitor of urease, to sheep lowered the concentration of ammonia in the rumen and increased nitrogen retention (Streeter et al., 1969).

Methane formation in the rumen can be inhibited using a variety of chemicals, the most potent being the halomethanes (Trei et al., 1971). Supplementing cattle and sheep diets containing 40-50% roughages with a hemiacetal of chloral and starch decreased methane formation in the rumen (Trei et al., 1970), improved the efficiency of energy utilization (Johnson, 1972a; Trei and Scott, 1971; Trei et al., 1972), and increased nitrogen retention (Johnson, 1974; Singh and Trei, 1972; Trei et al., 1973). Improved energy utilization or a more efficient use of rumen ammonia for microbial protein synthesis due to slower degradation of dietary protein in the rumen may be contributing factors to the increased nitrogen retention. In addition to suppressing methanogenesis the halomethanes partially block amino acid deamination (Chalupa, 1975) which may result in free amino acids bypassing rumen fermentation. Although published data relating changes in rumen metabolism to animal performance are limiting, this approach appears to offer potential for improving both the quality and quantity of nutrients passed to the absorption sites in the lower gut. However, the success of this method will depend on developing a feed additive that will control selected metabolic pathways of fermentation in the rumen without altering overall rumen metabolism.

Closure of the Esophageal Groove

Esophageal groove closure is a normal function in young ruminants that shunts liquids from the cardia to the reticulo-omasal orifice. Thus, rumen bypass of protein is a natural process in young ruminants, but this seldom occurs in older animals eating solid feeds. Closure of the groove is a conditioned reflex and the animal must be in an "excited" state to achieve closure (Orskov, 1972). Other factors suggested to affect esophageal groove closure are age, method of drinking, position of the animal while drinking, composition and temperature of the liquid, and site of delivery into the esophagus (Orskov, 1972). Salts of sodium, copper, silver, and zinc activate closure of the groove (Chalupa, 1975).

Closure of the esophageal groove can be used to bypass dietary protein in liquid solution or suspension to the abomasum of young and adult sheep (Orskov and Fraser, 1969; Orskov and Benzie, 1969; Orskov et al., 1970; Orskov, 1972). These studies have demonstrated that a number of proteins are more efficiently utilized when they escape degradation in the rumen. Although esophageal groove closure

has limitations for mature ruminants, from a practical consideration
it offers advantages for rearing young ruminants and for research to
establish amino acid requirements.

SUMMARY AND CONCLUSIONS

Animal performance is greatly influenced by the quantity of
dietary and microbial protein that passes to the small intestine.
Microbial protein synthesis in the rumen is rather constant and the
quantity of dietary protein that escapes rumen fermentation is largely
dependent on solubility of the protein. The performance of ruminant
animals has been improved by infusing high quality protein or amino
acids into the abomasum. Methods, other than infusion, used to protect proteins and/or amino acids from degradation in the rumen include: chemical treatment, analogs of amino acids, encapsulation of
amino acids, alteration of rumen metabolism, and closure of the esophageal groove. For such techniques to be successful, the nutrients
must escape rumen fermentation and be available for absorption in
the lower gut. Proper protection of protein and/or amino acids reduces the loss of nitrogen that occurs during rumen fermentation and
can increase the quantity and improve the quality of protein by
altering the distribution of individual amino acids available for
absorption postruminally. Thus, if protected proteins or amino acids
are fed, less total nitrogen may be required in the diet. The use of
less expensive nitrogen sources, such as urea, to meet the nitrogen
requirements for microbial protein synthesis and feeding high quality
protected protein or amino acids to supplement the microbial protein
passing to the small intestine appears to be the optimum method for
feeding ruminant animals in the future.

REFERENCES

Amos, H.E., D. Burdick and T.L. Huber. 1974. Effects of formaldehyde
    treatment of sunflower and soybean meal on nitrogen balance in
    lambs. J. Animal Sci. 38:702.

Balch, C.C. and R.C. Campling. 1965. Rate of passage of digesta through the ruminant digestive tract. In R.W. Dougherty (Ed.) Physiology of Digestion in the Ruminant. Butterworth Inc., Washington, D.C.

Barker, R.A., D.N. Mowat, J.B. Stone, K.R. Stevenson and M.G. Freeman. 1973. Formic acid or formic acid-formalin as a silage additive. Can. J. Animal Sci. 53:465.

Barry, T.N. 1970. The effect of feeding formaldehyde treated casein and lucerne meal to sheep on nitrogen metabolism and wool production. Proc. New Zealand Soc. Animal Prod. 30:216.

Barry, T.N. 1972. The effect of feeding formaldehyde treated casein to sheep on nitrogen retention and wool growth. New Zealand J. Agr. Res. 15:107.

Bassett, J.M., R.H. Weston and J.P. Hogan. 1971. Dietary regulation of plasma insulin and growth hormone concentrations in sheep. Aust. J. Biol. Sci. 24:321.

Beever, D.E., D.G. Harrison and D.J. Thomson. 1972. Determination of the quantities of food and microbial nitrogen in duodenal digesta. Proc. Nutr. Soc. 31:61A.

Belasco, I.J. 1972. Stability of methionine hydroxy analog in rumen fluid and its conversion in vitro to methionine by calf liver and kidney. J. Dairy Sci. 55:353.

Bird, P.R. and R.J. Moir. 1972. Sulphur metabolism and excretion studies in ruminants. VIII. Methionine degradation and utilization in sheep when infused into the rumen or abomasum. Aust. J. Biol. Sci. 25:835.

Black, J.L. 1971. A theoretical consideration of the effect of preventing rumen fermentation on the efficiency of utilization of dietary energy and protein in lambs. Brit. J. Nutr. 25:31.

Black, J.L. and D.E. Tribe. 1973. Comparison of ruminal and abomasal administration of feed on the growth and body composition of lambs. Aust. J. Agr. Res. 24:763.

Black, J.L., G.E. Robards and R. Thomas. 1973. Effects of protein and energy intakes on the wool growth of Merino wethers. Aust. J. Agr. Res. 24:399.

Blackburn, T.H. 1965. Nitrogen metabolism in the rumen. In R.W. Dougherty (Ed.) Physiology of Digestion in the Ruminant. Butterworth Inc., Washington, D.C.

Blaxter, K.L. and A.K. Martin. 1962. The utilization of protein as a source of energy in fattening sheep. Brit. J. Nutr. 16:397.

Boila, R.J. and T.J. Devlin. 1972. Effects of lysine infusion per abomasum of steers fed continuously. Can. J. Animal Sci. 52:681.

Broderick, G.A., T. Kowalczyk and L.D. Satter. 1970. Milk production response to supplementation with encapsulated methionine per Os or casein per abomasum. J. Dairy Sci. 53:1714.

Brown, D.C. and S.C. Valentine. 1972. Formaldehyde as a silage additive. I. The chemical composition and nutritive value of frozen lucerne, lucerne silage and formaldehyde-treated lucerne silage. Aust. J. Agr. Res. 23:1093.

Burgos, A. and H.H. Olson. 1970. Effects of 40 g of methionine hydroxy analog on yield and composition of milk. J. Dairy Sci. 53:647.

Burris, W.R., N.W. Bradley, J.A. Boling, A.W. Young, G.M. Hill and L.C. Pendlum. 1974. Postruminal infusion of lysine in steers fed a urea supplemented diet. J. Animal Sci. 39:234.

Burroughs, W., G.S. Ternus, A.H. Trenkle, R.L. Vetter and C.C. Cooper. 1970. Amino acids and proteins added to corn-urea rations. J. Animal Sci. 31:1037.

Chalmers, M.I., D.P. Cuthbertson and R.L.M. Synge. 1954. Ruminal ammonia formation in relation to the protein requirement of sheep. I. Duodenal administration and heat processing as factors influencing fate of casein supplements. J. Agr. Sci. 44:254.

Chalupa, W. 1972. Metabolic aspects of nonprotein nitrogen utilization in ruminant animals. Fed. Proc. 31:1152.

Chalupa, W. 1974. Amino acid nutrition of growing cattle. In Tracer Studies on Non-Protein Nitrogen for Ruminants. Int. Atomic Energy Agency, Vienna.

Chalupa, W. Rumen bypass and protection of proteins and amino acids. J. Dairy Sci. 58:1198 (1975).

Chalupa, W. and J.E. Chandler. 1972. Amino acid nutrition of ruminants. In Tracer Studies on Non-Protein Nitrogen for Ruminants. Int. Atomic Energy Agency, Vienna.

Chalupa, W., J.E. Chandler and R.E. Brown. 1972. Amino acid nutrition of growing cattle. Fed. Proc. 31:681.

Chalupa, W., J.E. Chandler and R.E. Brown. 1973. Abomasal infusion of mixtures of amino acids to growing cattle. J. Animal Sci. 37:339.

Clark, J.H. Lactational responses to postruminal administration of proteins and amino acids. J. Dairy Sci. 58:1178 (1975).

Clark, J.H., H.R. Spires and R.G. Derrig. 1973. Postruminal administration of glucose and Na-caseinate in lactating cows. J. Animal Sci. 37:340.

Clark, J.H., C.L. Davis and E.E. Hatfield. 1974. Effects of formaldehyde treated soybean meal on nutrient use, milk yield and composition and free amino acids in the lactating bovine. J. Dairy Sci. 57:1031.

Colebrook, W.F. and P.J. Reis. 1969. Relative value for wool growth and nitrogen retention of several proteins administered as abomasal supplements to sheep. Aust. J. Biol. Sci. 22:1507.

Cuthbertson, D.P. and M.I. Chalmers. 1950. Utilization of a casein supplement administered to ewes by ruminal and duodenal fistulae. Biochem. J. 46:xvii.

Danke, R.J., L.B. Sherrod, E.C. Nelson and A.D. Tillman. 1966. Effects of autoclaving and steaming of cottonseed meal for different lengths of time on nitrogen solubility and retention in sheep. J. Animal Sci. 25:181.

Derrig, R.G., J.H. Clark and C.L. Davis. 1974. Effect of abomasal infusion of sodium caseinate on milk yield, nitrogen utilization and amino acid nutrition of the dairy cow. J. Nutr. 104:151.

Devlin, T.J. and W. Woods. 1964. Nitrogen metabolism as influenced by lysine administration in and posterior to the rumen. J. Animal Sci. 23:872.

Devlin, T.J. and W. Woods. 1965. Nitrogen metabolism as influenced by lysine administration posterior to the rumen. J. Animal Sci. 24:878.

Dinius, D.A., R.R. Oltjen, C.K. Lyon, G.O. Kohler and H.G. Walker Jr. 1974. Utilization of a formaldehyde treated casein-safflower oil complex by growing and finishing steers. J. Animal Sci. 39:124.

Driedger, A. and E.E. Hatfield. 1972. Influence of tannins on the nutritive value of soybean meal for ruminants. J. Animal Sci. 34:465.

Egan, A.R. 1970. Utilization by sheep of casein administered per duodenum at different levels of roughage intake. Aust. J. Agr. Res. 21:85.

Ely, D.G., C.O. Little, P.G. Woolfolk and G.E. Mitchell Jr. 1967. Estimation of the extent of conversion of dietary zein to microbial protein in the rumen of lambs. J. Nutr. 91:314.

Emery, R.S. 1971. Disappearance of methionine from the rumen. J. Dairy Sci. 54:1090.

Faichney, G.J. 1971. The effect of formaldehyde-treated casein on the growth of ruminant lambs. Aust. J. Agr. Res. 22:453.

Faichney, G.J. 1972. Digestion by sheep of concentrate diets containing formaldehyde-treated peanut meal. Aust. J. Agr. Res. 23:859.

Faichney, G.J. 1974. The effect of formaldehyde treatment of a casein supplement on urea excretion and on digesta composition in sheep. Aust. J. Agr. Res. 25:599.

Faichney, G.J. and H.L. Davies. 1972. The effect of formaldehyde treatment of peanut meal in concentrate diets on the performance of calves. Aust. J. Agr. Res. 23:167.

Faichney, G.J. and H.L. Davies. 1973. The performance of calves given concentrate diets treated with formaldehyde. Aust. J. Agr. Res. 24:613.

Faichney, G.J. and R.H. Weston. 1971. Digestion by ruminant lambs of a diet containing formaldehyde-treated casein. Aust. J. Agr. Res. 22:461.

Ferguson, K.A. 1971. Method and food composition for feeding ruminants. U.S. Patent 3,619,200.

Ferguson, K.A., J.A. Hemsley and P.J. Reis. 1967. Nutrition and wool growth. The effect of protecting dietary protein from microbial degradation in the rumen. Aust. J. Sci. 30:215.

Fisher, L.J. 1969. Effect of methionine infusion on milk production and plasma-free amino acids of lactating cows. J. Dairy Sci. 52:943.

Fisher, L.J. 1972. Response of lactating cows to the intravenous infusion of amino acids. Can. J. Animal Sci. 52:377.

Gil, L.A., R.L. Shirley and J.E. Moore. 1973. Effect of methionine hydroxy analog on growth, amino acid content and catabolic products of glucolytic rumen bacteria in vitro. J. Dairy Sci. 56:757.

Glimp, H.A., M.R. Karr, C.O. Little, P.G. Woolfolk, G.E. Mitchell Jr. and L.W. Hudson. 1967. Effect of reducing soybean protein solubility by dry heat on the protein utilization of young lambs. J. Animal Sci. 26:858.

Goering, H.K. and D.R. Waldo. 1974a. Processing effects on protein utilization by ruminants. Proc. Cornell Nutr. Conf. p. 25.

Goering, H.K. and D.R. Waldo. 1974b. Protein value of heat- and formaldehyde-treated ruminant feeds. Proc. Md. Nutr. Conf. p. 52.

Goering, H.K., C.H. Gordon, R.W. Hemken, D.R. Waldo, P.J. Van Soest and L.W. Smith. 1972. Analytical estimates of nitrogen digestibility in heat damaged forages. J. Dairy Sci. 55:1275.

Goering, H.K., P.J. Van Soest and R.W. Hemken. 1973. Relative susceptibility of forages to heat damage as affected by moisture, temperature and pH. J. Dairy Sci. 56:137.

Gossett, W.H., T.W. Perry, M.T. Mohler, M.P. Plumlee and W.M. Beeson. 1962. Value of supplemental lysine, methionine, methionine analog and trace minerals on high urea fattening rations for beef steers. J. Animal Sci. 21:248.

Grass, G.M. and R.R. Unangst. 1972. Glycerol tristerate and higher fatty acid mixture for improving digestive absorption. U.S. Patent 3,655,864.

Griel, L.C., Jr., R.A. Patton, R.D. McCarthy and P.T. Chandler. 1968. Milk production response to feeding methionine hydroxy analog to lactating dairy cows. J. Dairy Sci. 51:1866.

Hale, G.D. and D.R. Jacobson. 1972. Feeding or abomasal administration of casein, gelatin, partially delactosed whey (PDW), or zein to lactating cows. J. Dairy Sci. 55:709.

Hale, G.D., D.R. Jacobson and R.W. Hemken. 1972. Continuous abomasal infusion of casein in lactating Holsteins fed urea supplemented diets. J. Dairy Sci. 55:689.

Hatfield, E.E. 1970. Selected topics related to the amino acid nutrition of the growing ruminant. Fed. Proc. 29:44.

Hatfield, E.E. 1973. Treating dietary proteins with tannins or aldehydes. In Effect of Processing on the Nutritional Value of Feeds. National Academy of Sciences, Washington, D.C.

Hedde, R.D., K.L. Knox, D.E. Johnson and G.M. Ward. 1974. Energy and protein utilization in calves fed via rumen by-pass. J. Animal Sci. 39:108.

Hemsley, J.A. 1967. Sodium chloride intake and flow through the rumen. Aust. J. Exp. Biol. Med. Sci. 45:39.

Hemsley, J.A., P.J. Reis and A.M. Downes. 1973. Influence of various formaldehyde treatments on the nutritional value of casein for wool growth. Aust. J. Biol. Sci. 26:961.

Henderickx, H. and J. Martin. 1963. In vitro study of the nitrogen metabolism in the rumen. Compt. Rend. Researches Sci. Ind. Agr. Bruxelles 31:1.

Hertelendy, F.,L.J.Machlin and D.M. Kipnis. 1969. Further studies on the regulation of insulin and growth hormone secretion in sheep. Endocrinology 84:192.

Hertelendy, F., K. Takahashi, L.J. Machlin and D.M. Kipnis. 1970. Growth hormone and insulin secretory responses to arginine in the sheep, pig and cow. Gen. and Comp. Endocrinology 14:72.

Hill, D.L. and C.H. Noller. 1963. The apparent digestibility of protein in low moisture silages. J. Animal Sci. 22:850.

Hogan, J.P. Quantitative aspects of nitrogen utilization in ruminants. J. Dairy Sci. 58:1164 (1975).

Hogan, J.P. and R.H. Weston. 1969. The effect of antibiotics on ammonia accumulation and protein digestion in the rumen. Aust. J. Agr. Res. 20:339.

Hogan, J.P. and R.H. Weston. 1970. Quantitative aspects of microbial protein synthesis in the rumen. In A.T. Philipson (Ed.) Physiology of Digestion and Metabolism in the Ruminant. Oriel Press Limited, England.

Holter, J.B., C.W. Kim and N.F. Colovos. 1972. Methionine hydroxy analog for lactating dairy cows. J. Dairy Sci. 55:460.

Hudson, L.W., H.A. Glimp, C.O. Little and P.G. Woolfolk. 1970. Ruminal and postruminal nitrogen utilization by lambs fed heated soybean meal. J. Animal Sci. 30:609.

Hughes, J.G. and G.L. Williams. 1971. The effect of formaldehyde treatment of protein supplements upon their in vitro fermentation and utilization by sheep. Proc. Nutr. Soc. 30:41A.

Hume, I.D. 1970. Synthesis of microbial protein in the rumen. 3. The effect of dietary protein. Aust. J. Agr. Res. 21:305.

Hungate, R.E. 1966. The Rumen and Its Microbes. Academic Press, New York.

Hutton, J.B. 1957. The effect of growth hormone on the yield and composition of cow's milk. J. Endocrinology 16:115.

Isaacs, J. and F.N. Owens. 1972. Protein soluble in rumen fluid. J. Animal Sci. 35:267.

Johnson, D.E. 1972a. Effects of a hemiacetal of chloral and starch on methane production and energy balance of sheep fed a pelleted diet. J. Animal Sci. 35:1064.

Johnson, D.E. 1972b. Heat increment of acetate and corn and effects of casein infusions with growing lambs. J. Nutr. 102:1093.

Johnson, D.E. 1974. Adaptational responses in nitrogen and energy balance of lambs fed a methane inhibitor. J. Animal Sci. 38: 154.

Jones, G.M. 1973. Performance of dairy cows fed propionic acid-treated high-moisture shelled corn rations for complete lactations. J. Dairy Sci. 56:207.

Judson, G.J. and R.A. Leng. 1973. Studies on the control of gluconeogenesis in sheep: effect of propionate, casein and butyrate infusions. Brit. J. Nutr. 29:175.

Kellaway, R.C., S.S.E. Ranawana, J.H. Buchanan and L.D. Smart. 1974. The effect of nitrogen source in the diet on milk production and amino-acid uptake by the udder. J. Dairy Res. 41:305.

Lindsay, D.B. and C. Dyke. 1974. The effect of casein and amino acids on glucose synthesis in sheep. Proc. Nutr. Soc. 33:39A.

Lindsay, D.B. and R.L. Williams. 1971. The effect of glucose entry rate of abomasal protein infusion in sheep. Proc Nutr. Soc. 30:35A.

Linton, J.H., T.C. Loughheed and I.R. Sibbald. 1968. Elevation of free methionine in bovine plasma. J. Animal Sci. 27:1168.

Linzell, J.L. and T.B. Mepham. 1974. Effects of intramammary arterial infusion of essential amino acids in the lactating goat. J. Dairy Res. 41:101.

Little, C.O. and G.E. Mitchell Jr. 1967. Abomasal vs. oral administration of proteins to wethers. J. Animal Sci. 26:411.

Little, C.O., W. Burroughs and W. Woods. 1963. Nutritional significance of soluble nitrogen in dietary proteins for ruminants. J. Animal Sci. 22:358.

Little, C.O., G.E. Mitchell Jr. and G.D. Potter. 1968. Nitrogen in the abomasum of wethers fed different protein sources. J. Animal Sci. 27:1722.

Machlin, L.J. 1973. Effect of growth hormone on milk production and feed utilization in dairy cows. J. Dairy Sci. 56:575.

MacRae, J.C., M.J. Ulyatt, P.D. Pearce and J. Hendtlass. 1972. Quantitative intestinal digestion of nitrogen in sheep given formaldehyde-treated and untreated casein supplements. Brit. J. Nutr. 27:39.

Mangan, J.L. 1972. Quantitative studies on nitrogen metabolism in the bovine rumen. Brit. J. Nutr. 27:261.

McAtee, J.W. and A. Trenkle. 1971. Metabolic regulation of plasma insulin levels in cattle. J. Animal Sci. 33:438.

McDonald, I.W. 1954. The extent of conversion of food protein to microbial protein in the rumen of sheep. Biochem. J. 56:120.

McDonald, I.W. and R.J. Hall. 1957. The conversion of casein into microbial proteins in the rumen. Biochem. J. 67:400.

McGilliard, A.D. 1972. Modifying proteins for maximum utilization in the ruminant. J. Amer. Oil Chem. Soc. 49:57.

Mepham, T.B. and J.L. Linzell. 1974. Effects of intramammary arterial infusion of non-essential amino acids and glucose in the lactating goat. J. Dairy Res. 41:111.

Miller, E.L. 1972. The digestion of formaldehyde treated groundnut meal before and after the abomasum of lambs. Proc. Nutr. Soc. 31:27A.

Mohanty, G.P., N.A. Jorgensen, R.M. Luther and H.H. Voelker. 1969. Effect of molded alfalfa hay on rumen activity, performance, and digestibility in dairy steers. J. Dairy Sci. 52:79.

Mowat, D.N. and K. Deelstra. 1972. Encapsulated methionine supplement for growing-finishing lambs. J. Animal Sci. 34:332.

Nelson, L.F. 1970. Amino acids for ruminants. Proc. Amer. Feed Manuf. Ass. Nutr. Council. p. 13.

Neudoerffer, T.S., D.B. Duncan and F.D. Horney. 1971. The extent of release of encapsulated methionine in the intestine of cattle. Brit. J. Nutr. 25:333.

Nimrick, K., E.E. Hatfield, J. Kaminski and F.N. Owens. 1970a. Qualitative assessment of supplemental amino acid needs for growing lambs fed urea as the sole nitrogen source. J. Nutr. 100:1293.

Nimrick, K., E.E. Hatfield, J. Kaminski and F.N. Owens. 1970b. Quantitative assessment of supplemental amino acid needs for growing lambs fed urea as the sole nitrogen source. J. Nutr. 100:1301.

RUMEN BYPASS OF PROTEIN AND AMINO ACIDS

Nimrick, K., A.P. Peter and E.E. Hatfield. 1972. Aldehyde-treated fish and soybean meals as dietary supplements for growing lambs. J. Animal Sci. 34:488.

Nishimuta, J.F., D.G. Ely and J.A. Boling. 1973. Nitrogen metabolism in lambs fed soybean meal treated with heat, formalin and tannic acid. J. Nutr. 103:49.

NRC. 1971. Nutrient requirements of domestic animals. No. 3. Nutrient requirements of dairy cattle. National Research Council, Washington, D.C.

Oltjen, R.R., W. Chalupa and L.L. Slyter. 1970. Abomasal infusion of amino acids into urea and soy fed steers. J. Animal Sci. 31:250.

Orskov, E.R. 1972. Reflex closure of the oesophageal groove and its potential application in ruminant nutrition. S. Afr. J. Animal Sci. 2:169.

Orskov, E.R. and D. Benzie. 1969. Using the oesophageal groove reflex in ruminants as a means of bypassing rumen fermentation with high-quality protein and other nutrients. Proc. Nutr. Soc. 28:30A.

Orskov, E.R. and C. Fraser. 1969. The effect on nitrogen retention in lambs of feeding protein supplements direct to the abomasum. Comparison of liquid and dry feeding and of various sources of protein. J. Agr. Sci., Camb. 73:469.

Orskov, E.R., C. Fraser and E.L. Corse. 1970. The effect on protein utilization of feeding different protein supplements via the rumen or via the abomasum in young growing sheep. Brit. J. Nutr. 24:803.

Orskov, E.R., C. Fraser and I. McDonald. 1971. Digestion of concentrates in sheep. 2. The effect of urea or fish-meal supplementation of barley diets on the apparent digestion of protein, fat, starch and ash in the rumen, the small intestine and the large intestine and calculation of volatile fatty acid production. Brit. J. Nutr. 25:243.

Orskov, E.R., C. Fraser and R. Pirie. 1973. The effect of bypassing the rumen with supplements of protein and energy on intake of concentrates by sheep. Brit. J. Nutr. 30:361.

Papas, A., G.A.B. Hall, E.E. Hatfield and F.N. Owens. 1974a. Response of lambs to oral or abomasal supplementation of methionine hydroxy analog or methionine. J. Nutr. 104:653.

Papas, A., E.E. Hatfield and F.N. Owens. 1974b. Responses of growing lambs to abomasal infusion of corn oil, starch, casein and amino acid mixtures. J. Nutr. 104:1543.

Pearson, R.M. and J.A.B. Smith. 1943. The utilization of urea in the bovine rumen. 3. The synthesis and breakdown of protein in the rumen ingesta. Biochemistry 37:153.

Peter, A.P., E.E. Hatfield, F.N. Owens and U.S. Garrigus. 1971. Effects of aldehyde treatments of soybean meal on in vitro ammonia release, solubility and lamb performance. J. Nutr. 101:605.

Pierson, D.C., R.D. Goodrich, J.C. Meiske and J.G. Linn. 1971. Influence of heat damage on haylage quality. J. Animal Sci. 33:296.

Polan, C.E., P.T. Chandler and C.N. Miller. 1970a. Methionine hydroxy analog: varying levels for lactating cow. J. Dairy Sci. 53:607.

Polan, C.E., P.T. Chandler and C.N. Miller. 1970b. Methionine analog effect on ruminant digestion. J. Animal Sci. 31:251.

Potter, G.D., J.W. McNeill and J.K. Riggs. 1971. Utilization of processed sorghum grain proteins by steers. J. Animal Sci. 32:540.

Ramirez, A. 1972. Deaminative activity of rumen microflora with molasses/urea diets. Rev. Cubana Cierc. Agr. 6:35.

Rattray, P.V. and J.P. Joyce. 1970. Nitrogen retention and growth studies with young sheep using two sources of formalin-treated protein. New Zealand J. Agr. Res. 13:623.

Reis, P.J. 1969. The growth and composition of wool. V. Stimulation of wool growth by the abomasal administration of varying amounts of casein. Aust. J. Biol. Sci. 22:745.

Reis, P.J. 1970. The influence of abomasal supplements of some amino acids and sulfur-containing compounds on wool growth rate. Aust. J. Biol. Sci. 23:441.

Reis, P.J. and W.F. Colebrook. 1972. The utilization of abomasal supplements of proteins and amino acids by sheep with special reference to wool growth. Aust. J. Biol. Sci. 25:1057.

Reis, P.J. and A.M. Downes. 1971. The rate of response of wool growth to abomasal supplements of casein. J. Agr. Sci., Camb. 76:173.

Reis, P.J. and P.G. Schinckel. 1961. Nitrogen utilization and wool production by sheep. Aust. J. Agr. Res. 12:335.

Reis, P.J. and P.G. Schinckel. 1963. Some effects of sulfur-containing amino acids on the growth and composition of wool. Aust. J. Biol. Sci. 16:218.

Reis, P.J. and P.G. Schinckel. 1964. The growth and composition of wool. II. The effect of casein, gelatin, and sulphur-containing amino acids given per abomasum. Aust. J. Biol. Sci. 17:532.

Reis, P.J. and D.A. Tunks. 1969. Evaluation of formaldehyde-treated casein for wool growth and nitrogen retention. Aust. J. Agr. Res. 20:775.

Reis, P.J., D.A. Tunks and A.M. Downes. 1973. The influence of abomasal and intravenous supplements of sulphur-containing amino acids on wool growth rate. Aust. J. Biol. Sci. 26:249.

Roffler, R.E., R.P. Niedermeier and B.R. Baumgardt. 1967. Evaluation of alfalfa-brome forage stored as wilted silage, low-moisture silage and hay. J. Dairy Sci. 50:1805.

Salsbury, R.L., D.K. Marvil, C.W. Woodmansee and G.F.W. Haenlein. 1971. Utilization of methionine and methionine hydroxy analog by rumen microorganisms in vitro. J. Dairy Sci. 54:390.

Satter, L.D. and R.E. Roffler. Nitrogen utilization and requirements in dairy cattle. J. Dairy Sci. 58:1219 (1975).

Schelling, G.T. and E.E. Hatfield. 1968. Effect of abomasally infused nitrogen sources on nitrogen retention of growing lambs. J. Nutr. 96:319.

Schelling, G.T., G.E. Mitchell Jr. and R.E. Tucker. 1972. Prevention of free amino acid degradation in the rumen. Fed. Proc. 31:681.

Schelling, G.T., J.E. Chandler and G.C. Scott. 1973a. Postruminal supplemental methionine infusion to sheep fed high quality diets. J. Animal Sci. 37:1034.

Schelling, G.T., C.R. Richardson, R.E. Tucker and G.E. Mitchell Jr. 1973b. Lamb responses to dietary methionine and oxyletracycline. J. Animal Sci. 37:356.

Schmidt, S.P., N.J. Benevenga and N.A. Jorgensen. 1973a. Effects of formaldehyde, glyoxal, or hexamethylenetetramine treatment of soybean meal on nitrogen utilization and growth in rats and in vitro rumen ammonia release. J. Animal Sci. 37:1238.

Schmidt, S.P., N.A. Jorgensen, N.J. Benevenga and V.H. Brungardt. 1973b. Comparison of soybean meal, formaldehyde treated soybean meal, urea and starea for steers. J. Animal Sci. 37:1233.

Schmidt, S.P., N.J. Benevenga and N.A. Jorgensen. 1974. Effect of formaldehyde treatment of soybean meal on the performance of growing steers and lambs. J. Animal Sci. 38:646.

Schwab, C.G. and L.D. Satter. 1973. Response of lactating dairy cows to the abomasal infusion of amino acids. J. Dairy Sci. 56:664.

Schwab, C.G. and L.D. Satter. 1974. Effect of abomasal infusion of amino acids on lactating dairy cows. J. Dairy Sci. 57:632.

Sharma, H.R. and J.R. Ingalls. 1973. Comparative value of soybean, rapeseed and formaldehyde-treated rapeseed meals in urea-containing calf rations. Can. J. Animal Sci. 53:273.

Sharma, H.R. and J.R. Ingalls. 1974. Effect of treating rapeseed meal and casein protein with formaldehyde on apparent digestibility and amino acid composition of rumen digesta and bacteria. Can. J. Animal Sci. 54:157.

Sharma, H.R., J.R. Ingalls and J.A. McKirdy. 1972. Nutritive value of formaldehyde-treated rapeseed meal for dairy calves. Can. J. Animal Sci. 52:363.

Sharma, H.R., J.R. Ingalls and R.J. Parker. 1974. Effects of treating rapeseed meal and casein with formaldehyde on the flow of nutrients through the gastrointestinal tract of fistulated Holstein steers. Can. J. Animal Sci. 54:305.

Sherrod, L.B. and A.D. Tillman. 1962. Effects of varying the processing temperatures upon the nutritive values for sheep of solvent-extracted soybean and cottonseed meals. J. Animal Sci. 21:901.

Sherrod, L.B. and A.D. Tillman. 1964. Further studies on the effects of different processing temperatures on the utilization of solvent-extracted cottonseed protein by sheep. J. Animal Sci. 23:510.

Sibbald, I.R., T.C. Loughheed and J.H. Linton. 1968. A methionine supplement for ruminants. Proc. 2nd World Conf. Animal Prod.

Singh, Y.K. and J.E. Trei. 1972. Influence of a methane inhibitor on nutrient digestibilities and nitrogen retention in lambs. J. Animal Sci. 34:363.

Smith, R.H. 1969. Reviews of the progress of dairy science. Nitrogen metabolism and the rumen. J. Dairy Res. 36:313.

Sniffen, C.J. 1974. Nitrogen utilization as related to solubility of NPN and protein in feeds. Proc. Cornell Nutr. Conf. p. 12.

Spechter, H.H. 1972. Postruminal casein infusion of urea-fed lactating cows. Ph.D. Dissertation, The University of Guelph, Guelph, Ontario, Canada.

Spires, H.R., J.H. Clark and R.G. Derrig. 1973. Postruminal administration of sodium caseinate in lactating cows. J. Dairy Sci. 56:664.

Stern, J.S., C.A. Baile and J. Mayer. 1971. Growth hormone, insulin and glucose in suckling, weanling and mature ruminants. J. Dairy Sci. 54:1052.

Streeter, C.L., R.R. Oltjen, L.L. Slyter and W.N. Fishbein. 1969. Urea utilization in wethers receiving the urease inhibitor, acetohydroxamic acid. J. Animal Sci. 29:88.

Tagari, H., I. Ascarelli and A. Bondi. 1962. The influence of heating on the nutritive value of soya-bean meal for ruminants. Brit. J. Nutr. 16:237.

Teichman, R., E.V. Caruolo and R.D. Mochrie. 1969. Milk production and composition responses to intravenous infusion of L-methionine. J. Dairy Sci. 52:942.

Thomas, P.C. 1973. Microbial protein synthesis. Proc. Nutr. Soc. 32:85.

Tillman, A.D. and K.S. Sidhu. 1969. Nitrogen metabolism in ruminants: rate of ruminal ammonia production and nitrogen utilization by ruminants. A review. J. Animal Sci. 28:689.

Trei, J.E. and G.C. Scott. 1971. Performance of steers on the methane inhibitor--HCS. J. Animal Sci. 33:301.

Trei, J.E., Y.K. Singh and G.C. Scott. 1970. Effect of methane inhibitors on rumen metabolism. J. Animal Sci. 31:256.

Trei, J.E., R.C. Parish, Y.K. Singh and G.C. Scott. 1971. Effect of methane inhibitors on rumen metabolism and feedlot performance of sheep. J. Dairy Sci. 54:536.

Trei, J.E., G.C. Scott and R.C. Parish. 1972. Influence of methane inhibition on energetic efficiency of lambs. J. Animal Sci. 34:510.

Trei, J.E., W. Chalupa, J.E. Chandler and R.E. Brown. 1973. Energy and amicloral additions to a fattening lamb ration. Fed. Proc. 32:899.

Tyrrell, H.F., D.J. Bolt, P.W. Moe and H. Swan. 1972. Abomasal infusion of water, casein or glucose in Holstein cows. J. Animal Sci. 35:277.

Valentine, S.C. and D.C. Brown. 1973. Formaldehyde as a silage additive. II. The chemical composition and nutritive value of lucerne hay, lucerne silage and formaldehyde and formic acid-treated lucerne silages. Aust. J. Agr. Res. 24:939.

Vik-Mo, L., R.S. Emery and J.T. Huber. 1974. Milk protein production in cows abomasally infused with casein or glucose. J. Dairy Sci. 57:869.

Wachira, J.D., L.D. Satter, G.P. Brooke and A.L. Pope. 1974. Evaluation of formaldehyde-treated protein for growing lambs and lactating cows. J. Animal Sci. 39:796.

Waldo, D.R. 1968. Symposium: nitrogen utilization by the ruminant, nitrogen metabolism in the ruminant. J. Dairy Sci. 51:265.

Waldo, D.R. 1973. Extent and partition of cereal grain starch digestion in ruminants. J. Animal Sci. 37:1062.

Waldo, D.R., L.W. Smith, R.W. Miller and L.A. Moore. 1969. Growth, intake and digestibility from formic acid silage versus hay. J. Dairy Sci. 52:1609.

Waldo, D.R., J.E. Keys Jr., L.W. Smith and C.H. Gordon. 1971. Effect of formic acid on recovery, intake, digestibility and growth from unwilted silage. J. Dairy Sci. 54:77.

Waldo, D.R., J.E. Keys Jr. and C.H. Gordon. 1973a. Preservation efficiency and dairy heifer response from unwilted formic and wilted untreated silages. J. Dairy Sci. 56:129.

Waldo, D.R., J.E. Keys Jr. and C.H. Gordon. 1973b. Formaldehyde and formic acid as a silage additive. J. Dairy Sci. 56:229.

Whitelaw, F.G., T.R. Preston and G.S. Dawson. 1961. The nutrition of the early-weaned calf. II. A comparison of commercial groundnut meal, heat-treated groundnut meal and fish meal as the major protein source in the diet. Animal Prod. 3:127.

Whiting, F.M., J.W. Stull, W.H. Brown and B.L. Reid. 1972. Free amino acid ratios in rumen fluid, blood plasma, milk and feces during methionine and methionine hydroxy analog supplementary feeding. J. Dairy Sci. 55:983.

Williams, A.J., G.E. Robards and D.G. Saville. 1972. Metabolism of cystine by Merino sheep genetically different in wool production. II. The responses in wool growth to abomasal infusions of L-cystine or DL-methionine. Aust. J. Biol. Sci. 25:1269.

Williams, L.R., F.A. Martz and E.S. Hilderbrand. 1970. Feeding encapsulated methionine supplement to lactating cows. J. Dairy Sci. 53:1709.

Wilson, G.F. 1970. The influence of protein supplements on milk yield and composition. Proc. Soc. Animal Prod. 30:123.

Wohlt, J.E. 1973. Nutritional significance of rations varying in soluble nitrogen and amino acid profile for the ruminant. M.S. Thesis. University of Maine, Orono.

Wohlt, J.E., C.J. Sniffen and W.H. Hoover. 1973. Measurement of protein solubility in common feedstuffs. J. Dairy Sci. 56:1052.

Wright, P.L. 1971. Body weight gain and wool growth response to formaldehyde treated casein and sulfur amino acids. J. Animal Sci. 33:137.

12

MUSHROOMS AS A SOURCE OF FOOD PROTEIN

Ralph H. Kurtzman

Western Regional Research Laboratory
Agricultural Research Service
U.S. Department of Agriculture
Berkeley, California

Mushrooms are a good source of protein. Normally, they contain from 19 to 40% protein on a dry weight basis. Most species contain all of the essential amino acids, and most of them are found in about the same proportions as in eggs. They are approximately equal to yeast in vitamin content, with the exception of thiamine. The cost of mushrooms is a function of labor costs. Modern mushroom culture produces more protein per unit area of land than any other form of agriculture. They may, therefore, become more available to the people of poor countries. Mushrooms can do much to alleviate protein and vitamin shortages.

INTRODUCTION

Mushrooms have far too often been regarded only as a delicacy. While there is no reason to malign their palability, it would be better to look upon them as a food that can do much to relieve protein deficiency in developing countries. They may contain as much as 40% protein on a dry weight basis and thereby, surpass many other foods, including milk. The apparent problem of high price is not what it appears to be and is not likely to be a problem in developing nations.

The price of mushrooms depends, to a very great degree, on the cost of labor (Ganney, 1973) and to a very small degree upon the value or general agricultural productivity of the land. In developing countries, labor is generally among the least expensive things and a very high proportion of the peasants earnings must be used to purchase food. Since a portion of almost every item Ganney (1973) lists is either labor, or things which can be replaced by labor, the price of labor is of greater importance than he indicates. In North America and Europe mushroom growing is a highly mechanized industry, while in Taiwan almost everything is done by hand labor. However, this has been no handicap to Taiwan, which has risen in a few short years from a very minor producer of *Agaricus bisporus*, the common commercial mushroom of the West, to the world's second largest producer. At the same time many other species are grown in Taiwan, while in North America and until recently in Europe, only *Agaricus bisporus* was grown commercially.

Land is often a limiting factor in the production of foods in developing countries. If the land used to grow the substrate for mushrooms is not considered, then land is of relatively little importance in mushroom culture. Current technology will allow over 125 pounds of mushrooms to be grown on a square foot of land every year (620 kg/m^2). That is based upon five crops per year, trays or shelves stacked five high, and a yield of five pounds per square foot (25 kg/m^2) of bed per crop (Schroeder et al., 1974). It also assumes that single story houses are used. It is unrealistic to think that one can use nearly all of one's land for mushroom cultivation since there is need for access, space for composting and various other functions. However, if caves, mines, or multi-story buildings are used, the concept of a square food of land becomes meaningless. With such facilities one can think in terms of simultaneous multiple use of the same land or astronomical yields per square foot of land.

Nor, is it unrealistic to disregard the land used to grow the substrate for mushrooms. Mushrooms are generally grown on wastes

from other forms of agriculture. Horse manure is the traditional
substrate for *Agaricus*, however, the basic requirements are ligno-
cellulose, nitrogen, some calcium, and other minerals. In Taiwan,
rice straw, fertilizers, and limestone are the primary ingredients
(Chiou et al., 1972). In the United States apparently most of the
nitrogen still comes from animal wastes, especially poultry manure,
but straw, corn cobs, and the like are important ingredients
(Schisler and Wuest, 1973).

A few mushrooms are so efficient at recovering nitrogen that
they can be grown on straw with no added nitrogen and yield as much
as 1.25 kg of fresh mushroom per kg of dry straw. They will, at
the same time, contain at least 1.4% protein, which would be 19%
protein on a dry weight basis (Kalberer and Kunsch, 1974).

Some mushrooms do require light; however, the quantity required is so small that it is likely that fluorescent lamps would
require less energy than windows (Gyurko, 1972). This is true
because unless the outdoor temperature was almost the same as that
used to grow the mushrooms, the exchange of heat through the
windows would have to be compensated by heating or cooling.

While general practice has by no means caught up with research,
in recent years we have learned to cultivate new species and have
bred new varieties of established species so that one can pick the
mushroom to fit the average conditions, rather than using elabo-
rate heating and cooling equipment. Edible species are known
which can be cultivated at temperatures from 0° to 40°C (32° to
105°F) (Kurtzman, 1975). The maintenance of an even temperature
and humidity, however, is of considerable importance.

The analysis of fungi for total protein is complicated by the
fact that they contain chitin (poly-acetylglucosamine) and chitosans (poly-glucosamine), which together with the nucleic acids
account for some of the nitrogen (Aronson, 1965). Thus, a Kjeldahl
nitrogen determination does not give a true indication of protein.
A variety of factors including maturation, and the particular
structure analyzed may affect the distribution of nitrogen between

307

the proteins, polysaccharides, and nucleic acids, as well as the total nitrogen (Chang, 1972). It is, therefore, not possible to be completely certain of the amount of protein in mushrooms. The composition of several commercially grown mushrooms are listed in Table 1. "Protein, wet weight" is a list of figures ranging from 6.25 x N down to that figure multiplied by two-thirds. The figures are generally not comparable. "Protein, dry weight" is far more comparable and is based on 6.25 x N, but includes the non-protein nitrogen as well. The amount of protein indicated on a dry weight basis places mushrooms below most animal meats, but well above most other foods, even animal products such as milk. In light of this, it is ironic that the United States has shipped large quantities of milk to developing nations to relieve protein deficiency, when those countries could have been taught to grow mushrooms and produce a continued supply of protein.

While some of the work on the nutritional value of mushrooms dates back many years (Mendel, 1898), most analyses of mushrooms have been inadequate to reflect the value of the protein. An examination of Table 2 indicates that there has been a great deal of discrepancy in these analyses. While the differences between species is not unexpected, the extreme differences within species are difficult to accept. Some of the essential amino acids of *Agaricus bisporus* (the common mushroom that most of the Western World consumes) vary by an order of magnitude and only two vary by less than a factor of two. The recalculation of the data of Seelkopf and Schuster (1957), may be the cause of part of the discrepancy. It can not account for the differences in the data from FAO (1970).

Of all the analyses of mushrooms shown in Table 2, only those of Doesburg and Meijer (1964) were carried out with reasonably modern methods of hydrolysis. While Doesburg and Meijer did not mention that they had done alkali hydrolysis for tryptophan, the high value for that amino acid indicates that they might have done so. They are, however, the only ones who used performic acid oxida-

MUSHROOMS AS A SOURCE OF PROTEIN

TABLE 1

Mushrooms, Percent Composition

	Moisture	Ash	Protein, wet weight	Fat, ether extract	Crude fiber	Protein, dry weight (total N x 6.25)
Agaricus bisporus [c]	89.7	0.82	4.88	0.20	0.38	47.4
Agaricus bisporus [d]	89.5	1.26	3.94	0.19	1.09	37.5
Agaricus bisporus [e]	90.4	0.9	2.7 [a]	0.30	0.80	45.0
Pleurotus sp. [f]	90.95	0.97	2.78 [b]	0.65	1.08	39.9
Pleurotus ostreatus [g]	92.47	--	2.15	--	--	30.0
Volvariella diplasia [h]	90.4	1.1	3.90	0.25	1.67	43.1
Volvariella volvacae [c]	88.4	1.46	4.99	0.74	1.38	43.0

[a] 6.25 x N x 2/3.

[b] Additional non-protein nitrogen, 0.14%.

[c] Chang (1973).

[d] Esselen and Fellers (1946)

[e] Watt and Merrill (1963).

[f] Zakia et al. (1963).

[g] Kalberer and Kunsch (1974).

[h] Zakia et al. (1971).

TABLE 2

Amino Acid Compositions of Mushrooms, Mg Amino Acid Per Gram Nitrogen

	Item #	Ile	Leu	Lys	Phe	Tyr	Cys	Met	Thr	Trp	Val
Agaricus bisporus, 1 sample[b]	1	140	230	280	130	120	33	29	170	64	160
Agaricus bisporus, 10 samples[c]	2	256	406	369	238	200	50	88	256	100	294
Agaricus bisporus, young caps[d]	3	61	221	409	176	219	421	90	278	661	164
Agaricus bisporus, old caps[d]	4	88	256	564	170	186	452	49	256	646	145
Agaricus bisporus, whole[d]	5	57	278	487	259	147	438	23	134	614	137
Lentinus edoes, whole[e]	6	226	362	181	272	181	--	91	272	--	272
Pleurotus ostreatus, "grey type"[f]	7	187	299	201	163	132	20	68	203	61	228
Pleurotus ostreatus, "Florida"[f]	8	186	273	175	151	129	20	63	185	43	216
Pleurotus sp.[g]	9	363	275	313	125	--	--	81	263	56	294
Volvariella diplasia[g]	10	344	219	268	306	100	144	56	263	69	425
Brewer's Yeast[b]	11	365	500	565	303	259	56	100	346	--	459
Eggs, chicken[b]	12	393	551	436	358	260	152	210	320	93	428

Table 2 (continued)

	Item #	Arg	His	Ala	Asp	Glu	Gly	Pro	Ser
Agaricus bisporus, 1 sample[b]	1	320	84	290	280	440	160	320	170
Agaricus bisporus, 10 samples[b,c]	2	312	125	331	575	775	256	256	275
Agaricus bisporus, young caps[d]	3	440	141	366	409	429	245	239	217
Agaricus bisporus, old caps[d]	4	482	106	284	437	363	266	202	192
Agaricus bisporus, whole[d]	5	468	143	425	405	569	209	200	167
Lentinus edodes, whole[e]	6	362	91	317	408	1404	226	226	271
Pleurotus ostreatus, "gray type"[f]	7	234	75	282	399	725	197	201	216
Pleurotus ostreatus, "Florida"[f]	8	214	16	315	395	623	191	188	190
Pleurotus sp.[g]	9	419	131	---	---	---	---	---	---
Volvariella diplasia[g]	10	256	131	---	---	---	---	---	---
Brewer's yeast[b]	11	313	156	422	678	669	300	241	365
Eggs, chicken[b]	12	381	152	370	601	796	207	260	478

Table 2 (continued)

	Item #	Total aromatic	Total S-containing	Total essential	Total amino acids
Agaricus bisporus, 1 sample[b]	1	250	62	1356	3470
Agaricus bisporus, 10 samples[bc]	2	438	138	2257	5162
Agaricus bisporus, young caps[d]	3	395	511	2700	---
Agaricus bisporus, old caps[d]	4	356	501	2912	---
Agaricus bisporus, whole[d]	5	406	461	2574	5162[a]
Lentinus edodes, whole[c]	6	453	---	---	5162[a]
Pleurotus ostreatus, "gray type"[f]	7	295	88	1562	3895
Pleurotus ostreatus, "Florida"[f]	8	280	83	1441	3618
Pleurotus sp.	9	---	---	---	---
Volvariella displasia	10	406	200	2194	---
Brewer's yeast[b]	11	562	156	3022	6166
Eggs, chicken[b]	12	618	362	3201	6446

[a]Assumed, other figures in item and items #3 and 4 calculated from this.

[b]FAO (1970).

[c]Doesburg and Meijer (1965).

[d]Seelkopf and Schuster (1957).

[e]Sugimori et al. (1971).

[f]Kalberer and Kunsch (1974).

[g]Zakia et al. (1963).

tion of the sulfur-amino acids. Their value for methionine reflects their careful work.

While the data in Table 2 is given in mg/g nitrogen, one should not expect the total to equal N x 6.25, since mushrooms and other fungi (including yeasts) have cell walls of chitin and chitosans as well as nucleic acids and other nitrogenous compounds. However, from the data in column #2 we might expect that N x 5.16 would be a minimum figure for mushroom proteins. It is to be expected that with the many manipulations required for amino acid analysis, low values due to loss are far more likely than values that are too high.

The ratio of the essential acids of mushrooms to those of eggs, based on the data in Table 2 are shown in Table 3. Because the values for the sulfur amino acids are undoubtedly low for all of the mushrooms except those reported by Doesburg and Meijer, they are not shown in Table 3 as individual amino acids. They are, however, included in the total values. The ratios of the amino acids of A. *bisporus* to those for egg make it appear to be a very fine source of essential amino acids although it is low in the sulfur amino acids. Shiitake, *Lentinus edodes*, the popular forest mushroom from Japan appears to be a somewhat poorer source of lysine, but well-balanced otherwise, *Pleurotus ostreatus*, the oyster mushroom, is also well-balanced. The poorest balanced of all of the mushrooms is apparently *Volvariella*, the paddy mushroom.

While much has been done in recent years to acclaim yeasts as the answer to the protein shortage, amino acids of brewer's yeast are not as well-balanced as those of mushrooms with the exception of *Volvariella*. Table 3 shows that only the amino acid ratios of *Volvariella* and brewer's yeast vary by more than $\pm$ 20% of the mean if tryptophan and the sulfur amino acids are disregarded. The sulfur amino acids also deviate more from the mean values for brewer's yeast than they do for A. *bisporus*.

The yeast analyses in Table 4 are on a dry weight basis and the mushrooms on a wet weight basis. Since mushrooms are 89 to 92%

Table 3

Comparison of Essential Amino Acids in Mushrooms to Those in Eggs.
Figures Expressed as the Ratios of Data From Table 2

	Ratio of items	Ile	Leu	Lys	Phe	Tyr	Thr	Trp
Agaricus bisporus	# 2/12	.655	.735	.822	.665	.769	.800	1.075
Lentinus edodes	# 6/12	.575	.655	.414	.758	.697	.850	---
Pleurotus ostreatus	# 7/12	.475	.543	.461	.538	.504	.635	.655
Volvariella diplasia	#10/12	.875	.399	.615	.854	.385	.821	.742
Brewer's yeast	#11/12	.928	.905	1.295	.845	.995	1.082	---

	Ratio of items	Val	Cys	Met	Total essential	Total amino acids
Agaricus bisporus,	# 2/12	.688	.329	.420	.705	.800
Lentinus edodes	# 6/12	.635	---	---	---	.800
Pleurotus ostreatus	# 7/12	.635	---	---	.489	.603
Volvariella diplasia	#10/12	.993	---	---	.685	---
Brewer's yeast	#11/12	1.071	.368	.477	.955	.943

Table 4

Vitamins in Mushrooms and Yeasts. Quantities Per 100 Gm

	Thiamine mg	Riboflavin mg	Niacin mg	Ascorbic acid mg	Vit. K	Pantothenic acid mg	Biotin mg	Pyridoxin mg	Folic acid mg	Vit. D i.u.
Torula yeast, dry[a]	14.01	5.60	44.4	trace	--	--	--	--	--	--
Brewer's yeast, dry	15.61	4.28	37.9	trace	--	--	--	--	--	--
Agaricus bisporus, fresh[a]	0.10	0.46	4.2	3.0	--	--	--	--	--	--
Agaricus bisporus, canned[a]	0.02	0.25	2.0	2.0	--	--	--	--	--	--
Agaricus bisporus, fresh[b]	0.12	0.52	5.85	8.6	+	2.38	0.018	(0.45)	(0.98)	--
Lentinus edodes, dry[c]	+	+	+	--	--	--	--	+	--	40000

+ = Present, no indication of quantity. -- = No data.

[a]Watt and Merrill (1963). [c]Mori (1974).

[b]Esselen and Fellers (1946).

315

water, as are many vegetables, the values for the mushrooms must be multiplied by about ten to be comparable to yeast. Also, while yeasts have a higher thiamine content, mushrooms have more ascorbic acid. Riboflavin and niacin contents of mushrooms and yeasts differ little. The data of Esselen and Fellers (1946) shown in Table 4 appear to be a collection of their highest rather than their average values. Their routine analyses appear to agree better with the results of Watt and Merrill (1963). Mushrooms contain a variety of other vitamins in addition to those most commonly indicated. While most fungi produce ergosterol, provitamin D, shiitake dried in the sun or under ultraviolet light contains up to 400 i.u. of vitamin D per gram of mushroom on a dry weight basis (Mori, 1974). Mori also makes broad claims for the health giving properties of this mushroom. Some special beneficial properties have also been claimed for the oyster mushroom (Yoshioka et al., 1972).

Even with the advantages of mushrooms, the comparison of mushrooms to yeasts may indeed be futile. It is hard to imagine anyone sitting down to a big dish of yeast which was not disguised in some manner. However, a dish of mushrooms is a gourmet's delight. Also, it is possible to grow mushrooms commercially with relatively simple equipment. The cultivation of yeast requires sophisticated and expensive fermentors.

In summary, mushrooms are a good source of protein. Conflicting reports of the food value of mushrooms have lead to confusion and resulting lack of confidence in the nutritional adequacy of this palatable food. A number of developing nations with protein deficient diets are producing mushrooms for export and import more expensive protein of no greater value.

LITERATURE CITED

Aronson, J. M. 1965. The cell wall. *In* The Fungi, eds. G. C. Ainsworth and A. S. Sussman, Vol. I, p. 49. Academic Press, New York.

MUSHROOMS AS A SOURCE OF PROTEIN

Chang, S.-T. 1972. The Chinese Mushroom. The Chinese University of Hong Kong, Hong Kong.

Chiou, C. M., S. Cheng, and H. H. Wang. 1972. Quality control of rice-straw composting for mushroom cultivation. Mushroom Sci. 8:343.

Doesburg, J. J. and A. Meijer. 1965. Analyse van Nederlandse blikconserven. II. Groente en vruchtenprodukten. Voeding 25: 258.

Esselen, W. B., Jr., and C. R. Fellers. 1946. Mushrooms for food and flavor. Mass. Agr. Expt. Sta. Bull., No. 434.

FAO. 1970. Nutritional studies no. 24. Amino Acid Contents of Foods and Biological Data on Proteins. Rome.

Ganney, G. W. 1973. Economics of mushroom growing, 1975. Mushroom J. 1973:352.

Gyurko, P. 1972. Die Rolle der Belichtung bei dem Anbau des Austernseitlings (Pleurotus ostreatus). Mushroom Sci. 8:461.

Kalberer, P. and U. Kunsch. 1974. Amino acid composition of the mushroom oyster (pleurotus ostreatus). Food Sci. Technol. 7:242.

Kurtzman, R. H., Jr. 1975. Summary of mushroom culture. Pakistan Agricultural Research Council, Karachi (in press).

Mendel, J. B. 1898. The chemical composition and nutritive value of some edible American fungi. Am. J. Physiol. 1:225.

Mori, K. 1974. Mushrooms as Health Foods. Japan Publications, Inc., Tokyo.

Schisler, L. C. and P. J. Wuest. 1973. A few practical tips on compost and the composting process. Mushroom News 21:(11)4.

Schroeder, M. E., L. C. Schisler, R. Sneisinger, V. E. Crowley, and W. L. Barr. 1974. Transport of MTDF trays at casing to conventional mushroom doubles. Mushroom News 22:(11)15.

Seelkopf, C. and H. Schuster. 1957. Qualitative and quantitative Aminosaurebestimmungen and einigen wichtigen Speisepilzen. Z. Lebensmittel-Unters. u.-Forsch. 106:177.

Sugimori, T., Y. Oyama, and T. Omichi. 1971. Studies of basidio-mycetes. I. Production of mycelium and fruiting body from noncarbohydrate organic substances. J. Ferment. Technol. 49:435.

Watt, B. K. and A. L. Merrill. 1963. Composition of Foods. Agricultural Handbook No. 8, U.S. Department of Agriculture, Washington.

Yoshioka, Y., T. Ikekawa, M. Noda, and F. Fukuoka. 1972. Studies on antitumor activity of some fractions from basidiomycetes. I. An antitumor acidic polysaccharide fraction of P. ostreatus Quel. Chem. Pharm. Bull. 20:1175.

317

Zadrazil, F. 1973. Anbauverfahren fur *Pleurotus florida* FovoSe. Der Champignon 13:(139).

Zakia, B., K. S. Srinivasan, and H. C. Srivastava. 1963. Amino acid composition of the protein from a mushroom. (*Pleurotus sp.*) Appl. Microbiol. 11:184.

Zakia, B., K. S. Srinivasan, and N. S. Singh. 1971. Essential amino composition of the protein of a mushroom. (*Volvariella diplasia.*) J. Food Sci. Technol. 8:180.

13

NUTRITIONAL EVALUATION OF ALFALFA LEAF PROTEIN CONCENTRATE

E. M. Bickoff, A. N. Booth, D. de Fremery, R. H. Edwards,
B. E. Knuckles, R. E. Miller, R. M. Saunders, and G. O. Kohler
Western Regional Research Laboratory
Agricultural Research Service
U.S. Department of Agriculture
Berkeley, California

The nutritive value of whole leaf protein concentrate (LPC) and of the green and white fractions prepared from alfalfa by the Pro-Xan and Pro-Xan II processes was evaluated by both chemical and biological methods. The amino acid patterns show that the white fraction contains sufficient amounts of the essential amino acids and in the proper balance to serve as a high quality food supplement. It has an amino acid score of 100 based on the provisional amino acid scoring pattern (FAO, 1973) and a protein digestibility of 99% by an in vitro assay.

The predicted high quality evaluation obtained by chemical means was confirmed by an in vivo protein digestibility of 99% and a protein efficiency ratio (PER) value equivalent to that of casein.

Both the PER and protein digestibility of the white protein fraction were influenced by a number of processing variables including pretreatment of the fresh alfalfa with bisulfite, employment of heat to coagulate the protein, use of a dilute acid wash to remove soluble, deleterious components, and drying methods and temperatures.

The green fraction was slightly lower in lysine and total

sulfur amino acids. The PER of this fraction was about 1.7. The first and second limiting amino acids for the rat are methionine and lysine, respectively.

INTRODUCTION

From a nutritional standpoint it has been shown that the vegetative growth of alfalfa contains satisfactory amounts of all the eight essential amino acids with the possible exception of methionine (Livingston et al., 1971). Leaf protein concentrates (LPC) have been reported to contain more lysine than the best high lysine corn, more methionine than soybean protein, and to compare favorably with animal proteins (Akeson and Stahmann, 1965). The isolation of this leaf protein for food was advocated by Pirie in the early 1940's (Pirie, 1942). More recently, Olatunbosun et al. (1972) and Kamalanathan et al. (1969) have reported results of feeding and acceptability trials incorporating LPC in human diets.

In 1947, this laboratory described a pilot plant procedure for obtaining LPC in bulk, free from the fibrous mass of green vegetation (Bickoff et al., 1947).

More recently, we developed a process for the preparation of whole leaf protein concentrate (the Pro-Xan process) (Kohler et al., 1968). This process was commercialized in 1969 for the preparation of a product which was employed primarily in poultry rations (Kohler and Bickoff, 1971). A somewhat similar process has been reported in Hungary (Hollo and Koch, 1971). It is possible to separate the whole leaf proteins into two fractions by differential heat coagulation (Subba Rau et al., 1969), and practical conditions for this separation were recently reported (de Fremery et al., 1973; Bickoff and Kohler, 1974). One of the products is a bland-tasting, off-white protein fraction more acceptable for human consumption. This product has recently been carried through pilot plant production at our laboratory (Edwards et al., 1973).

The present report evaluates the quality of pilot plant

ALFALFA LEAF PROTEIN CONCENTRATE

preparations of the several LPC products by chemical and biological methods. Studies have emphasized attempts to minimize any detrimental effects of the processing variables and to develop optimum processing conditions.

MATERIALS AND METHODS

The Pro-Xan processes for the preparation of LPC have been described completely elsewhere (Kohler et al., 1968; Knuckles et al., 1970; Kohler and Bickoff, 1971; Spencer et al., 1971; de Fremery et al., 1973; Edwards et al., 1973; Bickoff and Kohler, 1974). To obviate the need to consult this literature, a brief description of the processes and products is presented.

For purposes of this and future papers from this laboratory, the total heat coagulable protein of the press juice of fresh alfalfa plants is called Pro-Xan or whole leaf protein concentrate (whole LPC). When the protein is fractionated as in the Pro-Xan II process, a green protein fraction is obtained which is designated "green-fraction LPC" or "Pro-Xan II." This fraction is called chloroplastic protein by some although a part of the protein originally in the chloroplast is not included in this fraction and a portion of the true cytoplasmic protein is included. The light-colored protein fraction from the fractionation process is referred to as "white LPC" or "white protein," although some preparations may have a tan or grayish cast. It is a mixture of proteins from the cytoplasm and from subcellular bodies in the cytoplasm. A major fraction of the white protein is the enzyme ribulose diphosphate carboxylase (also known as Fraction I protein or 18 S protein) which comes from the chloroplasts during the maceration and pressing of the leaves (Siegel et al., 1972). For this reason we feel that the use of "cytoplasmic" and "chloroplastic" proteins for the fractionated products, as has been general practice in the past, should be abandoned.

Pilot Scale Preparation of Leaf Protein Concentrates

Whole LPC was prepared by heat coagulation of juice from freshly harvested, ammoniated alfalfa. The coagulated protein was separated from the serum, and drained. The drained material was then dried directly or pressed prior to drying.

Preparation of white LPC involves a protein fractionation and employs an initial mild heat treatment of the whole alfalfa juice, followed by centrifugation to remove the green protein fraction. This green fraction is then heated to temperatures above 85°C to form a curd which can be readily pressed and dried. The green-fraction LPC contains considerably less protein than whole LPC and is also considered most suitable as a feed-grade product because of its grassy flavor and green color.

The clear brown solution remaining after the removal of the green proteins is heated to 80°C to coagulate the white protein fraction. After thorough washing, the product may be spray-dried.

Bisulfite Addition

In a number of experiments, a solution of sodium metabisulfite was added to the chopped alfalfa as it was conveyed to the press. It was added at a rate equivalent to either 200 or 1000 ppm SO_2, based on the wet weight of the fresh alfalfa.

Drying of LPC Preparations

Studies were made of a number of different methods of drying, including freeze-drying, rotary air drying, vacuum drying, and forced air drying (Miller et al., 1972).

Washing of LPC Preparations

Washing was accomplished by resuspending one part of wet precipitate in 50 parts of acidified wash water. The precipitate was then recovered by filtration or centrifugation.

ALFALFA LEAF PROTEIN CONCENTRATE

IN VITRO EVALUATION OF NUTRITIVE VALUE

Amino Acid Score

To calculate the amino acid score, the content of each essential amino acid in the LPC is expressed as a percentage of the content of the same amino acid in the scoring pattern selected as the standard. For the laboratory rat, the standard employed was the amino acid scoring pattern described by Rama Rao et al. (1964). For the human, the standard employed was the 1973 provisional amino acid scoring pattern of the FAO (1973). The essential amino acid that shows the largest percentage is the limiting amino acid, and this percentage is called the amino acid score.

In Vitro Protein Digestibility

Protein digestibility was determined by the pepsin-trypsin method of Saunders et al. (1973). The protein was incubated in 0.1 N HCl with 5% of its weight of pepsin at 37°C for 48 hr, centrifuged, and washed. It was then reincubated with trypsin (0.5% of its weight) at pH 8 and 23°C for 16 hr, and the total solubilized nitrogen determined.

E/T Ratio

The E/T ratio is expressed as the content of total essential amino acids (in grams) per gram of nitrogen in the sample.

BIOLOGICAL EVALUATION OF NUTRITIVE VALUE

Protein efficiency ratio (PER) and in vivo protein digestibility were employed for the determination of biological value (AOAC, 1970; Saunders et al., 1973). For the feeding trials, groups of five weanling male rats, initial age 22 days (Sprague-Dawley strain), were housed in individual wire-bottom stainless steel cages and were provided feed and water ad libitum during the

4-week assay. The diets, including that of the casein control, were formulated to contain 10% protein (N x 6.25). Diets were adjusted to contain equal levels of moisture, fat, and fiber. From the 7th to the 14th day of the experiment, the feces were collected from each group and the weights and moisture and nitrogen contents were determined. Excreted fecal nitrogen values were corrected for metabolic fecal nitrogen. This was determined on a separate group of rats fed a 10% casein diet for 26 days and then fed a nitrogen-free diet for nine days during which fecal collections were made. In vivo nitrogen digestibility (%) was calculated as follows:

$$\text{Nitrogen Digestibility} = \frac{\text{N in feed} - (\text{N in feces} - \text{metabolic N})}{\text{N in feed}} \times 100$$

PER values were calculated as follows:

$$\text{PER} = \frac{\text{g gain / g N in feed (sample)}}{\text{g gain / g N in feed (casein)}} \times 2.5$$

CHEMICAL ANALYSES

Moisture, nitrogen, ash, crude fat, crude fiber, and nitrogen-free extract were determined by standard AOAC methods (AOAC, 1970). Soluble solids were determined by extracting 1 g of solids with 20 ml of distilled water in a shaker for 16 hr. Amino acids were determined by the ion exchange chromatography procedure of Kohler and Palter (1967) on a modified Phoenix amino acid analyzer (Model K-8000). Tryptophan was determined by the procedure of Lombard and de Lange (1965).

RESULTS

The composition of the various LPCs evaluated in the present study is presented in Table 1. The crude protein content of the whole LPC and the green-fraction LPC are in the range of 45-60%, whereas the white LPC is higher in protein but lower in fat, fiber,

and ash. The high ash in the green products may be reduced by a
dilute acid wash. Since the largest part of the lipid fraction
remains associated with the green products, less than 1% crude fat
is found in the white LPC.

In a recent review paper, Byers (1971) reports that the amino
acid composition of whole LPC from different species, including
alfalfa, is quite similar. The largest differences are in the
amounts of the S-containing amino acids and of lysine and proline.
Our results with whole LPC (Table 2) are in the range of those reported in this review. In a study of several plants (not including
alfalfa), Byers also reported that the so-called "cytoplasmic" and
"chloroplastic" proteins (designated by us, white LPC and green-
fraction LPC, respectively) have different compositions. However,
she did not present results on tryptophan and cystine. She found
less leucine and substantially more histidine and lysine in the
"cytoplasmic" than in the "chloroplastic" fraction. Our results on
green and white products confirm her observations on leucine, histidine, and lysine, but we find also that the white LPC is higher
in arginine, threonine, glutamic acid, cystine, and tyrosine, and
is lower in glycine, serine, isoleucine, and phenylalanine. Data
in Table 2 show that white LPC prepared from sulfite-treated
alfalfa contains higher levels of methionine and cystine.

The amino acid scores for rats and in vitro digestibilities
are shown in Table 3. The data indicate that total sulfur amino
acids and lysine are about equally limiting in all three products.
However, the score for the white LPC is substantially higher than
those for the green products. The digestibilities are higher than
those encountered by other workers in the field (Byers, 1971). The
value of the white LPC (97%) is comparable to egg and milk proteins.

The nutritional value of Pro-Xan and Pro-Xan II, prepared in
the pilot plant but dried and washed under different conditions, is
illustrated in Table 4. It is interesting to note that even though
Pro-Xan II contained less of the highly nutritious white LPC than
did Pro-Xan, the PER values and nitrogen digestibilities were essentially the same. Heating the centrifuge sludge to about 85°C, as

TABLE 1

Proximate Composition of Alfalfa LPC (Dry Basis)

Fraction	Nitrogen %	Crude protein[a] %	Fat %	Fiber %	Ash %	Nitrogen-free extract %	Soluble solids %
Whole LPC (Pro-Xan)							
Drained	8.64	54.00	6.52	1.24	14.68	23.56	24.8
Pressed	9.90	61.85	8.89	1.66	11.08	16.52	8.1
Green-fraction LPC (Pro-Xan II)	7.24	45.25	13.29	4.35	15.64	21.47	7.9
White LPC	14.19	88.69	<0.6	<1.0	0.39	9.32	0.3

[a]% N x 6.25.

TABLE 2

Amino Acid Composition of Alfalfa LPC[a]

Amino acid	Whole LPC		Green-fraction LPC	White LPC	
	Drained	Pressed		-HSO$_3$	+HSO$_3$[b]
Alanine	6.07	5.55	6.28	6.31	6.35
(Ammonia)	1.61	1.30	1.39	1.16	1.07
Arginine	6.17	5.99	6.14	7.46	7.98

Aspartic acid	10.44	9.43	10.27	10.69	10.04
Cystine	1.25	1.16	1.00	1.44	1.68
Glutamic acid	11.18	10.25	11.03	12.00	12.02
Glycine	5.21	4.88	5.71	5.12	5.52
Histidine	2.45	2.33	2.42	2.93	3.19
Isoleucine	5.24	4.94	6.19	5.46	5.28
Leucine	8.92	8.19	10.26	9.37	9.42
Lysine	6.31	6.18	5.88	6.54	6.43
Methionine	2.02	2.09	2.16	2.27	2.65
Phenylalanine	5.78	5.25	6.62	6.25	6.36
Proline	4.69	4.41	4.46	4.67	4.44
Serine	4.42	4.00	5.09	3.93	3.65
Threonine	5.01	4.81	4.71	5.76	5.70
Tryptophan	1.65	1.38	0.96	2.40	2.45
Tyrosine	4.58	4.09	4.54	5.43	5.63
Valine	6.41	6.25	6.99	7.19	6.91
% N recovered	91.92	85.20	92.61	96.82	97.65
E/T ratio	2.95	2.77	3.08	3.26	3.28

[a] Grams amino acid / 16 grams nitrogen.

[b] 1000 ppm SO_2 in the form of sodium metabisulfite was sprayed on the fresh alfalfa prior to juice expression.

TABLE 3

In Vitro Evaluation of Alfalfa LPC for Rats[a]

Amino acid	Rat amino acid scoring pattern[b]	Amino acid composition		
		Pro-Xan	Pro-Xan II	White LPC
Histidine	2.5	2.33	2.42	2.93
Isoleucine	5.5	4.94	6.19	5.46
Leucine	7.0	8.19	10.26	9.37
Lysine	9.0	6.18	5.88	6.54
Methionine	1.6	2.09	2.16	2.27
Methionine + cystine	5.0	3.25	3.16	3.71
Phenylalanine	4.2	5.25	6.62	6.25
Phenylalanine + tyrosine	7.2	9.34	11.16	11.68
Threonine	5.0	4.81	4.71	5.76
Tryptophan	1.1	1.38	0.96	2.40
Valine	5.5	6.25	6.99	7.19
In vitro digestibility (%)	--	88	87	97
Amino acid score[c]				
1st limiting amino acid	--	65(S)	63(S)	73(L)
2nd limiting amino acid	--	69(L)	65(L)	74(S)

[a]Grams amino acid / 16 grams nitrogen.

[b]Rama Rao et al., 1964.

[c]Letter in ( ) refers to limiting amino acid; S = total S-containing amino acids, L = lysine.

required in the process to coagulate the protein, caused no reduction in PER values, nor did acid washing of the freeze-dried products (Experiment 1). Freeze-dried and vacuum oven-dried samples had the highest PER values, the forced draft oven-dried samples had slightly lower values, and the rotary air-dried samples, with the highest drying temperatures, had the lowest PER values. No large changes in nitrogen digestibility were observed. These results tend to agree with those of earlier workers (Duckworth and Woodham, 1961; Henry and Ford, 1965; Shah et al., 1967; Buchanan, 1969; Woodham, 1971) in that drying at 100°C is harmful, the product of such treatment being much reduced in biological value. In our case, acid washing of the rotary air-dried sample brought the PER almost back to the value for freeze-dried material. Since an acid wash of the freeze-dried LPC had no effect on improving nutritional quality, it appears that the drying operation at high temperatures produces a growth-depressing factor which is soluble in dilute acid. Thus the precursor of this factor is probably present in the brown juice.

Working with rats, a number of workers have reported that methionine enhances the nutritive value of LPC (Duckworth and Woodham, 1961; Byers, 1971; Woodham, 1971). These observations were confirmed in the present investigation (Table 5). In Experiment 1, addition of methionine increased the corrected PER from 1.74 to 2.77. When lysine was added alone (Experiment 2), no growth enhancement resulted. However, when methionine was added in sufficient amounts, the further addition of lysine did produce additional growth response (Experiments 2 and 3), indicating that lysine was the second limiting amino acid.

Table 6 presents the results of amino acid supplementation on white LPC. The PER values for the unsupplemented materials are considerably higher than those for the green proteins which range from 1.6 to 1.8. Subba Rau et al. (1969) showed similar differences between the green and white protein fractions, but our PER values are higher than his for both products. The amino acid scores in Table 3 indicate that methionine and lysine are equally limiting for the rat in white LPC. In contrast to what might be expected from chemical scores, but in agreement with other workers (Shurpalekar et al., 1969; Hove et al., 1974; Myer and Cheeke, 1974), methionine produced a marked enhancement in the PER in the absence of lysine

TABLE 4

Effect of Processing Variables on Nutritive Value of Green Products

Experiment #	Dietary source of protein	Drying conditions	Subsequent wash	Weight gain g	PER[a] (corrected)	Nitrogen digestibility %
1	Casein	--	--	113	2.50a	99.6
1	Pro-Xan	Freeze-dried	--	64	1.68b	87.8
1	Pro-Xan	Freeze-dried	pH 3.5	63	1.67b	86.4
1	Centrifuge sludge	Freeze-dried	--	55	1.64b	83.1
1	Pro-Xan II	Freeze-dried	--	61	1.67b	85.1
1	Pro-Xan II	Freeze-dried	pH 3.5	72	1.83b	87.9
2	Casein	--	--	114	2.50a	100
2	Pro-Xan	Freeze-dried	--	55	1.63b	86.3
2	Pro-Xan	Forced air[b]	--	52	1.53b	85.5
3	Casein	--	--	98	2.50a	100
3	Pro-Xan	Freeze-dried	--	50	1.75b	86.8
3	Pro-Xan	Freeze-dried	pH 3.5	61	1.81b	89.1
3	Pro-Xan	Freeze-dried	pH 3.5[c]	58	1.78b	87.8
3	Pro-Xan	Rotary hot air[d]	--	38	1.14c	89.6
3	Pro-Xan	Rotary hot air[d]	pH 3.5	50	1.71b	94.3

[a]Within each experiment, means followed by the same letter are judged not significantly different at the 5% probability level.

[b]Sample dried at 80°C in forced draft oven for four hours.

[c]Sample dried at 60°C in vacuum oven after acid wash. All other acid-washed samples freeze-dried.

[d]Sample dried in rotary hot air drier; inlet temperature, 250°C, outlet temperature, 80°C.

ALFALFA LEAF PROTEIN CONCENTRATE

TABLE 5

Effect of Methionine and Lysine Supplementation on Nutritive Value of Whole LPC

Experiment #	Dietary source of protein	Methionine supplement %	Lysine supplement %	Weight gain g	PER[a] (corrected)	Nitrogen digestibility %
1	Casein	--	--	98	2.50b	101.2
1	Pro-Xan	--	--	57	1.74c	88.1
1	Pro-Xan	0.1	--	133	2.77a	87.8
2	Casein	--	--	100	2.50b	100
2	Pro-Xan	--	--	61	1.87c	85.4
2	Pro-Xan	--	0.3	54	1.70d	87.0
2	Pro-Xan	0.4	--	121	2.57b	88.6
2	Pro-Xan	0.4	0.3	143	2.86a	87.7
3	Casein	--	--	106	2.50b	99.6
3	Pro-Xan	--	--	73	1.84c	87.7
3	Pro-Xan	0.2	--	140	2.63b	87.7
3	Pro-Xan	0.2	0.3	161	2.83a	86.8
3	Pro-Xan	0.4	0.3	172	2.97a	88.0

[a]Within each experiment, means followed by the same letter are judged not significantly different at the 5% probability level.

TABLE 6

Effect of Methionine and Lysine
Supplementation on Nutritive Value of White LPC

Dietary source of protein	Methionine supplement %	Lysine supplement %	Weight gain g	PER[a] (corrected)	Nitrogen digestibility %
Casein	--	--	106	2.50d	99.6
White LPC	--	--	112	2.40de	98.7
White LPC	--	0.3	98	2.31e	98.2
White LPC	0.2	--	156	2.76c	97.8
White LPC	0.2	0.3	188	3.06b	98.7
White LPC	0.4	0.3	198	3.24a	98.6

[a]Means followed by the same letter are judged not significantly different at the 5% probability level.

supplementation. Since lysine supplementation alone produced no PER enhancement, it appears that methionine is the first limiting amino acid. However, lysine produced a supplementary response in white LPC which had been fortified with methionine, indicating that lysine is the second limiting amino acid.

Data in Table 7 demonstrate that addition of bisulfite during processing improves the nutritive value of white LPC. Bisulfite treatment of the fresh alfalfa prior to juice expression yields products with PER values greater than that of casein. This result is not unexpected, recalling that addition of bisulfite during processing increased the concentration of sulfur amino acids (Table 2). Data in Table 8 confirm that treatment with bisulfite during processing increased the PER values of white LPC. Supplementation of sulfite-treated and untreated products with methionine produced high PER values not significantly different from each other. This indicates that the effect of bisulfite treatment in increasing PER values is due to its protective effect on the sulfur amino acids. The bisulfite treatment is also effective in preventing the formation of colored oxidation products which tend to give a tan or brown color to the protein concentrate.

TABLE 7

Effect of Bisulfite Addition During Processing on Nutritive Value of White LPC

Experiment #	Dietary source of protein	pH of wash	Bisulfite level (ppm SO_2)	Weight gain g	PER[a] (corrected)	Nitrogen digestibility %
1	Casein	--	0	125	2.50a	99.8
1	White LPC	4.5	0	119	2.15b	95.6
1	White LPC	4.5	1000	160	2.57a	97.8
2	Casein	--	0	116	2.50a	101.8
2	White LPC	4.5	0	96	2.13b	96.2
2	White LPC	4.5	1000	139	2.54a	99.6
3	Casein	--	0	110	2.50b	100.1
3	White LPC	4.5	0	95	2.23c	97.0
3	White LPC	4.5	200	98	2.30c	97.3
3	White LPC	4.5	1000	160	2.84a	98.7
4	Casein	--	0	120	2.50a	100
4	White LPC	6.5	0	105	2.27b	96.9
4	White LPC	6.5	200	121	2.56a	97.6
4	White LPC	6.5	1000	141	2.58a	98.4

[a]Within each experiment, means followed by the same letter are judged not significantly different at the 5% probability level.

TABLE 8

Combined Effect of Methionine and
Bisulfite on Nutritive Value of White LPC

Dietary source of protein	Methionine supplement %	Bisulfite level (ppm SO_2)	Weight gain g	PER^a (corrected)	Nitrogen digestibility %
Casein	--	--	120	2.50b	100
White LPC	--	0	105	2.27c	96.9
White LPC	--	200	121	2.56b	97.6
White LPC	--	1000	141	2.58b	98.4
White LPC	0.2	0	178	2.91a	94.0
White LPC	0.2	200	165	2.92a	97.8
White LPC	0.2	1000	154	2.84a	98.6

[a]Means followed by the same letter are judged not
significantly different at the 5% probability level.

DISCUSSION

In the development of new protein sources, in vitro protein
digestibility and amino acid score (based on amino acid composition
and amino acid requirements) are useful initial screening procedures. However, these chemical tests are not sufficient in themselves. Biological testing is mandatory even when the food has
been prepared from raw material which has been eaten by man and
animals from earliest times. The possible presence of toxic or
growth-inhibitory components, whether caused by processing damage
or enrichment of trace toxins, also requires that tests on animals
be carried out.

In vitro and in vivo protein digestibilities of 97-99% and
chemical scores of 100 based on the provisional amino acid pattern
(FAO, 1973) predict that white LPC contains sufficient amounts of
the essential amino acids and in the proper balance to serve as a
high quality food (Table 9).

In earlier reports, rat growth and protein digestibility

TABLE 9

In Vitro Evaluation of Alfalfa LPC for Humans[a]

Amino acid	Adult amino acid scoring pattern[b]	Amino acid composition		
		Washed whole LPC	White LPC	Whole egg[c]
Isoleucine	4.0	5.42	5.28	6.29
Leucine	7.0	9.31	9.42	8.82
Lysine	5.5	6.21	6.43	6.98
Methionine + cystine	3.5	3.47	4.33	5.79
Phenylalanine + tyrosine	6.0	11.44	11.99	9.89
Threonine	4.0	4.95	5.70	5.12
Tryptophan	1.0	1.38	2.45	1.49
Valine	5.0	6.19	6.91	6.85
In vitro digestibility (%)	--	88	97	100
Amino acid score	--	99	100(117)	100(126)
1st limiting amino acid	--	Met + Cys	Lys	Leu

[a]Grams amino acid / 16 grams nitrogen.
[b]FAO, 1973.
[c]FAO, 1970.

studies have shown LPC to be superior to wheat, soybeans, and beef, and to approach that of milk protein (Akeson and Stahmann, 1965). The biological evaluation obtained for white LPC in the present study confirms the predictive high quality evaluation obtained by chemical means.

Our biological studies have shown that methionine supplementation of whole LPC or white LPC produced increased performance. Lysine supplements by themselves produced no response, but when added in addition to methionine they did produce a response. These

results would not be expected from the rat chemical scores which
indicate that lysine and sulfur amino acids are equally limiting.
We therefore conclude that the chemical scores are not predictive
in these samples. It should be pointed out that the performic acid
oxidation method for methionine and cystine determination includes
any preformed methionine sulfoxide, methionine sulfone, cystine
monoxide, cystine dioxide, cystenic acid, and cysteic acid which
might have been in the samples either originally or formed by
oxidation during preparation. Research at this laboratory using
photoelectron emission spectroscopy (ESCA) has shown that such
oxidized sulfur amino acids do indeed occur in these and other processed proteins in substantial amounts (Walker et al., Part 1).
Since rats and chicks cannot utilize cysteic acid or methionine
sulfone, and the partially oxidized forms are only partially
utilized as essential amino acids, the true chemical scores are
lower than those shown.

The results with sulfite strengthen the idea that methionine
and/or cystine is being lost during the processing steps. Sulfite
increases PER values and reduces the increment of gain obtainable
by methionine supplementation. The reason for the increases in
chemical assay values of methionine and cystine may be related to
the instability of the intermediately oxidized compounds to acid
during the performic acid oxidation and their stabilization by
sulfite. Further work will be necessary to clarify these questions.

Since nutritional requirements of weanling rats are considerably greater than that of man (Rama Rao et al., 1964; FAO, 1973),
translating these results to humans is difficult. Feeding trials
with humans are still required as the ultimate criterion of quality.
Limited studies by Waterlow (1962) and Olatunbosun et al. (1972)
with washed whole LPC demonstrate the value of its use as a protein-
rich supplement in the treatment of protein malnutrition of children.

Since white LPC would not be used as the sole protein source,
its true value must be assessed by its ability to make good the

TABLE 10

Comparison of Amino Acid Score and
E/T Ratio of Alfalfa LPC and Common Foods[a]

Protein	Amino acid score[b]	E/T ratio
FAO recommendation	100	2.25
Hen's egg, whole	100(126)	3.20
Beef muscle	100(101)	2.78
Cow's milk, untreated	95	2.95
Casein	91	3.21
Soybean seed	74	2.46
Rice, polished	66	2.39
Wheat, whole grain	53	2.05
Maize, whole meal	49	2.51
White LPC (sulfite-treated)	100(117)	3.28
Whole LPC (washed)	99	3.02

[a]Data for common foods from FAO (1970).

[b]Calculated according to the essential amino acid scoring pattern of FAO (1973).

deficiencies in other protein-containing foodstuffs. The excellence of the material as a complement for other protein sources is shown by its high content of essential amino acids as compared with other foods (see Table 10) and especially its high level of lysine. Rat tests showing such complementary effects have been reported for combinations of whole LPC with rice, corn, wheat flour, powdered milk, dried cod, and cassava (Miller, 1965; Eggum, 1970; Woodham, 1971). Amino acid scores (Table 10) show that white LPC from alfalfa, with an amino acid score of over 100, is nutritionally comparable with egg, meat, and milk in protein nutritional quality.

REFERENCES

Akeson, W.R. and M.A. Stahmann. 1965. Nutritive value of leaf protein concentrate, an in vitro digestion study. J. Agr. Food Chem. 13:146.

AOAC. 1970. Official Methods of Analysis (11th Ed.). Association of Official Agricultural Chemists, Washington, D.C.

Bickoff, E.M., A. Bevenue and K.T. Williams. 1947. Alfalfa has promising chemurgic future--a novel processing method is described. Chemurgic Digest. 6:213.

Bickoff, E.M. and G.O. Kohler. 1974. Preparation of edible protein of leafy green crops such as alfalfa. U.S. Patent No. 3,823,128.

Buchanan, R.A. 1969. In vivo and in vitro methods of measuring nutritive value of leaf protein preparations. Brit. J. Nutr. 23:533.

Byers, M. 1971. The amino acid composition of some leaf protein preparations. In N.W. Pirie (Ed.) Leaf Protein: Its Agronomy, Preparation, Quality and Use. International Biological Program Handbook 20. Blackwell, Oxford. p. 95.

de Fremery, D., R.E. Miller, R.H. Edwards, B.E. Knuckles, E.M. Bickoff and G.O. Kohler. 1973. Centrifugal separation of white and green protein fractions from alfalfa juice following controlled heating. J. Agr. Food Chem. 21:886.

Duckworth, J. and A.A. Woodham. 1961. Leaf protein concentrates. I. Effect of source of raw material and method of drying on protein value for chicks and rats. J. Sci. Food Agr. 12:5.

Edwards, R.H., R.E. Miller, D. de Fremery, B.E. Knuckles, E.M. Bickoff and G.O. Kohler. 1973. Abstract No. AGFD 78, 166th Meeting of the American Chemical Society. Chicago, Illinois.

Eggum, B.O. 1970. The protein quality of cassava leaves. Brit. J. Nutr. 24:761.

FAO Nutrition Studies No. 24. 1970. Amino acid content of foods and biological data on proteins. Rome, Italy.

FAO Nutritional Meetings Report Series No. 52. WHO Technical Report Series No. 522. 1973. Energy and protein requirements. Rome, Italy.

Henry, K.M. and J.E. Ford. 1965. The nutritive value of leaf protein concentrates determined in biological tests with rats and by microbiological methods. J. Sci. Food Agr. 16:425.

Hollo, J. and L. Koch. 1971. Commercial production in Hungary. In N.W. Pirie (Ed.) Leaf Protein: Its Agronomy, Preparation, Quality and Use. International Biological Program Handbook 20. Blackwell, Oxford. p. 63.

Hove, E.L., E. Lohrey, M.K. Urs and R.M. Allison. 1974. The effect of lucerne-protein concentrate in the diet on growth, reproduction and body composition of rats. Brit. J. Nutr. 31:147.

Kamalanathan, G., M.S. Usha and R.P. Devadas. 1969. Evaluation of acceptability of some recipes with leaf protein concentrates. J. Nutr. Dietetics. 6:12.

ALFALFA LEAF PROTEIN CONCENTRATE

Knuckles, B.E., R.R. Spencer, M.E. Lazar, E.M. Bickoff and G.O. Kohler. 1970. PRO-XAN process: incorporation and evaluation of sugar cane rolls in wet fractionation of alfalfa. J. Agr. Food Chem. 18:1086.

Kohler, G.O. and R. Palter. 1967. Studies on methods for amino acid analysis of wheat products. Cereal Chem. 44:512.

Kohler, G.O., E.M. Bickoff, R.R. Spencer, S.C. Witt and B.E. Knuckles. 1968. Wet processing of alfalfa for animal feed products. 10th Tech. Alfalfa Conference Proc., ARS-74-46. p. 71.

Kohler, G.O. and E.M. Bickoff. 1971. Commercial production from alfalfa in USA. In N.W. Pirie (Ed.) Leaf Protein: Its Agronomy, Preparation, Quality and Use. International Biological Program Handbook 20. Blackwell, Oxford. p. 69.

Kohler, G.O., H.G. Walker, D.D. Kuzmicky and S.C. Witt. Problems in analysis of sulfur amino acids in feeds and foods. See this volume.

Livingston, A.L., M.E. Allis and G.O. Kohler. 1971. Amino acid stability during alfalfa dehydration. J. Agr. Food Chem. 19:947.

Lombard, J.H. and D.J. de Lange. 1965. The chemical determination of tryptophan in foods and mixed diets. Anal. Biochem. 10:260.

Miller, D.S. 1965. Some nutritional problems in the utilization of nonconventional protein for human feeding. Recent Adv. Food Sci. 3:125.

Miller, R.E., R.H. Edwards, M.E. Lazar, E.M. Bickoff and G.O. Kohler. 1972. PRO-XAN process: air drying of alfalfa leaf protein concentrate. J. Agr. Food Chem. 20:1151.

Myer, R.O. and P.R. Cheeke. 1974. Protein quality evaluation of alfalfa protein concentrate with rats. Proc. West. Section Amer. Soc. Animal Sci. 25:166.

Olatunbosun, D.A., B.K. Adadevoh and O.L. Oke. 1972. Leaf protein: a new protein source for the management of protein calorie malnutrition in Nigeria. Nigerian Med. J. 2:195.

Pirie, N.W. 1942. Green leaves as a source of proteins and other nutrients. Nature. 149:251.

Rama Rao, P.B., H.W. Norton and B.C. Johnson. 1964. The amino acid composition and nutritive value of proteins. V. Amino acid requirements as a pattern for protein evaluation. J. Nutr. 82:88.

Saunders, R.M., M.A. Connor, A.N. Booth, E.M. Bickoff and G.O. Kohler. 1973. Measurement of digestibility of alfalfa protein concentrates by in vivo and in vitro methods. J. Nutr. 103:530.

Shah, F.H., Riaz-ud-Din and A. Salam. 1967. Effect of heat on the digestibility of leaf protein. I. Toxicity of the lipids and their oxidation products. Pakistan J. Sci. and Ind. Res. 10:39.

Shurpalekar, K.S., N. Singh and O.E. Sundaravalli. 1969. Nutritive value of leaf protein from lucerne (*Medicago sativa*): growth responses in rats at different protein levels and to supplementation with lysine and/or methionine. Indian J. Exp. Biol. 7:279.

Siegel, M.I., M. Wishnick and M.D. Lane. 1972. Ribulose-1,5-diphosphate carboxylase. *In* P.D. Boyer (Ed.) The Enzymes (3rd Ed.). Academic Press. vol. VI, p. 169.

Spencer, R.R., A.C. Mottola, E.M. Bickoff, J.P. Clark and G.O. Kohler. 1971. The PRO-XAN process: the design and evaluation of a pilot plant system for the coagulation and separation of the leaf protein from alfalfa juice. J. Agr. Food Chem. 19:504.

Subba Rau, B.H., S. Mahadeviah and N. Singh. 1969. Nutritional studies on whole-extract coagulated leaf protein and fractionated chloroplastic and cytoplasmic proteins from lucerne (*Medicago sativa*). J. Sci. Food Agr. 20:355.

Waterlow, J.C. 1962. The absorption and retention of nitrogen from leaf protein by infants recovering from malnutrition. Brit. J. Nutr. 16:531.

Woodham, A.A. 1971. The use of animal tests for the evaluation of leaf protein concentrates. *In* N.W. Pirie (Ed.) Leaf Protein: Its Agronomy, Preparation, Quality and Use. International Biological Program Handbook 20. Blackwell, Oxford. p. 115.

14

THE EFFECTS OF PROCESSING CONDITIONS ON
THE QUALITY OF LEAF PROTEIN

N. W. Pirie

Rothamsted Experimental Station
Harpenden, Hertfordshire, England

Amino acid analysis and experience on nonruminant herbivores suggest that leaf protein will be a useful food if not damaged during processing. Some members of the mixture loosely called leaf protein are conjugated with other substances, e.g., nucleic acids, lipids, and chlorophylls. All of them can form complexes with leaf components such as sugars, polyphenols, and unsaturated fatty acids. The dissociation of a preexisting complex and the prevention of the formation of one are often advantageous, but care is needed lest the pursuit of a desirable objective has other unwanted results. For example: some delay between making an extract and heat coagulation diminishes the amount of nucleic acid in the product but increases conjugation with polyphenols and so diminishes digestibility and availability of lysine and possibly the sulfur amino acids. Washing the coagulum at pH 4 makes filtration easy and removes any risk that alkaloids may be present, but, especially if protein was coagulated at the minimum temperature, increases the risk that photosensitizing pheophorbide will be made. Solvent extraction simplifies storage and removes color but also removes nutritionally valuable carotene and unsaturated fatty acids. The ideal preparative procedure will depend on the source of the leaf, the group of consumers for which the protein is intended, and the scale of intended consumption.

INTRODUCTION

Insofar as experience with animals is a valid guide, the use of leaves as a main, or even sole, food by nonruminant herbivores (such as rabbits and colobus monkeys) is evidence that extracted leaf protein (LP) should be a valuable human food. This expectation was reinforced by early amino acid analyses; it has been confirmed by more recent analyses (e.g., Byers, 1971). As would be expected from the number of different proteins that make up what is loosely called LP, there is little species variation. Differences in digestibility in vitro and in vivo have however been commented on. These claims need not be discussed until there is evidence that the preparations used were prepared and stored in exactly the same ways, and that the supposed differences between species are greater than differences between preparations made from the same species harvested at different ages. Methods for preparing LP in bulk are described elsewhere (Pirie, 1971, 1975).

pH OF EXTRACTION

Leaf protein separates more completely from leaf fiber if the pulp is made slightly alkaline; that has been agreed to for 50 years. There is disagreement over the advantage of adding alkali to a leaf pulp that is naturally at about pH 5.8 because, at increased pH, more pectic substances are extracted and contaminate the protein, the extract from many species would have to be reacidified before it would coagulate satisfactorily, and phenolic substances oxidize more rapidly. The relevance of the last point is discussed in the next section. On the other hand, carotene and xanthophyll are more readily oxidized in slightly acid conditions (Walsh and Hauge, 1953; Spencer et al., 1971; Arkcoll and Holden,

1973) and they are useful components of human and poultry food.

RAPIDITY OF COAGULATION AND SEPARATION OF THE COAGULUM

In leaves, some protein is associated with nucleic acids in
ribosomes, some with chlorophylls and lipids in chloroplasts, and
some is probably complexed in other ways. When pulping damages the
cells so that autolysis starts, these structures begin to dissoci-
ate. It had long been known that trichloroacetic acid (TCA) precipitates more nitrogen from leaf extracts than is precipitated by
boiling; Singh (1960) found that TCA precipitates nucleic acid as
well as protein whereas, unless heating is sudden, leaf ribonuclease destroys nucleic acid during heat coagulation. If there should
be concern over the amount of nucleic acid in LP made from a young
and actively growing crop, delay before coagulation and slow heating may be advisable.

Freshly made leaf extracts, cleared of chloroplast fragments
by high-speed centrifuging, are pale and quickly darken at the
surface. This is mainly because phenolic compounds are oxidized to
quinones; these can react with proteins. The agricultural aspects
of these processes are reviewed by Pierpoint (1971). It was obvious (Pirie, 1953, 1966) that this tanning process would interfere
with protein extraction and damage what protein was extracted.
This expectation arose both from general experience with leather
and from the observation (Bawden and Klezckowski, 1945) that there
is so much phenolic material in some leaves that extracts from them
contain no soluble protein. Tannins were incriminated by Hawkins
(1959) as the cause of the poor digestibility of lespedeza cuneata
hay and, conversely, were used by Delort-Laval and Zelter (1968) to
protect protein from microbial deamination in the rumen. Feeny
(1969) studied the diminished hydrolysis by trypsin of nettle leaf
protein complexed with oak leaf tannin. Complex formation at the
ε-amino group of lysine is an important feature of the tanning process; Allison et al. (1973) found good correlation among many

343

samples of LP between nutritive value, digestibility in vitro, and the amount of lysine in which the ε-amino group could be deaminated by nitrous acid.

Methionine reacts with o-quinone (Vithayathil and Murthy, 1972) and p-quinone reacts with other thioethers (Bosshard, 1972). There is no evidence for such reactions in the conditions to which LP is exposed during preparation, but they may happen, and in these conditions o-quinones react with cysteine (Roberts, 1959; Pierpoint, 1969). Because of the partial interchangeability of the sulfur amino acids, a reaction that makes cysteine unavailable could explain the better performance of rats when methionine is added to a diet containing LP which, according to chemical analysis, contains adequate methionine. Methionine sulfoxide is formed when leaf extracts are processed slowly (Pirie, 1970). It is sometimes assumed that this does not matter because free sulfoxide seems to be equivalent to methionine nutritionally. The formation of sulfoxide may however affect enzymic digestion, and nothing is known about the stereoisomerism (about the S atom) of sulfoxide formation and reduction.

Fully acetylated casein can still combine with quinones (Horigome, 1974). If this is the result of conjugation at peptide bonds, and if LP reacts similarly, digestibility would presumably be diminished. There is therefore good reason to expect that the more quickly a leaf extract is coagulated, and the more quickly the coagulum is removed from the fluid, the better. Results confirming this expectation have not yet been published fully but are adumbrated in the Rothamsted Experimental Station Report from 1969 to 1972.

It is unlikely that an extract could be made, coagulated, and filtered so quickly that there would be no reaction with tanning agents, but browning, and so presumably damage to the protein, can be prevented by adding sulfite during pulping and by diluting the extract before heat coagulation. There has been little systematic work on the choice of crops for LP production. When this work starts, the manipulation of genetics and husbandry so as to diminish the amount of phenolic and other tanning agents should be an important part of it. It is well known that they tend to increase with maturity (e.g., Milić, 1972); they are also increased by the stresses of cold and drought (Wong, 1973). When studying the extent to which tanning agents are responsible for either the poor extraction or the poor quality of some types of LP, it would be reasonable to use in the laboratory methods that could not be used in bulk preparation. For example: some extractions should be made with rigid exclusion of air (Cohen et al., 1956; Pirie, 1961), or in the presence of nicotine (Thung and van der Want, 1951; Thresh, 1956) or cysteine (Hageman and Waygood, 1959).

RATE AND INTENSITY OF HEATING

Some of the protein in leaf extracts coagulates at 50-60° and the coagulum contains almost all the chlorophylls (Rouelle, 1773; there is a translation in Pirie, 1971) and lipids; the rest of the protein coagulates at 70°. The way in which the total protein in an extract is distributed between these two fractions depends on the species, the pH at which the extract is heated, and the criteria (e.g., intensity of centrifugation) used as evidence for coagulation at the lower temperature. Usually 2/3 is in the first coagulum, loosely called "chloroplastic," and 1/3 in the second, loosely called "cytoplasmic" (Byers, 1967; Lexander et al., 1970). Byers (1971) studied the properties of a series of fractions sedimented from unheated extracts by different intensities of centrifugation and found resemblances between the more easily sedimented and the more easily coagulated fractions. Cytoplasmic protein may contain 15% N, whereas it is exceptional for the chloroplastic fraction to contain 10% even after extracting the pigments and other lipids from it. Cytoplasmic protein has consistently greater nutritive value and digestibility in vivo (Henry and Ford, 1965) and in vitro (Byers, 1967, 1971; Lexander et al., 1970) than

chloroplastic protein. These are real merits and it may be that
when LP is produced industrially it will be worthwhile separating
the nearly colorless cytoplasmic fraction because it could be presented as a food in more ways than the chloroplastic fraction.
But the separation is not simple enough to be regarded as a farm
operation and, if the chloroplastic fraction is relegated to animal
feed, the carotene would be lost.

Morrison and Pirie (1961) commented on the hard texture, which
facilitates filtration, of the coagulum produced by heating the extract to 70 or 80° in a few seconds. Sudden heating, for example
by injecting steam into a stream of extract continuously, also
minimizes enzymic changes. Heating to 70 or 80° does not inactivate all the enzymes and they may cause changes in the protein
during prolonged storage. With leaves such as lucerne (*Medicago
sativa*), which contains more chlorophyllase than most crops, heating to 100° is advisable. Otherwise, the enzyme splits phytol
from some of the chlorophyll and the resulting chlorophyllides
readily lose Mg to yield pheophorbides (Arkcoll and Holden, 1973).
Protein made from a lucerne extract heated slowly to 80° contained
enough pheophorbide to photosensitize rats (Lohrey et al., 1974;
Tapper et al., in press). This photosensitization is analogous to
hypericism caused by various plant pigments and would presumably
(Darwin, 1868) affect only animals with white patches and kept in
strong light, but it should be avoided if possible. Preparations
heated to 100° absorb atmospheric O_2 more slowly than those heated
to 70° (Shah, 1968), but there is so much nonenzymic oxidation when
dry material is stored without protection that this difference is
probably not significant. The only known disadvantage in heating
extracts to 100° rather than 80° is the extra consumption of steam.

REMOVAL OF WATER-SOLUBLE MATERIAL

Few proteins have any intrinsic flavor. In many parts of the
world dry leaf powders are used as flavoring agents. However, in

the initial phase of popularizing LP, as much of the leaf flavor as possible should be removed. Furthermore, some potential sources of LP, e.g., potato (*Solanum tuberosum*) haulm, contain toxic water-soluble material; others, e.g., lucerne, contain growth depressants (Peterson, 1950); and all contain reducing sugars. The details of the Maillard reaction, in which lysine is made unavailable by combination with reducing sugar, have been studied by Finot and Mauron (1972). For all these reasons, as much soluble material as is practicable should be removed from LP.

Coagulum containing 40% dry matter is easily made by pressing. If the residual water contains the amount of soluble material usually found in leaf extracts, about 7.5% of the dry matter of the LP will be this extraneous soluble material. A less adequately pressed coagulum may contain 80% of water; soluble material will then account for about 20% of the dry matter. Similarly, when a well-pressed coagulum is resuspended in so much water that there is only 1 g or less of soluble material per liter and pressed again until it contains only 60% of water, only 0.15% of the final cake will be soluble. The recommended standard is < 1% soluble material (Pirie, 1971). As already mentioned, the coagulum from a suddenly heated extract filters off easily; when resuspended in water at leaf pH, filtration is difficult. Filtration is easy if salt is added to the water or if the suspension is acidified to about pH 4. A cake made at pH 4 is more reliably free from alkaloids than one at about pH 6 and it has the keeping quality of cheese, sauerkraut, or pickles. On the other hand, the chlorophylls are completely converted to pheophytins through loss of Mg. The dull green is less attractive than the bright color of neutral LP, and the risk of pheophorbide formation is increased. There is more loss of carotene from acid LP and the unsaturated fatty acids in it are more rapidly oxidized. If LP is regarded as something to be made on the farm, these defects of acid washing must probably be accepted. If it is regarded as an industrial product, it could be washed by centrifugation or, if washed by acidification and filtration, the washed, pressed, and crumbled coagulum could be neutralized again by exposure to NH_3 vapor.

DRYING AND OTHER METHODS OF PRESERVATION

All the usual methods of preservation can be used with moist LP. It can be canned, or pickled with such agents as acetic acid and orange peel (Subba Rao et al., 1967). If air is excluded by pressing the acid dough into a jar, it keeps well if enough salt is mixed in to give 200 grams/liter in the aqueous phase. The merit of drying is that it obviates the need to transport water. It is an expensive process and introduces several complications. The need for drying should therefore be considered carefully in the light of the manner in which the protein will be used.

As with other proteins, the effects of drying LP depend on temperature, rate, and the nature of the other substances present. The discouraging results of early feeding experiments (e.g., Cowlishaw et al., 1956) were the result sometimes of drying at too high a temperature and sometimes of using inadequately washed lucerne protein still contaminated with the toxic saponin (Peterson, 1950). Using washed protein from rye (*Secale cereale*) with a Gross Protein Value (GPV) on chicks of 88 when dried at 42°, Duckworth and Woodham (1961) found that the GPV was only 65 when drying was at 94°. At first sight the results of Subba Rau and Singh (1970) seem to be in disagreement; they found that the nutritional value of lucerne LP in rats was the same whether it was dried in vacuo, at 40°, at 100°, or by solvent extraction. The probable explanation is that heating in the presence of moisture is harmful (Buchanan, 1969a) so that a small amount of material dried quickly in a current of air will be harmed less than a larger amount dried more slowly at the same temperature.

Although air drying at 40-50° seems to do little, if any, harm to the nutritive value of LP, it results in an unattractive, black, horny product that must be ground before use. A more attractive product, which is also more digestible in vitro and reconstitutes more easily into a free-flowing paste, can be made by evaporating water from the LP press-cake (about 40% dry matter) in a current of warm air in a tumble-drier until it contains only 20-30% water. It is then very easily ground finely and dries in a current of warm air without darkening or hardening (Arkcoll, 1969). Freeze-dried material is similar if water is added to the press-cake until it contains only about 25% dry matter and if it is then frozen completely within 2-3 minutes. This is easily managed by evaporative cooling in a unit, with an efficient heat exchanger (Pirie, 1964), which can freeze-dry batches containing several kilograms of LP. If the process of freezing occupies 30 minutes or more, or if a drier cake is frozen, the product will be darker and more granular.

All the species that have been carefully examined yield LP containing 20-30% of lipid; about 1/3 is extractable with ether or petrol ether and the remainder is extracted by a mixture of chloroform and methanol or by a mixture of alcohol and ether in the presence of a strong acid. Half or more of the lipid is doubly or trebly unsaturated (Lima et al., 1965; Buchanan, 1969b; Hudson and Karis, 1973). It would be premature to attach importance to apparent species differences in the ratios of the different fatty acids until more is known about the effects of age and manurial status or lipid composition and about the differing extents to which lipids combine with protein during storage after extraction. Three main types of change have to be considered when LP is heated during drying: effects of heat on the protein itself, effects on the lipid, and interaction between these two components of the preparation. Three main conditions influence these changes: temperature and time, access of oxygen, and the amount of water present. Buchanan (1969a, 1969b) dissociated these environmental conditions and measured the extractability of the lipids, the in vitro digestibility, and the nutritive value for rats. During storage for a few days at 100° or weeks at 60° with access of air, lipid became less readily extractable and the protein less digestible by papain.

Loss of digestibility was obvious in even 5 hours at 100° when LP was heated in sealed tubes so as to retain the water (about 9%) present in air-dry protein; when only 2.5% of water was present, several weeks were needed for the same loss. There was a similar loss of digestibility in the absence of oxygen, but solvent-extracted protein did not lose digestibility even in the presence of air and moisture. By solvent extraction after moist heating, digestibility and nutritive value were restored. Oxygen is absorbed by dry LP much more slowly in the dark than the light (Arkcoll, 1973) and absorption can be inhibited by antoxidants (Shah, 1968).

These changes in LP in the presence of air and in equilibrium with atmospheric moisture are an important reason for extracting the material with a lipid solvent; if prolonged storage is envisaged, extraction may be advisable. The alternative is to store it with protection from light and air after thorough drying. That would probably cost less than solvent extraction. Furthermore, the β-carotene and linolenic acid, which are valuable dietary components, would not be removed. The former is stable for 27 years in the absence of light and air (Zscheile, 1973) and there is so much in fresh LP that 2 or 3 grams per day would satisfy the human need for vitamin A.

CONCLUSION

If LP is being made on a farm or village scale for local use, the method of preparation must be kept simple. This means that leaf species will be preferred that contain little phenolic material and little chlorophyllase and that give neutral extracts. The extract should be heated quickly to promote easy filtration, but the coagulum need not be separated very quickly from the whey. If other components of the diet are expected to be rich in purines, it may be advisable to have some delay between making and coagulating the extract; delay is unnecessary if the protein is to be fed to animals because they have uricase. The product would either be used fresh or pickled so that it will keep for a few months without drying.

If factory production is envisaged there is scope for using leaves that are more acid or that contain more phenolic substances because pH can be manipulated and the coagulum can be separated from whey quickly. Coagulation could be done in two stages so as to make a pigmented and less digestible product for animal feed and a pale product for use in food. This would deprive people of the carotene. Factory-made material would probably either be judiciously dried in warm air or extracted with a water-miscible solvent so as to yield a dry product with a long shelf-life.

Clearly there is no simple answer to the question "How should leaf protein be made?". The answer depends on where, from what, and for whom it is being made.

REFERENCES

Allison, R.M., W.M. Laird and R.L.M. Synge. 1973. Notes on a deamination method proposed for determining "chemically available lysine" of proteins. Brit. J. Nutr. 29:51.

Arkcoll, D.B. 1969. Preservation of leaf protein preparations by air drying. J. Sci. Food Agr. 20:600.

Arkcoll, D.B. 1973. The preservation and storage of leaf protein preparations. J. Sci. Food Agr. 24:437.

Arkcoll, D.B. and M. Holden. 1973. Changes in chloroplast pigments during the preparation of leaf protein. J. Sci. Food Agr. 24:1217.

Bawden, F.C. and A. Klezckowski. 1945. Protein precipitation and virus inactivation by extracts of strawberry plants. J. Pom. Hort. Sci. 21:2.

Bosshard, H. 1972. Über die Anlagerung von Thioäthern an Chinone und Chinonimine in stark sauren Medien. Helv. Chim. Acta. 55:32.

Buchanan, R.A. 1969. In vivo and in vitro methods of measuring nutritive value of leaf protein preparations. Brit. J. Nutr. 23:533.

Buchanan, R.A. 1969. Effect of storage and lipid extraction on the properties of leaf protein. J. Sci. Food Agr. 20:359.

Byers, M. 1967. The in vitro hydrolysis of leaf proteins. II. The action of papain on protein concentrates extracted from different species. J. Sci. Food Agr. 18:33.

Byers, M. 1971. The amino acid composition and in vitro digestibility of some protein fractions from three species of leaves of various ages. J. Sci. Food Agr. 22:242.

Cohen, M., W. Ginoza, R.W. Dorner, W.R. Hudson and S.G. Wildman. 1956. Solubility and color characteristics of leaf proteins prepared in air and nitrogen. Science. 124:1081.

Cowlishaw, S.J., D.E. Eyles, W.F. Raymond and J.M.A. Tilley. 1956. Nutritive value of leaf protein concentrates. I. Effect of addition of cholesterol and amino acids. II. Effects of processing methods. J. Sci. Food Agr. 7:768 and 7:775.

Darwin, C. 1868. The variation of plants and animals under domestication. John Murray, London. 2:227 and 2:337.

Delort-Laval, J. and S.Z. Zelter. 1968. Improving the nutritive value of proteins by tanning process. Proc. 2nd World Conf. Animal Prod. Maryland, USA. 457.

Duckworth, J. and A.A. Woodham. 1961. Leaf protein concentrates. I. Effect of source of raw material and method of drying on protein value for chicks and rats. J. Sci. Food Agr. 12:5.

Feeny, P.P. 1969. Inhibitory effect of oak leaf tannins on the hydrolysis of proteins by trypsin. Phytochemistry. 8:2119.

Finot, P.A. and J. Mauron. 1972. Le blocage de la lysine par la réaction de Maillard. II. Propriétés chimiques des dérivés N-(désoxy-1-D-fructosyl-1) et N-(désoxy-1-D-lactulosyl-1) de la lysine. Helv. Chim. Acta. 55:1153.

Hageman, R.H. and E.R. Waygood. 1959. Methods for the extraction of enzymes from cereal leaves with especial reference to the triosephosphate dehydrogenases. Plant Physiol., Lancaster. 34:396.

Hawkins, G.E. 1959. Relationships between chemical composition and some nutritive qualities of lespedeza sericea hays. J. Animal Sci. 18:763.

Henry, K.M. and J.E. Ford. 1965. The nutritive value of leaf protein concentrates determined in biological tests with rats and by microbiological methods. J. Sci. Food Agr. 16:425.

Horigome, T. 1974. Nutritive value of N-acetylcasein and brown-colored N-acetylcasein. Chem. Abstr. 80:35952.

Hudson, J.F. and I.G. Karis. 1973. Aspects of vegetable structural lipids. I. The lipids of leaf protein concentrate. J. Sci. Food Agr. 24:1541.

Lexander, K., R. Carlsson, V. Schalen, A. Simonsson and T. Lundborg. 1970. Quantities and qualities of leaf protein concentrates from wild species and crop species grown under controlled conditions. Ann. Appl. Biol. 66:193.

Lima, I.H., T. Richardson and M.A. Stahmann. 1965. Fatty acids in some leaf protein concentrates. J. Agr. Food Chem. 13:143.

Lohrey, E., B.A. Tapper and E.L. Hove. 1974. Photosensitization of albino rats fed on lucerne-protein concentrate. Brit. J. Nutr. 31:159.

Milić, B.L. 1972. Lucerne tannins. I. Content and composition during growth. J. Sci. Food Agr. 23:1151.

Morrison, J.E. and N.W. Pirie. 1961. The large-scale production of protein from leaf extracts. J. Sci. Food Agr. 12:1.

Peterson, D.W. 1950. Some properties of a factor in alfalfa meal causing depression of growth in chicks. J. Biol. Chem. 183:647.

Pierpoint, W.S. 1969. o-Quinones formed in plant extracts: their reactions with amino acids and peptides. Biochem. J. 112:609.

Pierpoint, W.S. 1971. Formation and behavior of o-quinones in some processes of agricultural importance. Rep. Rothamsted Exp. Station for 1970. Pt. 2, 199.

Pirie, N.W. 1953. Large-scale production of edible protein from fresh leaves. Rep. Rothamsted Exp. Station for 1952. 173.

Pirie, N.W. 1961. The disintegration of soft tissues in the absence of air. J. Agr. Eng. Res. 6:142.

Pirie, N.W. 1964. Freeze-drying, or drying by sublimation. In D.W. Newman (Ed.) Instrumental Methods of Experimental Biology. Macmillan, New York.

Pirie, N.W. 1966. Leaf protein as a human food. Science. 152:1701.

Pirie, N.W. 1970. Biochemistry Department. Rep. Rothamsted Exp. Station for 1969. Pt. 1, 133.

Pirie, N.W. (Ed.). 1971. Leaf Protein: Its Agronomy, Preparation, Quality and Use. International Biological Program Handbook 20. Blackwell, Oxford.

Pirie, N.W. 1975. Methods and merits of fodder fractionation. In G. Debry (Ed.) Proc. 2nd Symp. Int. Alimentation et Travail. (In press).

Roberts, E.A.H. 1959. The interaction of flavonol orthoquinones with cysteine and glutathione. Chem. Ind. 995.

Rouelle, H.M. 1773. Observations sur les fécules ou parties vertes des plantes, et sur la matière glutineuse ou végéto-animale. J. de médicine, chirurgie, pharmacie etc. 40:59.

Shah, F.H. 1968. Changes in leaf protein lipids in vitro. J. Sci. Food Agr. 19:199.

Singh, N. 1960. Differences in the nature of nitrogen precipitated by various methods from wheat leaf extracts. Biochim. Biophys. Acta. 45:422.

Spencer, R.R., A.C. Mottola, E.M. Bickoff, J.P. Clark and G.O. Kohler. 1971. The PRO-XAN process: the design and evaluation of a pilot plant system for the coagulation and separation of the leaf protein from alfalfa juice. J. Agr. Food Chem. 19:504. See also Bickoff et al., this volume.

Subba Rao, M.S., N. Singh and G. Prasanappa. 1967. Preservation of wet leaf protein concentrates. J. Sci. Food Agr. 18:295.

Subba Rau, B.H. and N. Singh. 1970. Studies on nutritive value of leaf protein from lucerne (*Medicago sativa*). II. Effect of processing conditions. Indian J. Exp. Biol. 8:34.

Tapper, B.A., E. Lohrey, E.L. Hove and R.M. Allison. Photosensitivity from chlorophyll-derived pigments. (In press).

Thresh, J.M. 1956. Some effects of tannic acid and of leaf extracts which contain tannins on the infectivity of tobacco mosaic and tobacco necrosis viruses. Ann. Appl. Biol. 44:608.

Thung, T.H. and J.P.H. van der Want. 1951. Viruses and tannins. Tijdschr. Pl. Ziekt. 57:72.

Vithayathil, P.J. and G.S. Murthy. 1972. New reaction of *o*-benzoquinone at the thioether group of methionine. Nature New Biol. 236:101.

Walsh, K.A. and S.M. Hauge. 1953. Carotene: factors affecting destruction in alfalfa. J. Agr. Food Chem. 1:1001.

Wong, E. 1973. Plant phenolics. *In* G.W. Butler and R.W. Bailey (Eds.) Chemistry and Biochemistry of Herbage. Academic Press. 1:265.

Zscheile, F.P. 1973. Long-term preservation of carotene in alfalfa meal. J. Agr. Food Chem. 21:1117.

15

COTTONSEED PROTEIN PRODUCTS: VARIATION
IN PROTEIN QUALITY WITH PRODUCT AND PROCESS

Wilda H. Martinez

Southern Regional Research Center
Agricultural Research Service
U. S. Department of Agriculture
New Orleans, Louisiana

and

Daniel T. Hopkins

Ralston Purina Company
St. Louis, Missouri

Defatted cottonseed flour, glandless or deglanded (liquid
cyclone process), when properly processed has a protein efficiency
ratio (PER) very near that of casein. Heat and moisture introduced
after removal of lipids significantly decrease the PER. Fractionation of the various types of cellular proteins during isolate preparation will also produce significant changes both favorable and
unfavorable. Storage protein isolates are low in lysine and the
sulfur amino acids, and low in protein quality. The nonstorage
protein isolates are high in all the essential amino acids and very
high in protein quality (PER > 2.5). The degree of fractionation
of the seed proteins and consequently the nutritive value of the
isolate are dependent upon the extraction characteristics of the
flour and the isolation process. Chemical scores, calculated from
amino acid composition according to FAO (1973) and Alsmeyer et al.
(1974), were unsatisfactory for estimating PER except in very broad
terms.

- - - - - - - - - - - - - -

The quality of defatted cottonseed depends upon the level of physiologically active or "free" gossypol and the degree of impairment incurred by the protein during the defatting operations (Altschul et al., 1958; Martinez et al., 1967). Gossypol is a binaphthyl, dialdehyde, polyhydroxyl pigment which is highly reactive and deleterious to monogastric animals (Berardi and Goldblatt, 1969). All of the gossypol in the seed is in discrete extracellular glands (Boatner, 1948). During processing the glands usually are ruptured and gossypol is either removed with the oil or converted to a physiologically inactive form through interaction with other cellular constituents. Edible cottonseed protein products, approved by FDA, have a maximum of 0.045% "free" gossypol. (Code of Federal Regulations Title 21--Food and Drugs, Chapter 1, Subchapter B, Subpart D, Paragraphs 121, 1019 Modified cottonseed products intended for human consumption.)

The inherent protein quality of cottonseed is good. An early study by Eagle and Davies (1957) using a rat assay very similar to the AOAC procedure for PER (protein efficiency ratio) (AOAC, 1975) showed that protein quality of cottonseed defatted with butanone in the absence of heat equaled that of the soybean meal control (Table 1). Commercial processing operations to remove oil and inactivate gossypol, however, usually impair the protein quality. The data in Table 1 illustrate the fact that the degree of heat, moisture, and pressure used in the various operations of tempering or cooking of the kernels, expressing or extraction of the oil, and, when necessary, desolventization of the product, can produce a significant destruction of the essential amino acid lysine and a reduction in protein quality. The level of "free" gossypol encountered in these meals apparently did not affect rats fed at the 9% protein level. Since the reduction in protein quality is the sum of the effects of the specific operating conditions, no one commercial process can be cited over the other. The screw press operation, however, appears to offer the least latitude.

When cottonseed meats are heated prior to hexane extraction in the absence of added free moisture and pigment glands, little if any

TABLE 1

Nutritive and Chemical Characteristics of Cottonseed Meals

Meal	PER[b]	Lysine[c] (g/16 g N)	Gossypol (%)[c] Free	Gossypol (%)[c] Total
Soybean	1.98	--	--	--
Cottonseed				
Experimental[a]	2.13	4.3	0.02	0.24
Commercial process				
Solvent	1.82	3.9	0.28	0.96
Prepress solvent	1.77	3.9	0.04	0.75
Prepress solvent	1.74	4.0	0.02	0.75
Prepress solvent	1.33	3.4	0.04	1.00
Screw press--low speed	1.71	3.9	0.02	0.62
Screw press--low speed	1.26	3.6	0.05	1.10
Screw press--high speed	0.88	3.4	0.03	1.00

[a]Butanone extraction followed by air desolventization and 4 hr at 49.4°C (Eaves et al., 1952).

[b]Protein efficiency ratio: average of replicate experiments (Eagle and Davies, 1957).

[c]Unpublished data from Southern Regional Research Center. Total lysine analysis (Moore and Stein, 1951); gossypol analysis (AOAC, 1975).

effect on lysine or PER occurs (Table 2). In the study of Cross et al. (1970), glandless cottonseed kernels, i.e., the variety of cottonseed free of pigment glands and hence gossypol (McMichael, 1959), were heated to specific temperatures prior to flaking, hexane extraction, and desolventization. No effect was noted at temperatures up to 93°C. Only when the cellular contents were disrupted by flaking prior to heating to 108°C, as in the last trial, was there any indication of a reduction in lysine availability.

The application of heat following oil removal produces quite a different effect. If the cells of the seed are disrupted by flaking, the oil extracted with hexane, and the resultant material heated in the presence of moisture, as in certain desolventization procedures,

TABLE 2

Effect of Cooking Temperature of
Glandless Cottonseed Meats on Meal Characteristics[a]

Maximum cooking temperature of meats (°C)	EAF lysine[e] (g/16 g N)	28-day gain (g)	PER
26.1[b]	3.82	87	2.34
27.2[c]	3.88	90	2.37
64.4	3.88	90	2.35
76.6	3.86	91	2.35
93.3	3.82	91	2.35
108.9[d]	3.76	84	2.30
ANRC Casein		91	2.50

[a]Cross et al. (1970).

[b]Hexane extraction temperature, 25.5°C.

[c]Extraction temperature for this and all others, 48.9°C.

[d]Heated as flakes.

[e]Epsilon amino free lysine or "available" lysine.

one obtains the typical results of the browning reaction, namely the inactivation and destruction of lysine. Table 3 shows the expected reduction in nutritive index, available lysine, and total lysine contents with autoclaving (Martinez et al., 1961). When both lipids and carbohydrates are removed by successive hexane and 80% ethanol extraction, there is very little effect on nutritive value, demonstrating the importance of the alcohol-extractable fraction to the effects of processing.

A similar study, using the protein efficiency ratio method as the animal assay (Table 4), gave comparable results (Martinez et al., 1967). Removal of carbohydrates before autoclaving did not prevent a reduction in EAF (epsilon amino free or "available") lysine and PER, but the extent of the reduction was significantly

TABLE 3

Effect of Temperature on Defatted and
Alcohol-Extracted Glandless Cottonseed--Rat Repletion[a]

Cottonseed	Autoclaved[d] (min)	Lysine (g/16 g N)		Nutritive index
		EAF	Total	
Lipid extracted[b]	0	4.1	4.2	101
	20	3.7	3.7	76
	60	3.1	3.5	68
Lipid and carbo-hydrate extracted[c]	0	4.6	4.6	96
	20	4.3	4.3	101
	60	4.1	4.2	86

[a]Rat repletion procedure (Cabell and Earle, 1954).

[b]Ambient hexane extraction and air desolventization.

[c]Hexane followed by 80% aqueous ethanol and air desolventization (Martinez et al., 1961).

[d]121°C, 15 lb pressure.

TABLE 4

Effect of Temperature on Defatted and
Alcohol-Extracted Glandless Cottonseed--PER

Cottonseed	EAF lysine (g/16 g N)	Weight gain (g)	PER[d]
Lipid extracted[a]	3.7	75.3	2.26[b,c]
Autoclaved[b]	3.4	49.7	1.52[e]
Lipid and carbohydrate extracted[c]	4.1	79.2	2.11[b,c]
Autoclaved[b]	3.8	63.2	1.78[d]
Soybean meal	--	65.1	2.06[c]
ANRC Casein	--	80.2	2.50[a]

[a]Ambient hexane extraction and air desolventization.

[b]20 min, 121°C, 15 lb pressure.

[c]Hexane followed by 80% aqueous ethanol and air desolventization.

[d]PERs without a common letter differ significantly at P = 0.01 (Duncan's multiple range test). From Martinez et al. (1967).

less. It should be noted that, again in this study, the PER of the defatted glandless flour was numerically, but not statistically, greater than that of the soybean meal (see Table 1).

Subsequent engineering research has provided another cottonseed product, the liquid cyclone process (LCP) flour, with which the inherently high quality of cottonseed protein can be demonstrated. In the liquid cyclone process (Figure 1) the meats are milled and the intact pigment glands, cell wall fragments, and clusters of cells are separated from the subcellular proteinaceous particulates by differential centrifugation in hexane followed by subsequent removal

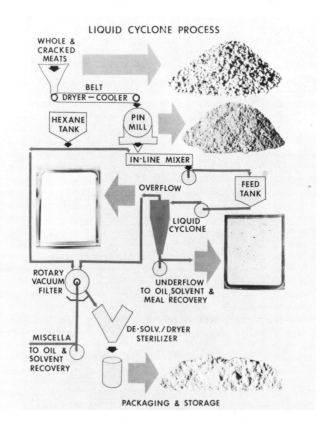

FIG. 1. Flow diagram of the liquid cyclone process. Courtesy of Homer K. Gardner Jr.

of the oil-rich miscella and desolventization of the flour (Gardner et al., 1973). This flour is termed deglanded to differentiate it from the product derived from genetically glandless cottonseed.

As in the solvent extraction process, desolventization, the operation that could cause the greatest heat damage to the protein, is critical in the liquid cyclone process. The LCP flour prepared in the pilot plant was desolventized at 93.3°C under a slight vacuum with nitrogen sparge. The glandless flour was prepared by hexane extraction of conditioned (70°C) flakes in a pilot-plant scale Crown Iron Works continuous, countercurrent extractor. Solvent was then removed in a Schneckens type unit at an exit temperature of 70°C. Under these conditions there was no appreciable reduction in available lysine.

A series of animal assays (Hopkins et al., 1973) using a slightly modified PER procedure was recently carried out to evaluate the protein quality of both types of cottonseed flours and the isolates prepared from them by the selective precipitation (Figure 2) (Martinez et al., 1970), selective extraction (Figure 3) (Berardi et al., 1969), and classical procedures (Figure 4) (Martinez et al., 1970). Composition of the control diet used in these assays is given in Table 5. Composition of the cottonseed flours and isolates and yield of isolates from the various processes are shown in Table 6. Test diets were formulated with the cottonseed protein products to furnish a level of 10% protein (N x 6.25). All diets were kept isocaloric by adjusting the corn oil and ground cellulose contents to insure similarity in total levels of fat and crude fiber plus ash. Except where noted, each diet was fed to 10 individually caged, weanling rats for 28 days. Protein efficiency ratios were calculated by procedures outlined by AOAC (1975).

Table 7 contains results from three separate evaluations of the cottonseed flours. In the first experiment, the deglanded flour gave an anomalous result. In the second, the PER of the glandless flour was less than expected. The third experiment produced statistically comparable results for the two flours and the casein control.

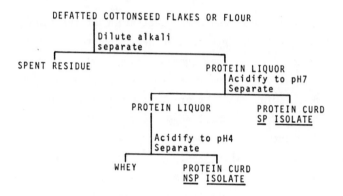

FIG. 2. Flow diagram of the selective precipitation procedure. SP, storage protein; NSP, nonstorage protein.

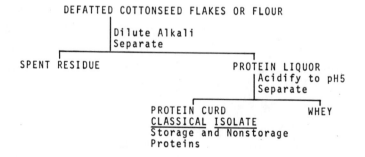

FIG. 3. Flow diagram of the selective extraction procedure. SP, storage protein; NSP, nonstorage protein.

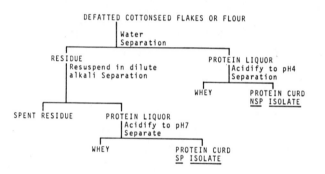

FIG. 4. Flow diagram of the classical procedure.

TABLE 5

Composition of Control Diet

Ingredient	%
Sucrose	68.82
Casein	11.11
Corn oil	9.97
Ground cellulose	4.86
Mineral mixture[a]	4.23
Vitamin mixture[b]	1.00
Ethoxyquin	0.01

[a]Furnishes to the diet: $CaHPO_4 \cdot 2H_2O$, 3.00%; NaCl, 0.5%; $KHCO_3$, 0.40%; $MgSO_4$, 0.24%; ferric citrate, 0.03%; $MnCO_3$, 0.05%; $ZnCO_3$, 0.008%; $CuCO_3 \cdot Cu(OH)_2$, 0.002%; $NaIO_3$, 0.0001%; Na_2SeO_3, 0.00001%.

[b]Adds the following quantities to each kg of diet: Vitamin A, 20,000 IU; Vitamin D_3, 2,000 USP; Vitamin E, 100 IU; menadione sodium bisulfite, 2 mg; thiamine HCl, 10 mg; riboflavin, 10 mg; niacin, 50 mg; pyridoxine HCl, 10 mg; Ca D Pentothenate, 20 mg; Vitamin B_{12}, 10 μg; folic acid, 2 mg; biotin, 0.5 mg; choline chloride, 1.5 g; BHT, 20 mg.

Neither the environmental or physical conditions of the rats, nor any one factor of the diets, accounted for the variation between these experiments.

Values in the third study for the LCP flour are of the same magnitude as those reported by Olson (1973), namely, 2.51 to 2.67 corrected to casein at 2.50. These data substantiate the observation that a properly processed cottonseed flour can equal casein in nutritive value when fed as a sole source of protein.

The nutritive quality of protein isolates from defatted oilseed flours is usually lower than the starting material. Fractionation of proteins and processing conditions are two of the factors contributing to the loss (Wolf and Cowan, 1971). The results of nutritional evaluation of cottonseed isolates are given in Table 8 (Hopkins et al., 1973). All isolates were prepared and spray dried on pilot-plant scale. As expected, the classical isolate was

TABLE 6

Preparation, Composition, and Yield of Cottonseed Protein Products

Process[a]	Product	Composition (%)				Yield (%)	
		Protein	Fat	Fiber	Ash	Wt	N
Cottonseed flours							
S	Glandless-B	59.6	1.6	2.9	7.2		
LCP	Deglanded-C	64.6	0.8	2.8	7.4		
	Deglanded-D	64.8	1.0	3.4	7.9		
	Deglanded-E	62.6	1.0	2.8	7.3		
	Deglanded-F	63.8	0.6	9.1			
Nonstorage protein isolate							
SP	Glandless-B	76.2	5.2	0.0	5.0	13	17
	Deglanded-C	77.5	4.1	0.6	6.4	12	17
SE	Glandless-B	86.2	2.8	0.2	5.9	6	8
	Deglanded-C	85.0	2.4	1.2	3.5	5	11
Storage protein isolate							
SP	Glandless-B	99.4	0.4	0.2	2.0	29	47
	Deglanded-C	100.0	0.6	0.7	2.9	34	47
SE	Glandless-B	103.1	0.8	0.1	1.4	25	44
	Deglanded-C	101.2	--	0.6	1.8	37	58
Classical isolate							
C	Glandless-A[b]	92.5	0.8	0.7	3.8	45	73

[a]S, solvent extracted; LCP, liquid cyclone process; SP, selective precipitation; SE, selective extraction; C, classical isolation.

[b]Solvent extracted under semicommercial conditions in a Crown extractor and desolventizer-toaster (DT) unit with exposure to a minimum of steam; exit temperature 67°C (Smith, 1970).

TABLE 7

PER Assay of Cottonseed Flours

Cottonseed flours	Average (g/rat/28 days)[b]		PER[b]
	Consumed	Gained	
Experiment 1			
Glandless-B	354[b]	88[a]	2.30[a]
Deglanded-C	268[a]	59[b]	1.92[b]
ANRC Casein	300[a]	81[a]	2.50[a]
Experiment 2			
Glandless-B	399[c]	98[a,b]	2.17[b]
Deglanded-C	398[c]	106[b]	2.34[a,b]
Deglanded-D	356[b]	100[a,b]	2.46[a]
Deglanded-E	334[a,b]	93[a,b]	2.43[a]
ANRC Casein[a]	317[a]	90[a]	2.50[a]
Experiment 3			
Glandless-B[a]	332[a]	88[a]	2.54[a]
Deglanded-F	325[a]	92[a]	2.70[a]
ANRC Casein[a]	346[a]	89[a]	2.50[a]

[a]20 rats per treatment.

[b]Means without a common letter differ significantly at P < 0.05 as computed by Duncan's multiple range test (Steel and Torrie, 1960).

manifestly lower in PER than the cottonseed flour. The data do suggest, however, that the classical isolate from cottonseed is equal to or better than other vegetable protein isolates (FAO, 1970).

Isolate procedures such as the selective extraction or selective precipitation procedures, designed specifically to fractionate seed proteins, have marked effects, both favorable and unfavorable, on nutritional quality (Table 8). The PER of the minor, nonstorage protein (NSP) isolate increased materially in comparison with flour whereas the major storage protein (SP) isolate decreased. Both the extent of fractionation of the proteins and the resultant nutritional quality of the isolate depend upon the extraction characteristics of

TABLE 8

PER Assay of Cottonseed Isolates

Experiment[a]	Cottonseed flour	Classical isolate	Protein efficiency ratio (PER)[b],[c]			
			Nonstorage protein isolate		Storage protein isolate	
			Selective precipitation	Selective extraction	Selective precipitation	Selective extraction
1	Glandless-A	2.18[b]	3.14[a]	2.23[b]		
2	Glandless-A	2.02[b]	3.16[a]	2.32[d]	1.46[c]	1.38[c]
3	Glandless-B		3.05[d]	3.02[d]	1.50[a,b]	1.33[a]
	Deglanded-C		2.80[c,d]	2.68[c]	1.30[a]	1.66[b]

[a]Experiment 1 conducted according to the standard PER procedure (AOAC, 1970). Experiments 2 and 3 conducted according to modified procedure (see text).

[b]Corrected to casein at 2.50[de].

[c]Means without a common letter differ within each experiment significantly at P < 0.05 as computed by Duncan's multiple range test (Steel and Torrie, 1960). Statistical comparisons should not be made between experiments.

the flour, which are determined by the defatting operation, and the isolation process (see Table 8, nonstorage protein isolates, Glandless-A versus Glandless-B and Glandless-B versus Deglanded-C).

The advent of nutritional labeling and recent government requirements for equalizing finished food products in terms of the quality-quantity relationship have added new emphasis to the continuing search for less costly and time-consuming methods of analysis for protein quality. One method which has received considerable attention, evaluation, and modification is the FAO/WHO chemical or amino acid score (FAO, 1973), which estimates protein quality by comparing amino acid composition of the protein with a reference pattern of amino acids (Table 9). Using a more recent approach, also based on amino acid content (Alsmeyer et al., 1974), amino acid analyses and PER values of a series of meat products were used to determine the mathematical relationships between PER and specific amino acids by multiple regression analysis (Table 9). The predictive ability of both methods was evaluated for cottonseed protein products. Amino acid composition was determined by the automated Moore and Stein procedure (Spackman et al., 1958). A modifided enzymatic digestion-colorimetric procedure was used to determine tryptophan (Research 900, Checkerboard Square Plaza, St. Louis, Missouri). All amino acid values were within the ranges studied by Alsmeyer et al. (1974).

Table 9 indicates that the equations developed with animal protein data, when applied to animal and vegetable protein combinations, are not appropriate for vegetable protein alone. With the cottonseed and soybean flours, values from Equation 1 closely approximate observed PER values, but agree neither in numerical number nor relationship between the flours. The FAO scores imply the proper relationship, but fail to denote the close biological response between casein and cottonseed flours. Although cottonseed flours score higher than soybean, cottonseed provides only three amino acids (tryptophan, phenylalanine, and tyrosine) in quantities equal to or in excess of the pattern, whereas soybean flour provides all in excess except two (total sulfur amino acids and threonine). This fact is especially important to blending proteins in a food product.

367

TABLE 9

Calculated Evaluation of Nutritive Quality

Parameter	FAO/WHO pattern[a]	Casein	Flours		
			Soybean	Cottonseed	
				Glandless	Deglanded
PER					
Observed		2.50	2.19[e]	2.42	2.48
Calculated[a]					
Equation 1			2.73	2.02	2.00
Equation 2			2.75	2.03	2.04
Equation 3			1.76	1.05	1.43
Amino acid score[b]		91[d]	69	74	73
Amino acids (mg/g of protein)[c]					
Isoleucine	40	54	47	30	30
Leucine	70	165	79	57	56
Lysine	55	81	62	42	41
Methionine and cystine	35	32*	24*	26*	26
Phenylalanine and tyrosine	60	110	90	84	80
Threonine	40	47	39	30	29*
Tryptophan	10	16	13	13	13
Valine	50	67	51	44	44

TABLE 9 (continued)

| Parameter | Nonstorage protein isolates | | | |
| | Selective precipitation | | Selective extraction | |
	Glandless	Deglanded	Glandless	Deglanded
PER				
Observed	3.05	2.80	3.02	2.68
Calculated[a]				
Equation 1	3.06	2.73	2.39	2.28
Equation 2	3.03	2.69	2.35	2.25
Equation 3	2.77	2.11	1.36	1.24
Amino acid score[b]	95	100	87	85
Amino acids (mg/g of protein)[c]				
Isoleucine	42	40	37	37
Leucine	81	76	68	66
Lysine	57	61	66	68
Methionine and cystine	33*	35	39	38
Phenylalanine and tyrosine	93	90	82	88
Threonine	43	43	35*	34*
Tryptophan	16	13	16	14
Valine	58	54	49	48

TABLE 9 (continued)

| Parameter | Storage protein isolates | | | |
| | Selective precipitation | | Selective extraction | |
	Glandless	Deglanded	Glandless	Deglanded
PER				
Observed	1.50	1.30	1.33	1.66
Calculated[a]				
Equation 1	2.29	2.14	2.33	2.17
Equation 2	2.31	2.17	2.34	2.20
Equation 3	1.64	1.49	1.33	1.56
Amino acid score[b]	54	54	51	54
Amino acids (mg/g of protein)[c]				
Isoleucine	35	33	35	34
Leucine	64	60	66	61
Lysine	33	32	31	32
Methionine and cystine	19*	19*	18 *	19*
Phenylalanine and tyrosine	98	93	98	94
Threonine	29	28	28	29
Tryptophan	11	12	11	12
Valine	51	50	52	50

[a]Alsmeyer et al. (1974). Equation 1: PER = -0.684 + 0.456 (Leu) - 0.047 (Pro). Equation 2: PER = -1.816 + 0.435 (Leu) - 0.105 (Tyr). Equation 3: PER = -1.816 + 0.435 (Met) + 0.780 (Leu) + 0.211 (His) - 0.944 (Tyr).

[b]FAO (1973).

$$\text{Amino acid score} = \frac{\text{mg of amino acid in 1 g of test protein}}{\text{mg of amino acid in reference pattern}} \times 100.$$

[c]N x 6.25 except for casein, N x 6.38. *Most limiting amino acid.

[d]Amino acid composition from FAO (1970).

[e]PER and amino acid data from Kellor (1973). Calculated PER values determined with unpublished data.

With the nonstorage protein isolates, values from Equation 1 reasonably approximate observed PERs for the selective precipitation isolates, but are very poor for the selective extraction isolates. These results illustrate the highly weighted importance in these equations of the leucine content of the protein. With the storage protein isolates, which are low in protein quality and have a rather different amino acid profile, Equation 3 rather than Equation 1 provides the more reasonable estimate of the observed PER. Here again, small differences in leucine content produce marked changes in calculated PER which conflict with observed PER. (See glandless storage protein isolates, selective precipitation versus selective extraction, Table 9.) However, the only instance where the predictive equation consistently met the criteria of acceptance set by Alsmeyer et al. (1974), namely ± 0.2 PER, was in the use of Equation 3 with storage protein isolates.

The amino acid scores for the cottonseed isolates reflect the broad difference in nutritive value between storage and nonstorage protein isolates. They do not, however, reflect the significant differences in observed PER within a specific type of isolate, as can be seen in Table 9 (nonstorage protein isolates, selective extraction, glandless versus deglanded, or storage protein isolates, deglanded, selective precipitation versus selective extraction). To achieve a greater degree of predictability the score should reflect differences in more than just the "most limiting amino acid" (FAO, 1973).

Amino acid data for the nonstorage protein isolates clearly show that different proteins are isolated by the two procedures. The data, however, do not provide concise evidence of the importance of the extraction characteristics of the flour to the composition of the isolate and its resultant nutritive value (Table 9, selective extraction, glandless versus deglanded). It is possible that the small differences in several amino acids (leucine, methionine and cystine, threonine, and valine) combine to produce a significant difference in PER with a high quality protein. However, the amino acid complement of the storage protein isolates does not explain observed differences in PER.

The inversion of the predictive equations which gave the closest estimate of the observed PER with the type of protein (nonstorage protein isolate, Equation 1; storage protein isolate, Equation 3) suggests that Equation 1 may be more suitable for high quality proteins and Equation 3 for low quality proteins. This premise, however, is not supported by data from either Table 9 or Alsmeyer et al. (1974), who noted that all three equations failed to predict PER for some products. These results imply that specific equations may be required for each type of protein product, or more probably, that these data merely reflect the limited variation in amino acid profile of the proteins used in establishing the equations. The use of a wider variety of proteins with distinctly different amino acid profiles (e.g., meat, cheese, fish, and vegetable proteins) might provide regression equations that would more effectively predict the PER of protein products.

NOTE

Reference to a company or product does not imply approval or recommendation by the U.S. Department of Agriculture over others not mentioned.

REFERENCES

Alsmeyer, R.H., A.E. Cunningham and M.L. Happich. 1974. Equations predict PER from amino acid analysis. Food Technol. 28:34.

Altschul, A.M., C.M. Lyman and F.H. Thurber. 1958. Cottonseed meal. In A.M. Altschul (Ed.) Processed Plant Foodstuffs. Academic Press, New York.

AOAC. 1970. Official Methods of Analysis (11th Ed.). Association of Official Agricultural Chemists, Washington, D.C.

AOAC. 1975. Official Methods of Analysis (12th Ed.). Association of Official Agricultural Chemists, Washington, D.C.

Berardi, L.C. and L.A. Goldblatt. 1969. Gossypol. *In* I.E. Liener (Ed.) Toxic Constituents of Plant Foodstuffs. Academic Press, New York.

Berardi, L.C., W.H. Martinez and C.J. Fernandez. 1969. Cottonseed protein isolates: two-step extraction procedure. Food Technol. 23:75.

Boatner, C.H. 1948. Pigments of cottonseed. *In* A.E. Bailey (Ed.) Cottonseed and Cottonseed Products. Wiley, New York.

Cabell, C.A. and I.P. Earle. 1954. Comparison of the rat repletion method with other methods of assaying the nutritive value of proteins in cottonseed meals. J. Agr. Food Chem. 2:787.

Cross, D.E., D.T. Hopkins, E.L. D'Aquin and E.A. Gastrock. 1970. Experiments with solvent extraction of glandless cottonseed and glanded cottonseed. J. Amer. Oil Chem. Soc. 47:4A.

Eagle, E. and D.L. Davies. 1957. Feed value and protein-quality determinations on cottonseed meals. J. Amer. Oil Chem. Soc. 34:454.

Eaves, P.H., L.J. Molaison, C.L. Black, A.J. Crovetto and E.L. D'Aquin. 1952. A comparison of five commercial solvents for extraction of cottonseed. J. Amer. Oil Chem. Soc. 29:88.

FAO Nutrition Studies No. 24. 1970. Amino acid content of foods and biological data on proteins. Rome, Italy.

FAO Nutritional Meetings Report Series No. 52. WHO Technical Report Series No. 522. 1973. Energy and protein requirements. Rome, Italy.

Gardner, H.K. Jr., R.J. Hron Sr. and H.L.E. Vix. 1973. Liquid cyclone process for edible cottonseed flour production. Oil Mill Gaz. 78:13.

Hopkins, D.T., J.R. Norris and W.H. Martinez. 1973. Cottonseed protein isolation. 4. Nutritional evaluation. 33rd Ann. Mtg. Inst. Food Technol., Miami. (Abstr.).

Kellor, R.L. 1973. Defatted soy flour and grits. Proc. World Soy Protein Conf. p. 77A.

Martinez, W.H., V.L. Frampton and C.A. Cabell. 1961. Effects of gossypol and raffinose on lysine content and nutritive quality of proteins in meals from glandless cottonseed. J. Agr. Food Chem. 9:64.

Martinez, W.H., L.C. Berardi, V.L. Frampton, H.L. Wilcke, D.E. Greene and R. Teichman. 1967. Importance of cellular constituents to cottonseed meal protein quality. J. Agr. Food Chem. 15:427.

Martinez, W.H., L.C. Berardi and L.A. Goldblatt. 1970. Potential of cottonseed: products, composition and use. Proc. Third Int. Cong. Food Sci. Technol. (SOS/70) p. 248.

McMichael, S.C. 1959. Hopi cotton: a source of cottonseed free of gossypol pigments. Agron. J. 51:630.

Moore, S. and W.H. Stein. 1951. Chromatography of amino acids on sulfonated polystyrene resins. J. Biol. Chem. 192:663.

Olson, R.L. 1973. Evaluation of LCP cottonseed flour. Oil Mill Gaz. 77:7.

Smith, K.J. 1970. Glandless cottonseed. What is its future in the cotton industry's markets? Oil Mill Gaz. 74:20.

Spackman, D.H., W.H. Stein and S. Moore. 1958. Automatic recording apparatus for use in the chromatography of amino acids. Anal. Chem. 30:1190.

Steel, R.G.D. and J.H. Torrie. 1960. Principles and Procedures of Statistics. McGraw-Hill Book Co., Inc., New York.

Wolf, W.J. and J.C. Cowan. 1971. Soybeans as a food source. Crit. Rev. Food Technol. 2:81.

16

NUTRITIONAL QUALITY OF SEVERAL PROTEINS AS AFFECTED BY HEATING IN THE PRESENCE OF CARBOHYDRATES

J. E. Knipfel

Research Station
Research Branch, Agriculture Canada
Swift Current, Saskatchewan

H.G. Botting and J. M. McLaughlan
Foods and Nutrition Division
Health Protection Branch
Health and Welfare Canada
Ottawa, Ontario

An investigation of the effects of carbohydrate-heat interactions upon nutritive value of casein, soy and egg proteins was undertaken with rats. Weight gains and food intake of rats fed egg protein were reduced more rapidly by autoclaving, regardless of carbohydrate presence, than were those of casein or soy fed rats. NPR of egg rapidly decreased with heating to approximately the same value as soy, while casein remained at a higher NPR value throughout the heating period in the presence of carbohydrates. Digestibility of egg protein was reduced more severely than that of casein or soy. The presence of glucose, fructose, or sucrose with the autoclaved proteins appeared to reduce nutritive value more than autoclaving alone, while starch and cellulose had little effect upon nutritive value. Autoclaving (in the presence or absence of carbohydrates) induced losses in nutritive value of the test proteins which were suggested to be composite of reduced palatability (lowered amino acid intake), depressed protein digestibi-

lity (decrease in total amino acids absorbed), and reduced availability of the limiting amino acid for growth (accentuation of specific amino acid deficiency). The relative importance of these
factors appeared to vary considerably with the different proteins
studied.

INTRODUCTION

The nutritional quality of a protein depends upon the total
amounts of amino acids present in the protein, the relative proportions of the constituent amino acids (pattern of amino acids),
and the degree to which the animal can liberate and utilize the
amino acids from the protein (amino acid availability). Nutritional
availabilities of amino acids in foodstuffs have been examined by
numerous investigators and in many instances have not been considered to be seriously limiting factors to protein nutritional
value.

Subjection of proteins to various types of processing may
result in substantial decreases in amino acid availabilities.
Heating of proteins has been shown (Miller et al., 1965; Ford and
Salter, 1966; Narayana Rao and McLaughlan, 1967) to reduce availability of lysine in particular, with the severity of heat damage
dependent upon both the duration and temperature of heating, and
upon the presence of other compounds in the heated material.

Different proteins have been observed (Ford, 1962; Osner and
Johnson, 1968) to vary widely in their susceptibility to heat
damage, suggesting that the total amounts of, and pattern of amino
acids available to the animal after heating may be of more importance than the absolute availability of one particular amino acid.
While a large number of studies have been undertaken to assess the
effects of heating upon protein nutritive value, there is limited
knowledge regarding comparative susceptibilities of different proteins to loss of nutritive value when heated in the presence of
different carbohydrates. The present investigation was designed to

EFFECT OF HEAT AND CARBOHYDRATES ON PROTEIN QUALITY

study the effects of carbohydrate presence upon changes in nutritive value of casein, soy protein, and egg protein when these proteins were subjected to varying intervals of heating.

MATERIALS AND METHODS

Each of the proteins was extracted with three washings of 2-propanol to remove residual lipid and was freeze-dried prior to further treatment. The proteins were thoroughly mixed with 10% (w/w) of carbohydrates to give the protein-carbohydrate mixtures shown in Table 1. Each mixture was subsampled into porcelain-coated steel trays to a 2 cm depth, which were autoclaved (121°C) for the time intervals indicated in Table 1. Upon cooling, the mixtures were ground to pass a 1 mm screen in a laboratory mill and incorporated into rat diets. The diets contained: protein (N X 6.25) 10%; purified cellulose, 5%; corn oil, 5%; minerals (USP XIV), 4%; vitamins (Morrison et al., 1961), 1%; cornstarch to make 100%.

Eight male weanling Wistar rats (55-60 g initial body weight) were fed each diet individually in screened bottom cages for a 14-day period in a randomized block design (Table 1). Food consumption and weight gains were recorded. Feces were collected for the duration of the test period. On day fourteen, the rats were fasted from 1700 hour until 0900 hour on day fifteen. Food cans were replaced and the animals were sacrificed six hours later. Blood was collected in heparinized tubes following decapitation, red blood cells were removed by centrifugation, and the plasma was deproteinized for analyses of free lysine and methionine levels as described by McLaughlan et al. (1963). Protein Efficiency Ratios (PER) and Net Protein Ratios (NPR) were calculated as outlined by Campbell (1963). Apparent Digestibility of Crude Protein (DCP) was determined from total protein intake and excretion data during the test period, based upon Kjeldahl nitrogen contents of feed and feces.

Table 1.

Experimental Design[a]

Carbohydrate	Protein	Duration (min) of heating (121°C)					
		0	20	60	140	300	1280
None	Casein						
	Egg						
	Soy						
Glucose	Casein						
	Egg						
	Soy						
Fructose	Casein						
	Egg						
	Soy						
Sucrose	Casein						
	Egg						
	Soy						
Starch	Casein						
	Egg						
	Soy						
Cellulose	Casein						
	Egg						
	Soy						

[a]The design was replicated four times with two animals per replicate.

Best fit curves relating the various criteria of nutritive value to the duration of autoclaving were determined by polynomial regression analyses (Steel and Torrie, 1960) for each protein-carbohydrate mixture.

EFFECT OF HEAT AND CARBOHYDRATES ON PROTEIN QUALITY

RESULTS

Food Intake

Casein and soy intake by rats decreased in similar fashions as
the duration of autoclaving increased, when these proteins were
heated alone or with glucose, sucrose, or starch (Figure 1).
Fructose addition to soy caused a more rapid initial reduction in
intake than occurred when fructose and casein were heated, while
cellulose incorporaton in the mixture resulted in a greater decrease
initially in casein intake than in soy intake as autoclaving period
increased (Figure 1). At more extended durations of heating, however, these initial differences were eliminated. The addition of
glucose to casein or soy caused a more rapid reduction in food
intake with increased autoclaving time than did the other carbohydrates (Figure 1), although food intake increased at more extended
heating times. Intake of egg was reduced more rapidly and to a
greater degree by autoclaving than was that of casein or soy,
regardless of the carbohydrate included in the mixture (Figure 1),
but also appeared to increase as the autoclaving period became
greatly extended.

Weight Gain

As the duration of autoclaving increased, weight gains of rats
fed egg in all carbohydrate treatments decreased to zero or negative value within 140 min of heating (Figure 2). When starch or
cellulose was added to egg, greatest weight losses were observed
at 300 min of autoclaving (Figure 2). Weight gains on the remaining egg-carbohydrate treatments were not further reduced by
autoclaving durations greater than 140 min (Figure 2). More rapid
initial reductions in weight gains of rats fed casein occurred when
glucose, fructose, sucrose or cellulose was added prior to heating,
than when casein was heated alone or with starch (Figure 2). At
the most extended duration of autoclaving, however, weight gains
on all casein-carbohydrate mixtures except sucrose were not markedly

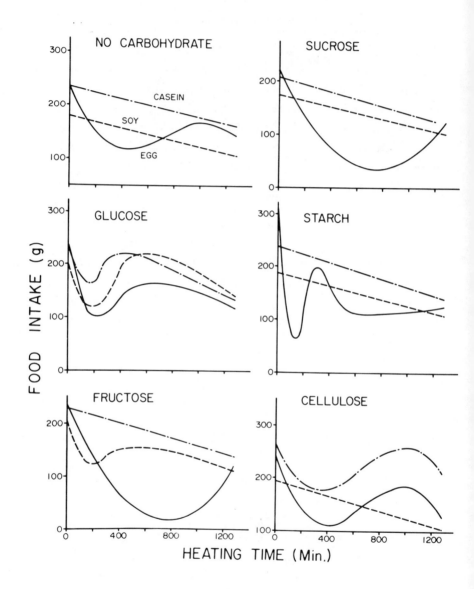

FIG. 1. Food intake of rats fed diets containing heated protein-carbohydrate mixtures.

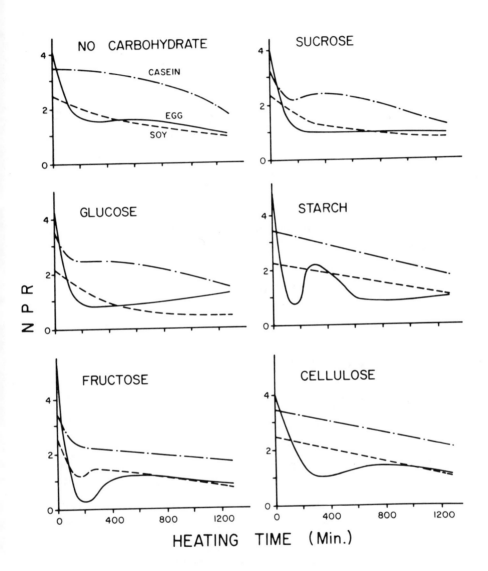

FIG. 2. Weight gains of rats fed diets containing heated protein carbohydrate mixtures.

different (Figure 2). Weight gains of soy-fed animals were reduced more rapidly by the inclusion of glucose, fructose, or sucrose, than by the remaining treatments (Figure 2).

Net Protein Ratio

Since PER is meaningful only when growth occurs, NPR was calculated to determine whether the proteins subjected to heat damage might make a contribution to maintenance of the animal even though not supporting growth. In all cases, the proteins did supply nutritive value above that of a nonprotein diet (Figure 3). NPR of egg was the most rapidly reduced by heating in all carbohydrate treatments, with NPR of soy decreasing to values close to that of heat treated egg as the autoclaving period was extended (Figure 3). The NPR of casein was reduced more rapidly when the simple sugars were incorporated into the autoclave mixture (Figure 3) but even after the most extended durations of heating the NPR of casein was approximately as high as that of soy prior to autoclaving.

Apparent Digestibility of Crude Protein

Egg DCP was dramatically reduced very rapidly with autoclaving, regardless of the carbohydrate treatment imposed (Figure 4). The extent of decrease in DCP was greatest for the simple sugar and cellulose treatments. DCP of casein was affected to a relatively minor extent by heating alone or in the presence of starch or cellulose (Figure 4), with a more rapid decrease in digestibility occurring when glucose, fructose or sucrose was heated with the casein. DCP of soy appeared to be lowered somewhat more rapidly than was that of casein when heated alone or with cellulose (Figure 4), and when heated with starch the soy decrease paralleled that of casein. Fructose or sucrose addition to soy caused a more pronounced and more rapid decrease in DCP than for any of the other carbohydrate treatments (Figure 4).

EFFECT OF HEAT AND CARBOHYDRATES ON PROTEIN QUALITY

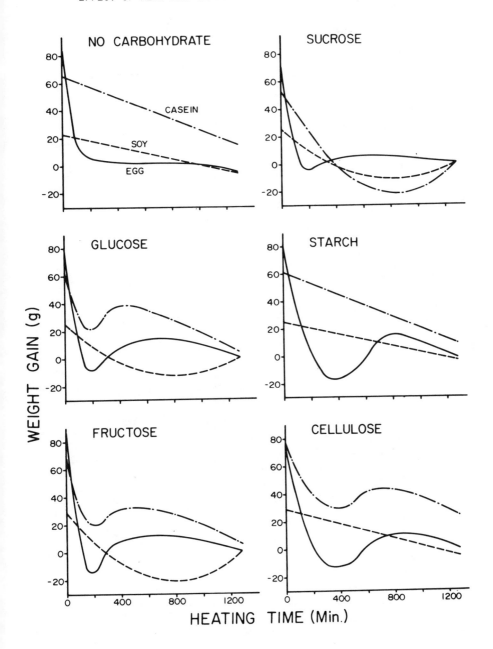

FIG. 3. Net Protein Ratios (NPR) as affected by heating of protein-carbohydrate mixtures.

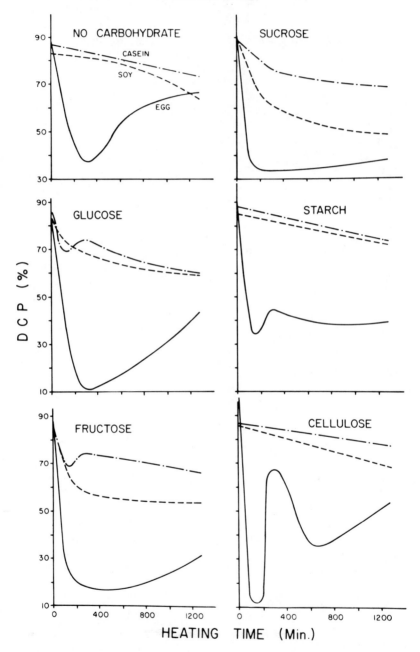

FIG. 4.   Digestibility of Crude Protein (DCP) as affected by heating of protein-carbohydrate mixtures.

EFFECT OF HEAT AND CARBOHYDRATES ON PROTEIN QUALITY

Plasma Amino Acid Levels

Plasma lysine levels from rats fed casein, casein plus starch, or casein plus cellulose remained relatively stable until the longest duration of autoclaving (1280 min, Figure 5). The addition of glucose, fructose or sucrose resulted in a progressive decrease in plasma lysine as the heating period was extended (Figure 5). A similar pattern of behavior was apparent for plasma methionine concentrations of rats fed casein (Figure 5). With soy, changes in plasma lysine were less evident than observed for casein, although glucose, fructose or sucrose addition appeared to reduce plasma lysine more readily than did the other carbohydrate treatments (Figure 5). Methionine concentrations in the plasma of rats fed soy mixtures tended to decrease to a minor extent as the duration of autoclaving increased (Figure 4). Decreasing plasma lysine concentrations with increased duration of autoclaving occurred for all egg-carbohydrate mixtures (Figure 5), with glucose, fructose, and sucrose causing the most rapid reductions. Plasma methionine concentrations were markedly reduced within 140 min of autoclaving by addition of glucose, fructose or sucrose with more gradual decreases in plasma methionine levels of rats fed the remaining egg-carbohydrate treatments also occurred (Figure 5).

Rats fed unheated casein mixtures showed higher levels of plasma lysine than did those fed soy or egg mixtures, and only after extended durations of heating were plasma lysine levels of casein fed rats reduced below 50 μM/100 ml plasma. Feeding the remaining two proteins resulted in plasma lysine concentrations of approximately the same magnitude when unheated, while autoclaving reduced plasma lysines of egg fed rats more rapidly than of soy fed rats (Figure 5).

Plasma methionine concentrations of rats fed casein or egg diets were initially of the same order of magnitude (Figure 5) but those of egg fed rats were reduced more quickly and to lower levels than those of casein fed animals.

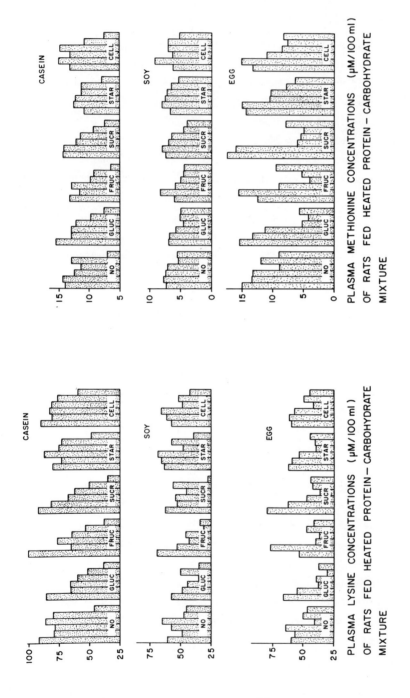

FIG. 5. Plasma lysine and methionine concentrations as influenced by duration of heating of protein-carbohydrate mixtures. The following durations of autoclaving, within each protein-carbohydrate mixture, were used: 0, 20, 60, 140, 300, 1280 min.

EFFECT OF HEAT AND CARBOHYDRATES ON PROTEIN QUALITY

DISCUSSION

Animal performance criteria indicated that casein and soy usually responded in similar manners to the effects of heating in the presence of various carbohydrates, while egg was much more susceptible to heat damage than the other two proteins. Kelly and Scott (1968) reported that autoclaving egg white alone for 30 min reduced weight gains of chicks to 15% of that of control birds, and suggested that a 50% reduction in protein quality would occur with as little as 10 min of autoclaving. The nutritive value of casein heated alone at 100-105°C for eight hours (Greaves et al., 1938) was unaffected, but at higher temperatures heat damage did occur, with the extent of damage proportional to duration of heating. Cogan et al. (1968) showed no reduction in weight gains, food consumption, or PER of rats fed isolated soy proteins which had been roasted for 30 min at 120°C, although the available lysine and methionine levels were reduced to some extent by roasting. As pointed out by Bender (1968), changes in animal performance such as weight gains, food intake, and PER will be affected only when a change in the degree of limitation of the first limiting amino acid occurs. Several investigations (Rao et al., 1963; Narayana Rao and McLaughlan, 1967) have shown lysine to be more subject to reductions in availability caused by heating and/or carbohydrate presence than is methionine. Proteins with lysine as first limiting amino acid might, therefore, be subject to more severe reductions in nutritive value than would those deficient in methionine. Chemical scores of the proteins examined in this study revealed that casein and soy were limiting in methionine (and/or cystine) while egg contained excess sulfur amino acids with lysine as the first limiting amino acid. In this situation, the more severe reductions in nutritive value of egg caused by heat and/or carbohydrate treatments could have been predicted from determination of the first limiting amino acid in these proteins.

Further investigation of the predictability of susceptibility
to heat damage from knowledge of amino acid limitations in proteins
should be untaken.

While severe reductions in lysine availability may have
accounted for a portion of the reduced performance of rats fed
heated egg-carbohydrate mixtures, other factors were also involved.
Reduced food intakes of rats fed heated egg mixtures were more
severe than for casein or soy fed rats, and cannot be attributed
solely to reduced amino acid availability since other workers
(Regier and Tappel, 1956; Carpenter et al., 1957) observed losses
in palatability of heated proteins with only minor concurrent
changes in nutritive value. In the present study, food intake was
reduced progressively as the duration of autoclaving increased for
all proteins and likely accounted for at least a portion of the
reduction in weight gains.

The digestibility of egg protein was severely and rapidly
reduced by heating regardless of carbohydrate presence, with
casein and soy digestibilities less markedly affected. These
losses in protein digestibility imply losses in availability of
several amino acids rather than only of lysine, and may be indicative of changes in the protein structure other than those associated with the intensively investigated Maillard reaction between
lysine and reducing sugars. Carpenter et al. (1962) and Miller
et al. (1965) demonstrated losses of several amino acids with
heating of fish products. Osner and Johnson, (1968) suggested as
a generalization that as long as temperature did not exceed 100°C
and the period of heating was no more than about hour, little
damage to proteins occurs. In light of the variation in protein
response to heating observed in this study, such generalizations
may be questioned.

Inclusion of glucose, fructose, or sucrose with the autoclaved proteins caused more rapid reductions in nutritive value

than did the polysaccharides. Miller et al. (1965) demonstrated more rapid losses in availability of lysine, methionine and tryptophan when 10% glucose was added to cod muscle prior to heating. Karel and Labuza (1968) showed that sucrose could be hydrolyzed to provide glucose to effect the Maillard reaction, while Fleming et al. (1968) suggested glucose and fructose to react similarly with lysine.

The polysaccharides would require hydrolysis to provide glucose for reaction, thus any effects on performance due to starch or cellulose may have been a result of residual reducing sugar presence.

Plasma lysine and methionine concentrations and the changes occurring in those concentrations with autoclaving gave an indication of amino acid limitations and availabilities as previously proposed by Smith and Scott (1965) and Narayana Rao and McLaughlan (1967). The quantitative aspects of the changes in plasma lysine and methionine and their relationships to animal performance remain unclear.

The results of this investigation have demonstrated that generalizations regarding the effects of heat and carbohydrate presence upon protein nutritional quality are not valid. While reductions in availability of certain amino acids undoubtedly occur as a result of heating, and the presence of carbohydrate may accentuate the effect, such reductions may not be reflected in animal performance unless the reduction results in a more severe limitation of the first limiting amino acid (Bender, 1968).

In proteins having as the first limiting amino acid one which is relatively stable to autoclave temperature, the overall digestibility of the protein, i. e., the pattern of available amino acids, and palatability of the diet may be of more importance to performance characteristics than would be the availability of the first limiting amino acid.

LITERATURE CITED

Bender, A. E. 1968. Factors affecting the nutritive value of protein foods. *In* "Proceedings International Biological Programme (IBP) and Wenner-Gren Symposium. Pergammon Press, Toronto, Ontario, 1970, p. 319.

Campbell, J. A. 1963. Methodology of Protein Evaluation. Publication No. 21, American University of Beirut, Beirut, Lebanon.

Carpenter, K. J., G. M. Ellinger, M. I. Munro and E. J. Roilfe. 1957. Fish products as protein supplements. Brit. J. Nutr. 11:162.

Carpenter, K. J., C. B. Morgan, C. H. Lea and I. J. Parr. 1962. Chemical and nutritional changes in stored meal. 3. Effect of heating at controlled moisture contents on the binding of amino acids in freeze-dried herring press cake and in related model systems. Brit. J. Nutr. 16:451.

Cogan, U., A. Yaron, Z. Birk and G. Zimmerman. 1968. Effect of processing conditions on the value of isolated soybean proteins. Agric. Food Chem. 16:196.

Fleming, M., K. J. Parker and J. C. Williams. 1968. Aspects of the chemistry of the browning reaction of reducing sugars. I.S.S.C.T. Proceedings (13th Congress) :1782.

Ford, J. E. 1962. A microbiological method for assessing the nutritional value of proteins. 2. The measurement of "available" methionine, leucine, isoleucine, arginine, histidine, tryptophan and valine. Brit. J. Nutr. 16:409.

Ford, J. E., and D. N. Satter. 1966. Analysis of enzymically digested food proteins by Sephadex-gel filtration. Brit. J. Nutr. 20:843.

Greaves, E. O., A. F. Morgan and M. K. Loveen. 1938. Effect of amino acid supplements and of variations in temperature and duration of heating upon the biological value of heated casein. J. Nutr. 16:115.

Karel, M. and T. P. Labuza. 1968. Nonenzymatic browning in model systems containing sucrose. Agric. Food Chem. 16:717.

Kelly, M. and H. M. Scott. 1968. Autoclaving time in relation to the nutritional quality of dried egg white. Poult. Sci. 47: 850.

McLaughlan, J. M., F. J. Noel, A. B. Morrison and J. A. Campbell. 1963. Blood amino acid studies. IV. Some factors affecting plasma amino acid levels in human subjects. Can. J. Biochem. 41:191.

EFFECT OF HEAT AND CARBOHYDRATES ON PROTEIN QUALITY

Miller, E. L., K. J. Carpenter and C. K. Milner. 1965. Availability of sulfur amino acids in protein foods. 3. Chemical and nutritional changes in heated cod muxcle. Brit. J. Nutr. 19: 547.

Morrison, A. B., E. J. Middleton and J. A. Campbell. 1961. Blood amino acid studies. II. Effects of dietary lysine level, sex and growth rats on plasma-free lysine and threonine levels in the rat. Can. J. Biochem. Physiol. 39:1675.

Narayana Rao, M. and J. M. McLaughlan. 1967. Lysine and methionine availability in heat casein-glucose mixtures. JAOAC 50(3):704.

Osner, R. C. and R. M. Johnson. 1968. Nutritional changes in proteins during heat processing. J. Fd. Technol. 3:81.

Rao, M. N., H. Sreenivas, M. Swaminathan, K. J. Carpenter and C. G. Morgan. 1963. The nutritionally availably lysine and methionine of heated casein-glucose mixtures. J. Sci. Food Agric. 14:544.

Regier, L. W. and A. L. Tappel. 1956. Freeze-dried meat. III. Nonoxidative deterioration of freeze-dried beef. IV. Factors affecting the rate of deterioration. Food Res. 21:630.

Smith, R. G. and H. M. Scott. 1965. Use of free amino acid concentrations in blood plasma in evaluating the amino adequacy of intact proteins for chick growth. I. Free amino acid patterns of blood plasma of chicks fed unheated and heated fishmeal proteins. J. Nutr. 86:37.

Steel, R. G. D. and J. H. Torrie. 1960. Principles and procedures of statistics. McGraw-Hill Inc., Toronto, Ontario.

391

17

THE ASSESSMENT OF THERMAL PROCESSING
ON WHEAT FLOUR PROTEINS
BY PHYSICAL, CHEMICAL, AND ENZYMATIC METHODS

L. P. Hansen, P. H. Johnston, and R. E. Ferrel

Western Regional Research Laboratory
Agricultural Research Service
U.S. Department of Agriculture
Berkeley, California

Commercial thermal processing of flour products induces protein changes that sometimes decrease the nutritional value of the product. Methods were developed to assess flour protein changes in a model system under controlled conditions of temperature, moisture, and time in a range used by commercial processors. Flour (Hard Red Winter Wheat--1st clears) was processed in a closed heat exchanger designed to control processing parameters of temperature (108, 150, and 174°C), moisture (13-33%), and time (2, 5, and 10 min). High processing temperatures in our model system produced protein break-down to peptides. With the production of the heat-produced peptides, lysine, arginine, and cystine contents were reduced. The enzymatic digestion rates of pepsin and trypsin on heat-treated flour proteins were decreased and the specific release of lysine and arginine by trypsin-carboxypeptidase-B was impaired. Similar observations have been made on high temperature commercial products--puffed wheat, wheat granules, wheat flakes, and bread crust. Low temperature pro-cessed products--wheat shreds and bread crumb--had minimal protein damage and correspondingly higher protein efficiency ratio (PER) values than the high temperature products.

INTRODUCTION

The worldwide utilization of wheat for food is based largely on its easy growth and storage properties. Cereals (wheat, rice, and corn) provide 49% of the total world supply of edible protein. The rest is supplied by roots, pulses, oilseeds, and nuts (17.9%), meat and poultry (12.9%), dairy products (11.3%), vegetable and fruit (3.5%), fish (3.4%), and eggs (1.8%), according to the Food and Agricultural Organization of the United Nations (Abbott, 1966). The poorer people in the world are necessarily more dependent on low-cost cereal products to meet their protein requirements than the middle-income and wealthy.

Although wheat plays a major role in feeding the world community, it cannot be used without some kind of processing. Wheat is used primarily in bread and breakfast cereal-type foods. New thermal processing methods such as extrusion, microwave heating, puffing, and spray drying that use high-temperature/short-time processing conditions have been widely adopted. Protein concentrates from wheat millfeeds and flours (Fellers et al., 1966, 1969), usable in high-protein, low-cost foods, can be processed using these methods. Wheat protein concentrate from millfeeds is currently used in a Wheat Soy Blend (WSB) in export programs of the U.S. Department of Agriculture (1972) to developing countries. However, protein changes in wheat due to thermal processing and their consequential nutritional effects have not yet been adequately explored.

A model system, using wheat flour to determine the effects of thermal processing on flour proteins, was designed to control the processing parameters of temperature, time, and moisture in a range used by commercial processors. In our study, commercially heat-treated products were selected which had a wide range of low to high heat treatments applied to them. The protein changes found in the commercial products were compared with those found in flour proteins in the model system. The assessment of thermal processing on proteins of wheat flour and in commercial products was determined by physical, chemical, and enzymatic methods and correlated with the nutritional values of the products obtained by rat PER evaluations.

THERMAL PROCESSING AND WHEAT FLOUR PROTEINS

EXPERIMENTAL PROCEDURE

Flour Heat Treatment

Hard red wheat flour (first clears, ash content 0.93%, N content dry basis 2.74%) was processed by Johnston et al. (1971) in a reversed heat exchanger in the model system. The flour sample (186 g total) at the stated moisture content was heated at the specified temperature and time (Table 1) in a stainless steel container with 21 individual tubes (0.95 cm i.d. x 16.5 cm) (Figure 1) and then water cooled.

The protein methodology presented is or will be described in detail in papers published by Hansen et al. (1972a, b; also one in press).

Urea Solubility of Flour Proteins

Proteins were extracted from a 500-mg flour sample with a 10-ml buffer solution (3 M urea-0.01 M phosphate, pH 7.0), shaken for 2 hr at 5°C, and centrifuged. Protein (0.03 µl supernatant aliquot) was measured at 500 nm by the procedure of Lowry et al. (1951).

Gel Filtration

An aliquot (4 ml) of the urea-phosphate-solubilized proteins was chromatographed on a Sephadex G-100 column (Pharmacia) and eluted with 3 M urea-0.01 M phosphate, pH 7.0, at ambient temperature. Peaks were detected by their 280 nm absorbance.

Amino Acid Analyses

Flour (60 mg) was heated under vacuum in 10 ml 6 N HCl ±1°C for 24 hr as described by Hansen et al. (in press). Cystine, cysteine, and methionine were performic acid-oxidized by the procedure of Moore (1963) prior to acid hydrolysis. Amino acid content of the acid hydrolysates was determined by a modification of the procedure of Spackman et al. (1958).

TABLE 1

Processing Conditions for Hard Red Wheat Flour

Moisture %	108°C			150°C			174°C		
		Time (minutes)			Time (minutes)			Time (minutes)	
	Heat[a]	Hold[b]	Come-down[c]	Heat[a]	Hold[b]	Come-down[c]	Heat[a]	Hold[b]	Come-down[c]
12.7	6.9	2	0.8	6.8	2	1.3	9.1	2	1.4
		5			5			5	
		10			10			10	
23.8	5.6	2	1.0	4.9	2	1.3	5.3	2	1.4
		5			5			5	
		10			10			10	
33.1	3.8	2	1.0	5.5	2	1.2	5.0	2	1.0
		5			5			5	
		10			10			10	

[a] Interval from time steam enters retort until processing temperature was achieved. Average times taken from time-temperature curves.

[b] Time at processing temperatures.

[c] Average time interval from end of holding time until room temperature was achieved.

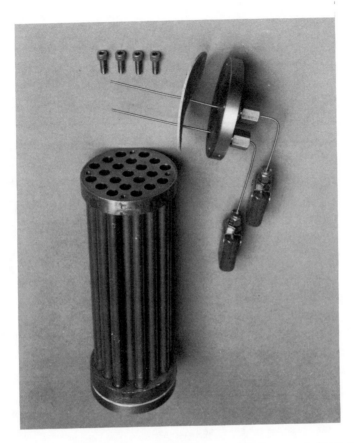

FIG. 1. The stainless steel heat-processing container and thermocouples used in thermal processing wheat flour in the model system.

Enzyme Assays

The initial rates of pepsin or trypsin digestion of unheated and heated proteins were determined by a modified procedure of Anson (1938). In the enzyme assays for lysine and arginine availability, the unheated and heated flour proteins were digested with trypsin for 5 hr at 37°C, followed by carboxypeptidase-B digestion for 15 hr at 37°C. Amino acid content of the digest was determined by a modified procedure of Spackman et al. (1958). All enzymes used were highly purified hog commercial preparations.

Commercial Products

Breakfast cereals (puffed wheat, wheat granules, wheat flakes, and wheat shreds) were purchased from a grocery supermarket. Puffed wheat is made from wheat kernels, heated to high temperatures (>260°C) in pressurized vessels. The fast temperature drop results in the sudden expansion of water in the interstices of the granule with the formation of the puffed product. Wheat granules are made of a dough (wheat, malted barley flour, salt, dry yeast, and water). The dough is held at 26°C for 4.5-5 hr, baked for 2 hr at 204°C, fragmented, and toasted. Wheat flakes, made from whole grains, are tempered (26°C for 24 hr), steamed until temperature reaches 95°C, cooked (149°C for 90 min), roller-flattened, and dried (138-154°C). Wheat shreds, made from whole grain, are cooked (100°C for 1 hr), tempered, shredded, and dried (121°C for 30-60 min). Information on the cereal technology is taken from Matz (1970).

Bread, similar to some commercial bread formulas, was prepared by our baking laboratory staff. The dough contained hard red wheat flour (approximately 70% extraction, untreated, ash content 0.42%, N content dry basis 2.25%), sugar, shortening, water, salt, potassium bromate, malt, and yeast. After fermentation, the dough was baked for 25 min at 219°C. Bread was separated into crumb and crust fractions and freeze-dried.

Protein methodology used for commercial products was the same as that described for the hard red wheat flour in the model system.

PER Determinations

Rats (male, weanling Sprague-Dawley strain) were fed diets calculated to contain 10% of the specified protein for a 28-day period.

RESULTS AND DISCUSSION

Urea Solubility of Flour Proteins

Most of the protein ($\cong$73%) from the unheated flour (control) was solubilized by the urea-phosphate solution. However, this solution did not solubilize the acetic acid-insoluble gel proteins. These proteins, constituting approximately 27% of the total flour proteins, have been characterized by Mecham et al. (1972) and Cole et al. (1972). The flour proteins including the gel proteins were solubilized with 1 N NaOH. Sodium hydroxide-solubilized protein gave an absorbance (500 nm) of 0.882 for a 0.03-ml aliquot.

Protein solubility in urea for all heat-treated flours at the specified moistures was affected by the heat treatment, as shown in Figure 2. A comparison of flours at 13, 24, and 33% moisture levels processed at 108°C showed the lowest moisture level flour (13%) was the least affected by the heat treatment as measured by protein urea

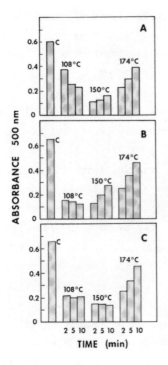

FIG. 2. Effect of thermal processing on flour protein solubility in 3 M urea-0.01 M phosphate, pH 7.0, as measured by the Lowry procedure. A: 13% moisture content flour. B: 24%. C: 33%. C is control-unheated flour at specified moisture before processing.

solubility. At 150°C 2-min flour processing there was a marked decrease in protein solubility in urea at all moisture levels compared to the unheated samples. At 174°C, the protein solubility showed a linear increase as a function of time for all moisture levels. The 13% moisture flour had the lowest rate of solubility change (absorbance 500 nm/min) at this temperature.

Gel Filtration

Gel filtration on Sephadex G-100 of urea-solubilized proteins from heated and unheated flours was used to determine the relative molecular weight changes of the proteins as a result of processing. Four peaks were obtained for the unheated proteins as shown in the chromatogram (Figure 3A). Peak I contained mostly glutenins, peak II mostly gliadins, peake III mostly globulins and albumins, and peak IV mostly peptides. Peak I appearing at the front has a molecular weight calculated to be 100,000; peak II, 51,200; peak III, 31,000; and peak IV, 2,000.

The effects of thermal processing on flour proteins are shown in Figure 3B. At 108°C, 13% moisture, peak I area had increased indicating that the lower molecular weight proteins had aggregated. The gliadin fraction (peak II area) showed some decrease. The albumin and globulin fraction (peak III area) showed a substantial decrease. The peptide fraction (peak IV area) showed little change. The effect of processing became more pronounced at 150°C where peak I area had decreased, the albumin and globulin peak III was absent, and a slight increase in the peptide peak IV was noted. At 174°C, there was a substantial breakdown of the proteins to peptides (peak IV).

Gel filtration can be used to measure processing effects on proteins with different flour moisture levels (Figure 4A). The effect of time of processing on flour proteins can be studied by this method also (Figure 4B). Peak IV, the peptide fraction, can be used to monitor protein breakdown from thermal processing by integrating the peak IV area.

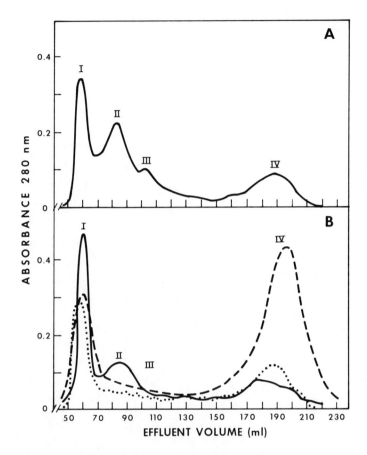

FIG. 3. Sephadex G-100 chromatography of urea-phosphate-solubilized proteins of heated and unheated flours. A: unheated flour proteins (13% moisture level flour). B: heated flour proteins; ——————— 13-108-2 (% moisture-°C-min); .... 13-150-2; — — — — — 13-174-2.

Amino Acid Analyses

Amino acid destruction in the flour samples by the heat treatments is shown in Figure 5. Lysine, arginine, and cystine-cysteine had significant losses due to thermal treatments. Flour moisture content appeared to exert a greater influence on cystine-cysteine destruction than on arginine and lysine. Little destruction (25% or less) of the other amino acids was found for the flour processed

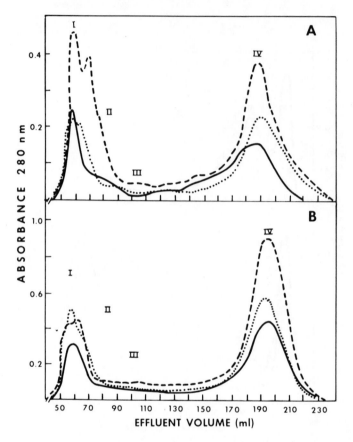

FIG. 4. A: effect of flour moisture content during processing;
————— 13-150-10 (% moisture-°C-min); .... 24-150-10; — — — — —
33-150-10. B: effect of holding time of processing; ————— 13-
174-2; .... 13-174-5; — — — — — 13-174-10.

at the maximum temperature (174°C) and time (10 min) studied.

The Food and Agricultural Organization of the United Nations
(1965) recommends the use of the essential amino acid content of
whole egg as a reference standard for other proteins because of its
high PER value (3.8) and complete digestibility. The chemical score
for unprocessed and processed flour proteins is shown in Table 2.
The chemical scores decreased as processing temperatures increased,
as shown by the lysine values. Cystine, which was not limiting in
the unheated flours, did become limiting at 174°C.

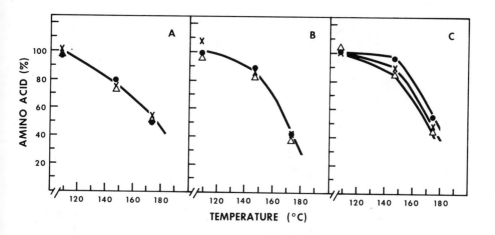

FIG. 5. Effect of processing temperatures on specific amino acids. A: Lysine. Unheated flour, 2.10 g/16 g N = 100%. B: Arginine, 3.68 g/16 g N. C: Cysteic acid, 2.84 g/16 g N. ● 13% moisture. × 24% moisture. Δ 33% moisture.

Enzyme Assays

The aim of in vivo digestion is the breakdown of food proteins by the endopeptidases, such as pepsin, trypsin, and chymotrypsin to polypeptides. The polypeptides are then further broken down to amino acids by the exopeptidases, which cleave the amino acids from the ends of the peptide chain. In this study, the initial breakdown of the flour proteins to polypeptides by pepsin and trypsin has been examined to determine if the start of protein degradation in the digestive process has been affected by the heat treatment. Carboxypeptidase-B, a lysine-releasing enzyme found in the pancreatic juice, was investigated because of the prime importance of lysine in the nutritional studies of flour, since it is the limiting amino acid in wheat products.

The initial rates of pepsin digestion of processed and unprocessed flour proteins are shown in Table 3. In general, the pepsin digestion rates of heated protein decreased as processing temperature and time increased. Pepsin present in the stomach gastric juice begins the protein cleavage to polypeptides in vivo by hydrolyzing peptide bonds containing tyrosine and phenylalanine.

TABLE 2

Effect of Thermal Processing on the Chemical Score of Hard Red Wheat Flour

Amino acid	Egg (mg amino acid/g N)	Wheat flour (33% moisture)			
		Unheated %	108°C-10 min %	150°C-10 min %	174°C-10 min %
Isoleucine	393	55.2	53.9	56.2	54.7
Leucine	551	77.3	76.2	78.8	77.5
Lysine	436	31.4[a]	30.1[a]	22.0[a]	15.4[a]
Methionine	210	67.6	68.1	59.5	58.6
Cystine	152	108.6	113.2	92.8	47.4
Phenylalanine	358	83.8	82.4	84.9	82.7
Tyrosine	260	71.9	58.9	70.4	68.5
Threonine	320	50.6	50.0	53.1	48.8
Valine	428	59.6	57.9	60.3	59.4

[a]Essential amino acid content is expressed as a percentage of the egg standard. The lowest percentage (underlined) is the chemical score. Block and Mitchell (1946).

THERMAL PROCESSING AND WHEAT FLOUR PROTEINS

TABLE 3

Effect of Processing on
Pepsin Digestion Rates of Flour Proteins

Processing conditions				
Temperature, °C	Moisture, %	2 min	5 min	10 min
		Digestion rates[a]		
108	13	67	68	31
	24	36	34	44
	33	53	53	44
150	13	59	51	56
	24	34	35	25
	33	46	46	18
174	13	41	41	40
	24	55	63	43
	33	43	46	48

[a]Based on rate constants [least squares analyses of increased absorbance (660 nm) as a function of time (min)]. The digestion rate of unheated flour proteins by pepsin was taken as 100.

Trypsin continues the digestion of food proteins to polypeptides in the large intestine. Initial digestion rates of heated proteins by trypsin were also inversely related to increasing processing temperatures (Table 4). The digestion reactions of peptide bonds of proteins by trypsin-carboxypeptidase-B (TCB) is shown in Figure 6. Trypsin cleaves only lysyl or arginyl peptide bonds so that the resulting peptides have a lysyl or arginyl terminal carboxyl group. The tryptic-formed peptides are cleaved by carboxypeptidase-B, which is specific for C-terminal basic groups--lysine or arginine. To test lysine availability, unprocessed flour proteins were incubated with trypsin in Tris-chloride buffer, pH 8.0, for 5 hr at 37°C, followed by carboxypeptidase-B digestion for 16 hr. The results of TCB digestion of unprocessed flour proteins are shown in Figure 7. Lysine was 70% released; arginine 79% released; histidine 20% released; and the other amino acids less than 21% released.

TABLE 4

Effect of Processing on
Trypsin Digestion Rates of Flour Proteins

Temperature, °C	Moisture, %	Processing conditions		
		2 min	5 min	10 min
		Digestion rates[a]		
108	13	96	94	86
	24	51	46	50
	33	70	65	50
150	13	30	17	25
	24	24	34	20
	33	36	39	36
174	13	23	31	14
	24	26	28	17
	33	37	18	37

[a]Based on rate constants [least squares analyses of increased absorbance (660 nm) as a function of time (min)]. The digestion rate of unheated flour proteins by trypsin was taken as 100.

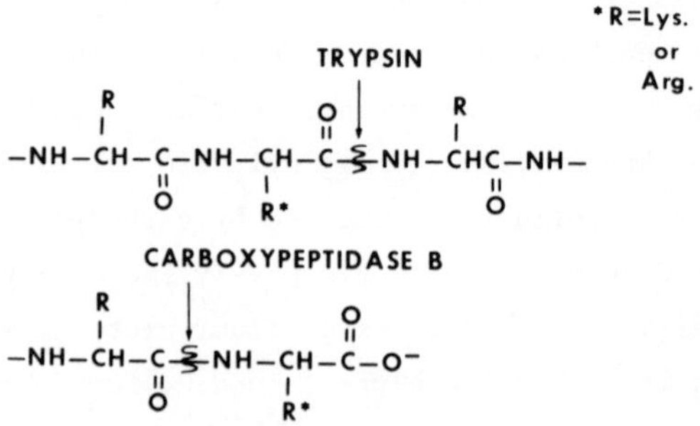

FIG. 6. Digestion reactions of peptide bonds of flour proteins by trypsin-carboxypeptidase-B.

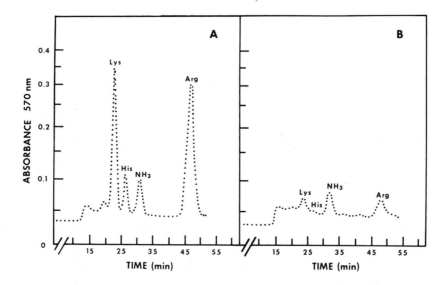

FIG. 7. A: Chromatogram (amino acid analysis) of trypsin-carboxypeptidase-B digest of unheated flour proteins. B: Chromatogram (amino acid analysis) of trypsin digest of unheated flour proteins.

Flour proteins digested with trypsin alone for 21 hr at 37°C showed that lysine and arginine release was slow in the absence of carboxypeptidase-B (Figure 7B). Both enzymes are highly specific with respect to their substrate requirements. Trypsin-carboxypeptidase-B digestion chromatograms of flour processed at 108, 150, and 174°C, respectively, are shown in Figure 8. Lysine and arginine release from flour proteins processed at 150 and 174°C was less compared to unheated flour proteins. The low-temperature flour heat treatment (108°C) showed a small increase in lysine and arginine release compared to unheated flour proteins. The decrease in lysine and arginine released by TCB from heat-treated flour proteins (150 and 174°C) is probably due to destruction of these amino acids, possibly by Maillard reactions (sugars reacting with the basic groups of proteins). Basic amino acids such as lysine and arginine in proteins would be especially sensitive to Maillard reactions at high processing temperatures because of their available basic groups.

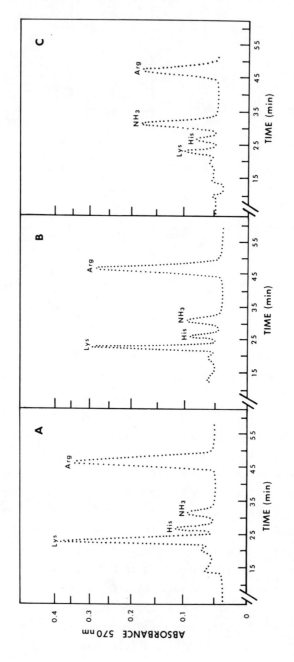

FIG. 8. Chromatograms (amino acid analyses) of trypsin-carboxypeptidase-B digestion of flour proteins processed at A (108°C), B (150°C), and C (174°C), respectively, for 2 minutes.

THERMAL PROCESSING AND WHEAT FLOUR PROTEINS

Lysine and arginine released by acid hydrolyses are compared with the enzymatic release (Table 5). Enzyme release of the amino acids was much slower than the acid release at various processing temperatures. The amino acid content, as measured by acid hydrolysis of a flour product, may not be indicative of the amount of amino acid available to the consumer.

Commercial Products

The products studied together with maximum processing temperatures for ready-to-eat cereals (Matz, 1970) and for bread crust and crumb (Walden, 1955) are listed in Table 6. Protein content for commercial products is conventionally determined by the Kjeldahl method for nitrogen (N% multiplied by a factor, F, to obtain protein content). Our Kjeldahl determinations by an AOAC method (1965) (Table 6) agreed with the protein contents stated on the commercial product labels. The nutritional values of the products based on PER determinations did not correlate well with protein content (Kjeldahl method) but gave a good inverse correlation with maximum processing

TABLE 5

Comparison of Enzymatic and
Acid Hydrolysis of Wheat Flour Proteins

Amino acid	Hydrolysis	Processing conditions[a]			
		Control	108°C- 2 min	150°C- 2 min	174°C- 2 min
		Amino acid available, %			
Lysine	TCB	70	81	59	13
Lysine	6 *N* HCl	100[b]	100	92	58
Arginine	TCB	79	92	77	44
Arginine	6 *N* HCl	100[b]	100	100	96

[a]13% moisture flour.

[b]Acid hydrolysate amino acid values of unheated flour taken as 100%.

TABLE 6

Effect of Processing Temperatures on the Nutritional Values of Cereal Products

Product	Maximum processing temperature °C	Protein[a] (N x F) %	Weight gain[b] g	PER[c]	Digestibility[d] (N) %
Puffed wheat	>260[e]	14.98[g]	-10	-0.87 ± 0.09	69
Wheat granules	204[e]	10.72[g]	6	0.36 ± 0.11	80
Wheat flakes	149[e]	10.55[g]	8	0.46 ± 0.10	72
Wheat shreds	121[e]	10.72[g]	44	1.67 ± 0.15	75
Bread crust[h]	175[f]	12.14[g]	10	0.62 ± 0.09	85
Bread crumb[h]	100[f]	13.62[g]	32	1.36 ± 0.08	88
Wheat flour		11.06[g]	23	1.11 ± 0.07	89
Casein			125	3.27 ± 0.08	94

[a]Based on nitrogen Kjeldahl determinations. F = 5.83 for puffed wheat, wheat flakes, and wheat shreds. F = 5.70 for wheat granules, flour, bread crust, and bread crumb.

[b]Weight gain = total weight - initial weight.

[c]PER = gain in rat weight (g) / protein intake (g).

[d]Digestibility = [(N intake - fecal N) / (N intake)] x 100.

[e]Applied temperature (Matz, 1970).

[f]Inner temperature (Walden, 1955).

[g]As is moisture basis.

[h]Freeze-dried.

410

temperatures. Protein thermal damage was not measurable by Kjeldahl
N determinations. Commercial products, which included the bran part
of the wheat kernel (puffed wheat, wheat flakes, and wheat shreds)
had protein, which was not readily digested in the gastrointestinal
tract, and therefore, not completely absorbed or utilized by the rat
as evidenced by lower digestibility values listed in Table 6.
Thermal processing resulted in a small decrease in in vivo digestibility of the commercial cereal products.

In our model system, Sephadex G-100 chromatography of urea-
phosphate-solubilized, heat-treated proteins showed an increase in
the peptide fraction (peak IV) with increasing processing temperatures. Similarly, peak IV for ready-to-eat cereal products increased with increasing processing temperature (Figure 9). Puffed
cereal with the highest maximum processing temperature (>260°C) had
the largest amount of protein breakdown to peptides as indicated by
peak IV area of the cereals examined. Wheat shreds, with the lowest
processing temperature (121°C), had the least amount of protein

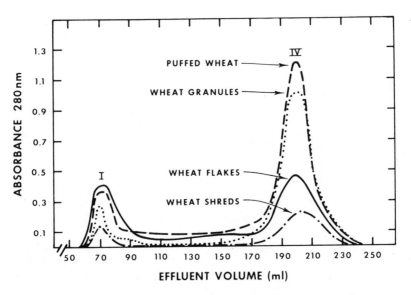

FIG. 9. Sephadex G-100 chromatography of urea-phosphate-
solubilized proteins of commercial cereal products.

breakdown with the smallest peak IV area. Bread crumb, bread crust, and bread flour exhibited a similar trend on chromatography of its urea-phosphate-solubilized proteins (Figure 10). The crust with a higher temperature (175°C) showed more protein thermal breakdown than bread crumb with an internal temperature of 100°C as measured by the peak IV area. The chromatography profile of bread flour proteins solubilized by urea-phosphate was similar to the profile obtained of first clears wheat flour (Figure 3A).

The value of any protein method for nutritional purposes can be evaluated to the extent results with the food products correlate with data obtained from biological assays. A comparison of lysine released by enzymatic (TCB) and acid hydrolyses of commercial wheat products with biological assays (PER) is given in Table 7. Both methods gave decreased lysine values with increasing processing temperatures. However, in the enzymatic hydrolysis (TCB), lysine values were more closely correlated with PER for products treated at high temperatures (puffed wheat, wheat granules, and wheat flakes)

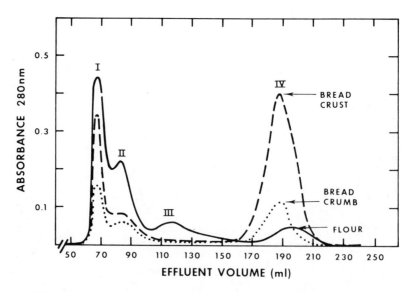

FIG. 10. Sephadex G-100 chromatography of urea-phosphate-solubilized proteins from flour used in bread making, bread crumb, and the bread crust.

TABLE 7

Lysine Released from Proteins by Acid and Enzymatic Hydrolyses of Cereal Products

Product	Maximum processing temperature °C	PER	Lysine 6 N HCl g/16 g N	Lysine TCB μmoles/ml
Puffed wheat	>260[a]	-0.87 (0)[c]	1.25 (53)	0.11 (17)
Wheat granules	204[a]	0.36 (32)	1.62 (69)	0.23 (35)
Wheat flakes	149[a]	0.46 (41)	1.74 (74)	0.30 (46)
Wheat shreds	121[a]	1.67 (150)	2.61 (112)	0.57 (86)
Bread crust	175[b]	0.62 (56)	1.47 (63)	0.43 (65)
Bread crumb	100[b]	1.36 (122)	2.32 (99)	0.73 (111)
Wheat flour[d]		1.11 (100)	2.34 (100)	0.66 (100)
Correlation coefficient with PER	0.88		0.96	0.90

[a] Applied temperature.
[b] Inner temperature.
[c] Negative PER taken as 0.
[d] Flour--unheated product taken as standard for comparison purposes.

413

than results obtained from acid hydrolyses. Evidently, enzyme digestion conditions (temperature, time, pH) are more closely related to in vivo conditions in the gastrointestinal tract than the acid digestion conditions.

In conclusion, there are critical temperatures that determine protein changes in wheat flour and wheat flour products such as protein aggregation, peptide formation, and amino acid destruction. Our results show that to maintain the nutritive value (PER) of the raw material of the wheat product, product temperature should not exceed 125°C. Bread would, therefore, appear to be a good vehicle for protein concentrates, since the internal crumb temperature does not exceed 100°C, where protein changes would be minimal.

ACKNOWLEDGMENTS

The authors thank Mrs. Imogene Simpson for helpful technical assistance, Mrs. Amy Noma for amino acid analyses, Dr. Michael Gumbmann and Miss Dorothy Robbins for PER determinations, and Mr. Max Hanamoto and Mrs. Kazuko Nishita for the bread baking.

Mention of firm names or trade products does not imply that they are endorsed or recommended by the U.S. Department of Agriculture over other firms or similar products not mentioned.

REFERENCES

Abbott, D.C. 1966. Protein supplies and prospects. *In* World Protein Resources. Advances in Chemistry Series, No. 57. American Chemical Society, Washington, D.C.

Anson, M.L. 1938. The estimation of pepsin, trypsin, papain, and cathepsin with hemoglobin. J. Gen. Physiol. 22:79.

AOAC. 1965. Official Methods of Analysis (10th Ed.), 2.042-2.043. Association of Official Agricultural Chemists, Washington, D.C.

Block, R.J. and H.H. Mitchell. 1946. The correlation of the amino acid composition of proteins with their nutritive value. Nutr. Abstr. and Rev. 16:249.

THERMAL PROCESSING AND WHEAT FLOUR PROTEINS

Cole, E.W., H. Ng and D.K. Mecham. 1972. Gradient ultracentrifugation of the acetic acid-insoluble proteins of wheat flour. Cereal Chem. 49:68.

FAO. 1965. Protein requirements. Report of a joint FAO/WHO expert group. Food and Agricultural Organization, Rome, Italy.

Fellers, D.A., A.D. Shepherd, N.J. Ballard and A.P. Mossman. 1966. Protein concentrate by dry milling of wheat millfeeds. Cereal Chem. 43:715.

Fellers, D.A., P.H. Johnston, S. Smith, A.P. Mossman and A.D. Shepherd. 1969. Process for protein-starch separation in .wheat flour. Food Technol. 23:560.

Hansen, L.P., P.H. Johnston and R.E. Ferrel. 1972a. Effects of hydrothermal processing on wheat flour proteins. Cereal Science Today. 17:266. (Abstr.).

Hansen, L.P., P.H. Johnston and R.E. Ferrel. 1972b. Action of digestive enzymes on hydrothermally processed wheat flour proteins. Cereal Science Today. 17:266. (Abstr.).

Hansen, L.P., P.H. Johnston and R.E. Ferrel. Heat-moisture effects on wheat flour. I. Physical-chemical changes of flour proteins resulting from thermal processing. Cereal Chem. (In press).

Johnston, P.H., R.E. Ferrel, L.P. Hansen and D.A. Fellers. 1971. Studies on the hydrothermal processing of wheat. Cereal Science Today. 16:308. (Abstr.).

Lowry, O.H., N.J. Rosebrough, A.L. Farr and R.J. Randall. 1951. Protein measurement with the Folin phenol reagent. J. Biol. Chem. 193:265.

Matz, S.A. 1970. Manufacture of breakfast cereals. *In* Cereal Technology. Avi Publishing Co., Westport, Connecticut.

Mecham, D.K., E.W. Cole and H. Ng. 1972. Solubilizing effect of mercuric chloride on the "gel" protein of wheat flour. Cereal Chem. 49:62.

Moore, S. 1963. On the determination of cystine as cysteic acid. J. Biol. Chem. 238:235.

Spackman, D.H., W.H. Stein and S. Moore. 1958. Automatic recording apparatus for use in chromatography of amino acids. Anal. Chem. 30:1190.

USDA. 1972. Purchase of wheat soy blend for use in export programs. U.S. Department of Agriculture. Agricultural Stabilization and Conservation Service. Announcement WSB-3.

Walden, C.C. 1955. The action of wheat amylases on starch under conditions of time and temperature as they exist during baking. Cereal Chem. 32:421.

18

EFFECTS OF PROCESSING ON THE NUTRITIVE VALUE
OF WSB-SKIM MILK MIXTURES FOR INFANTS

F. Monckeberg, E. Yanez, and D. Ballester

Departamento de Nutricion y Tecnologia de los Alimentos
Universidad de Chile
Santiago, Chile

and

C. O. Chichester and Tung-Ching Lee

Department of Food and Resource Chemistry
University of Rhode Island
Kingston, Rhode Island

In Chile, a high percentage of the infant population is malnourished, mainly as a result of poor protein intake. At one year
of age, almost 30% of Chilean children show some degree of malnutrition and this percentage is increased gradually in later years so
that at six years of age, almost 60% of the children are malnourished.

The present study reports the development of a protein-rich mixture called "Fortesan" which can replace milk for infants and be used
as a supplement to protein supplied by daily meals in preschool and
older children. It also reports the investigation of the optimal
processing conditions, the chemical analysis, the biological studies
for both rats and infants, and the acceptability test of Fortesan
in a province of Chile.

The WSB mixture was processed first in a Wenger X-25 extrusion
unit in order to gelatinize the starch and give the mixture characteristics of an instant product. Second, the milk powder was added in
order to improve the amino acid profile and the biological quality

of the protein. Third, 5% cocoa powder was added to simulate chocolate flavor. The finished product called Fortesan was assayed for
its biological quality in rats. Results showed that Fortesan gave
a protein efficiency ratio (PER) value of 2.65 compared to 2.87 for
casein. Net protein utilization (NPU) was 70 compared to 72 for
casein. Fortesan was also tested in 8 normal infants. In all of
the infants, the increase in weight and height was normal or better
than normal. Acceptability was normal and no digestive disorders
were noted. Fortesan was further tested on 8 severely undernourished
infants of the marasmic type. The results indicated that the digestibility and protein quality of Fortesan were good.

INTRODUCTION

In Chile, as in most developing countries, various investigations have indicated that a high percentage of the infant population
is malnourished (Monckeberg, 1967). At one year of age, almost 30%
of Chilean children show some degree of malnutrition and this percentage is increased gradually in later years so that at six years of
age, almost 60% of the children are malnourished. As a result of
this malnutrition, growth is altered and retarded, the capacity for
resisting infection is diminished, and intellectual capacities are
affected, damaging a child permanently.

The nutritional deficiencies in the diet of the Chilean child
are many and varied; they include calories, vitamins, minerals, and
proteins. The latter, however, is the principal limiting factor,
especially for proteins of animal origin.

Furthermore, there is a great gamut of limitations associated
with the conditions of the socio-economic underdevelopment of Chile
which hinder the positive aspects of the milk program. Among these
we mention:

1) the low level incomes in the homes that receive the milk
powder, making it difficult for everyone to obtain an adequate diet.
The milk designed originally for the child is therefore consumed by
all members of the family group.

NUTRITIVE VALUE OF WSB-SKIM MILK MIXTURES FOR INFANTS

2) bad environmental sanitary conditions, plus low cultural and educational levels result in easy contamination of the milk which in turn causes digestive disorders, conditions that aggravate malnutrition.

3) high incidence of intolerance to the lactose in milk in the low socio-economic groups.

One way to provide high quality protein to young children is through use of a protein-rich mixture that can replace milk for infants and be a supplement to protein supplied by the daily meals of preschool and older children.

Considering all of the factors mentioned, it has become essential that a milk substitute be produced which can be utilized and possess the following characteristics:

1) it must provide an adequate quality and quantity of proteins.

2) it must contain the least amount of lactose possible.

3) the carbohydrates present must be perfectly digestible and produce no digestive disorders.

4) it must be really consumed by the child and not diverted to other uses.

5) its cost must be lower than that of milk powder.

6) the principal raw materials must be readily available in Chile.

The present study reports the development of such a protein-rich mixture named "Fortesan" which fulfilled the above requirements. It also reports the investigation of the optimal processing conditions, the chemical analyses, the biological quality studies for both rats and infants, and the acceptability testing of Fortesan in a province of Chile.

MATERIALS AND METHODS

The WSB mixture was supplied by CARE. The dried skim milk was a commercial sample containing 36.6% protein.

A) Chemical analysis: ash, protein, and fat were determined by the Association of Official Agricultural Chemists method. The calorie content of all samples was calculated by using the factors.

B) Studies in rats: the biological quality of the materials was measured by NPUC (net protein utilization count) in rats, according to the method of Miller and Bender (1955) and by PER (protein efficiency ratio) according to the method of Campbell (1957).

C) Studies in infants and children: detailed description in text.

RESULTS AND DISCUSSION

Study of the Habits and Beliefs about Foods

It is necessary to first study the food habits and beliefs of a social group in order to achieve the ultimate goal of consumption of the test food by preschool children. For example, it is important to know the acceptability of a test food by the preschool children. However, it is perhaps more important to know the acceptability of the food by their mothers or guardians. It is possible to prepare a food that would be perfectly accepted by the child, but if the mother does not consider it to be adequate, the chance for getting the food to the child is very little. Furthermore, it is also important to know the food habits of the adult so as to avoid their consumption of those foods distributed specifically for the child.

In order to study the feeding habits of the population, the province of Curico was selected. Curico is considered to be typical of the Central Zone of Chile in which 80% of the population of the country is concentrated. Five hundred families were selected for this study; half as representative of urban populations and the other half as representative of rural populations. The following conclusions were obtained from the answers to a questionnaire which had been sent to each family.

A) Both in rural and urban zones, breast feeding was extraordinarily short, so that as an average, at 3 months of age, only 20% of the infants were receiving mother's milk. The reasons for this behavior were so varied that it would be difficult to draw any conclusions for this study.

B) To replace mother's milk, cow's milk was given (powdered milk distributed by the National Health Service of the Chilean Government). Between 3 and 5 months of age, a high percentage of the mothers added some kind of flour to the milk because the mothers believe that at this age milk is not an adequate food. Some of them added toasted wheat flour. The majority of mothers however buy various commercial products composed of wheat flour or corn flour plus some vitamins. This habit was observed in almost 96% of the families, in all socio-economic levels. The habit is so popular that most of the mothers stated that the product they added to the milk is more important than the milk itself. If given the alternative of eliminating one of the two ingredients, they would eliminate the milk, not the flour. However, if asked which they preferred to be distributed by the National Health Service, milk or flour, the majority preferred milk. Further analyzing showed that this preference was due to the fact that milk could be consumed by all members of the family, whereas this is not true of the flour because the mothers believe that flour is only for children. It was also noted that almost all of the mothers stated that their children liked the taste of toasted wheat flour.

C) Between 9 months and 1 year of age, a majority of the children ate twice a day with the diet the same as the rest of the family. In addition, twice a day, they drank cow's milk, or flours, or a mixture of both. It was shown that 70% of the diets were insufficient in protein supply, especially in animal proteins, in terms of the requirement for this age group.

D) On questioning the mothers as to which type of flour they preferred from a list of different products available on the market, they indicated a preference for the most expensive ones and those with better packaging. On questioning them as to which flavor they preferred, the majority of mothers indicated that their children liked the taste of chocolate and toasted wheat flour.

E) On questioning the mothers as to whether their children were well nourished or undernourished, 97% answered that their children were well nourished and indicated that this question irritated them. On the other hand, on questioning as to whether the child of their neighbor was well nourished or undernourished, 52% replied that their neighbor's child was undernourished.

F) On questioning the mothers as to why the flours were good for the children, the answers generally coincided: the children grew strong and healthy because they developed strong bones because the children gained more weight.

From the above study of the habits and beliefs of a typical population, very valuable information was obtained and was utilized in working up the program later developed.

In the first place it was obvious that it was important to utilize the habit of the flours, together with the belief that these had a high nutritive value. As we have indicated, the mothers believe that at 4 months of age, something should be added to the milk to make it more nutritious. For this reason it was decided to prepare a formula that consisted of milk (25%) and flours (wheat and soya, 75%) with dual objectives: the mother would receive the milk enriched with flour and in a form ready to give to the child. At the same time, providing milk with flour reduced the possibility of adult consumption, in accordance with the habit of the population to consider this food solely for the child and not to be utilized in other ways.

For a formula containing only 25% milk, the concentration of lactose in this formula would be decreased and at the same time the cost is reduced in relation to milk. Finally, the milk produced in Chile would be sufficient to contribute all the necessities of the program of milk distribution without the necessity of importing milk from abroad.

This formula would be for children no less than 6 months of age. Otherwise, it could have the possibility of replacement of mother's milk which obviously is not desirable. On the other hand, it would

not be advisable to give it to children beyond 7 years of age since
it would not provide sufficient caloric requirements for that age
group.

The product should have an optimum packaging and labelling so
that it could have maximum acceptability. The idea was to pack it
in tin cans with a label emphasizing the contents to the mothers
and that the product would make children grow strong and healthy.
For this reason the name "Fortesan" was selected. It was also
obvious that one could not overemphasize the product as one designed
to combat malnutrition, since no mother likes to admit that her child
could be in such a condition. Thus, the product should tend to
elevate the social status of the consumer.

The flavors which would seem to be the most acceptable to the
child are toasted wheat flour and/or chocolate.

Basic Studies of the Product Named Fortesan

One of the fundamental requirements that should be considered
for the preparation of this product is that the raw materials be
produced or obtainable in Chile. A test was made through a formula
which contained powdered milk, deodorized fish flour, protein of
sunflower, and wheat flour. The study of this product ("Leche
Alim") including the basic biological studies on animals and humans,
and the tests of acceptability in kindergartens, urban and rural
populations have been reported by Yanez et al. (1969) previously.
The prime materials of this product can be produced in Chile. The
resources of the sea permit the fabrication of up to a million tons
of fish flour per year. However, the process of deodorization has
not yet been totally determined and in the best of cases, the in-
stallation of a plant and its operation will take some years yet.

With reference to sunflowers, Chile reaches a production of
15,000 tons of sunflower presscake per year. Once extracted, the
protein is perfectly usable for human consumption with the advantage
that it contains a high level of methionine. However, all of the
sunflower presscake is utilized as animal feed at the present time;

the extraction process for human consumption elevates the cost.

For the above cited reasons, alternate basic ingredients were investigated for the preparation of Fortesan, especially soy flour which has been widely used in human consumption. Chile produces approximately 5000 tons annually, at present, and there is no reason why this production cannot be raised substantially. In order to accelerate the investigation in its early developmental stage, a mixture of soy and wheat flour (WSB, allocated by CARE, in which the soy has been previously treated and its toxic factors eliminated) was used to initiate the study.

A study was conducted first to determine the biological value of WSB both in experimental animals as well as infants of 2 months of age. WSB has the following composition:

> 73.3% bulgur wheat
>
> 20.0% defatted soy flour
>
> 4.0% soy oil
>
> 2.6% vitamins and minerals

Biological Value of the Protein in WSB

The NPU in rats was determined by the Miller and Bender method (1955) giving a value of 62, which is lower than that obtained with casein under equal conditions (NPU 70).

Biological Value of the Protein Tested in Infants of 2 Months of Age

The objective of the tests was to study the biological value and digestibility of the protein in humans. Small infants were chosen less than 4 months of age because their speed of growth is maximum and the necessity for protein of good quality is very high. At the same time the digestibility and tolerance are lessened. These conditions constitute the maximum requirements for the protein mixture to be tested. Four children were selected whose ages ranged between 1-3 and 3-4 months and they were fed exclusively with WSB plus corn oil (2%) and a mixture of vitamins and minerals to cover the deficit. As a control, 3 children of similar ages received

NUTRITIVE VALUE OF WSB-SKIM MILK MIXTURES FOR INFANTS

cow's milk in such a dilution that the caloric protein and fat contributions were similar. The result was not satisfactory in that the children who were receiving WSB, with a protein contribution superior than 4.5 grams protein per kilo per day, were not gaining weight satisfactorily so that the test was suspended after ten days and only milk was continued.

From these results it was concluded that the protein from the mixture of soy and wheat flours had an acceptable biological value but not an optimum NPU (62) and that it was not capable of promoting normal growth if it were used as the sole source of protein in infants who received 4.5 grams of protein per kilo per day. The digestibility of the protein also was not optimum in these children. The acceptability studied in preschool age children in kindergartens was good, but those who prepared it complained that the product did not dissolve well and sedimentation was very rapid. To use it, the following modifications had to be made:

1) Addition of 25% milk powder, thus considerably increasing the amino acid score.

2) Treatment of the WSB with an extrusion process. A product was obtained after extrusion that dissolved better in water and remained permanently suspended for hours. In addition, the process of extrusion hydrolyzed the starch to dextrins and disaccharides (maltose and isomaltose) which makes it much more digestible, especially in small infants who find starch difficult to digest.

The optimal processing conditions used in our experimental Wenger X-25 extruder are as follows:

retention time	10-12 seconds
maximum temperature	115-120°C
inlet moisture	24%

The extruded product was then dried and ground to 80 mesh.

3) Addition to the WSB mixture of 5% cocoa to give it a chocolate flavor. Thus, the formula for "Fortesan" is as follows:

70%	WSB/extruded
25%	powdered fat-free milk
5%	powdered cocoa

In chemical analysis, the formula had the following composition:

23% protein

4% fats

6.6% ash

(345 calories/100 grams)

The vitamin content of "Fortesan" (100 grams) is as follows:

Vitamin B_1	0.57 mg
Vitamin B_2	0.80 mg
Vitamin B_6	0.12 mg
Vitamin B_{12}	traces
Vitamin A	1.170 IU
Vitamin D	140 IU
Vitamin E	1.0 IU
Niacin	4.2 mg

The mineral content of "Fortesan" (100 grams) is as follows:

Calcium	800 mg
Phosphorus	450 mg
Iron	7.4 mg
Iodine	38 mg

This formula was easy to prepare in tepid water and it remained suspended in water for more than 8 hours. The flavor was a mixture between toasted wheat flour and chocolate.

Study of the Biological Quality of Fortesan in Rats

The PER value was determined by the Campbell method (1957) and the NPU by the Miller and Bender method (1955) at a level of 10% protein calories, comparing it to casein as a control.

Fortesan	2.65 (PER)	70 (NPU)
Casein	2.87 (PER)	72 (NPU)

With these results, it could be concluded that the biological value of Fortesan was similar to that observed in the casein.

NUTRITIVE VALUE OF WSB-SKIM MILK MIXTURES FOR INFANTS

Study of the Biological Quality of Fortesan in Infants

Eight normal infants were selected whose ages ranged between 2 and 4 months and during the study they were hospitalized in a Metabolism Unit. During the period of 20 days, they were fed with Fortesan as the only source of protein, prepared in the following manner:

For each 100 ml: Fortesan 10 g

Sugar 10 g

Corn oil 2 g

This mixture gives 91 calories per 100 ml. The infants received 130 calories per kilo per day and 3 grams of protein per kilo per day for the 20-day period. At the beginning and end of the experiment, the following tests were made: urinalysis, urocultive, hemograma, proteineimia, corotinemia, sedimentation rate, and flocculation test.

Both at the beginning and end of the experiment, all the laboratory examinations showed normal values. In Figure 1, it is shown that the weight curve of the eight infants studied suggests that weight increase was normal or better than normal. During the 20-day period, growth averaged 1.4 cm, which was also normal for their age groups. Acceptability was good and no digestive disorders were noted; the infants always had normal stools.

The results of this experiment were considered very positive since the growth and increase in weight was equal to that observed

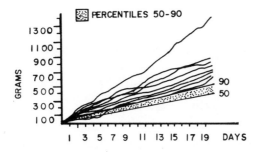

FIG. 1. Weight increment of eight normal children fed Fortesan as the only protein source.

in infants fed with cow's milk and even superior under equal conditions (3 grams of protein per kilo per day).

A second experiment was performed on severely undernourished
infants of the marasmic type. It is known that treatment of this
type of infant is very difficult, including treatment with milk,
owing to the disturbed metabolism of the individual. This makes
adequate utilization of the different nutrients difficult and there
is a high susceptibility to digestive disturbances. These patients
present difficulties in the intestinal absorption of the lactose
and also in the absorption of fatty acids. The test of Fortesan
in the treatment of infants with severe marasmic malnutrition was
interesting because if this formula is capable of "curing" an infant with this type of malnutrition, it would signify that its
digestibility is very good and that the protein is of good quality.

Eight infants were chosen whose ages ranged between 4 and 11
months and who showed signs of severe malnutrition, with weight
60% less than what it normally should be at their particular ages.
Weight at the time of the experiment fluctuated between 2.7 and 5.1
kilograms. The experiment began with the administration of skim
milk to which rape seed oil and sunflower oil were added, during a
period of 15 days. At the end of 15 days, all of the infants
received Fortesan to which corn oil had been added. During the
period that they received cow's milk or Fortesan, metabolism
balances of 5-days duration were realized.

The Fortesan was prepared as shown in Table 1.

TABLE 1

Preparation of Fortesan (100 ml)

Item	Grams	Protein	Fats	Carbohydrates	Calories
Fortesan mixture	12.0	2.9	0.2	7.0	--
Corn oil	3.5	--	3.5	--	--
Maltose dextrose	6.0	--	--	6.0	--
Total		2.9	3.7	13.0	97

NUTRITIVE VALUE OF WSB-SKIM MILK MIXTURES FOR INFANTS

This mixture, as with the milk, was administered ad libitum during the entire period of 15 days, observing that the total ingestion varied between 130 and 150 ml per kilo per day so that the caloric ingestion was approximately 130 calories per kilo per day, while the protein ingestion was approximately 4.1 grams per kilo per day.

With both diets, the control diet (milk), as well as Fortesan, had excellent acceptability. The average weight gain during the control period was from 6.7 grams per kilo per day with the control diet, and 5.7 grams per kilo per day with Fortesan. The difference was not significant and in both cases, it could be considered a good weight gain for this type of patient.

The results of the nitrogen balance studies can be seen in Table 2. By expressing retained nitrogen as a percentage of absorbed nitrogen, 20% was retained for the control diet (skimmed milk) and 37% was retained for Fortesan. The difference for the retained nitrogen was statistically very significant ($p < 0.001$).

The result of the fats balance studies can be seen in Table 3.

Also, in the group fed Fortesan, one observes a better absorption of fats and a high percentage of fat retention. One cannot draw a definite conclusion from this difference, since the type of oil used in the control group (rape seed oil and sunflower oil) was different than the oil used with Fortesan (corn oil). However, it

TABLE 2

Nitrogen Balance Study of Fortesan and Control Diet

Item	Control diet	Fortesan
	mg per kilo per day	
Nitrogen ingestion	528	610
Nitrogen excretion	110	133
Nitrogen absorbed	418 (79%)	477 (78%)
Nitrogen urine	333	300
Nitrogen retained	85 (16%)	177 (29%)

429

TABLE 3

Fats Balance Study of Fortesan and Control Diet

Item	Control diet	Fortesan
	g per kilo per day	
Fat ingestion	4.9	4.6
Fat excretion	1.0	0.31
Fat absorbed	3.9	4.2
Percentage of absorption	80%	93%

is necessary to note that a better absorption of fats did occur among those malnourished infants who received Fortesan. The results of this experiment indicate that Fortesan is a good mixture which can be tolerated and digested by undernourished infants. The percentage of retention of nitrogen is better than that of milk, which demonstrates the excellent quality of Fortesan as a protein source.

Acceptability Tests of Fortesan in the General Population

An acceptability test of Fortesan in the Province of Curico was conducted for 9 months. Approximately 1,400 children from 1 to 6 years of age were selected to receive Fortesan, while the control group of 350 children of the same age group received only powdered milk. The children gathered in those places at which Fortesan was distributed each 40 days and they were examined, weighed, and measured. The mothers of the children received two cans of Fortesan, with instructions for preparation. Taking advantage of the program, on distribution day, the mothers gathered to discuss the subject of nutrition. A program for house visits was developed to assure that the mothers were following instructions properly with respect to the preparation and use of Fortesan and to provide additional information on nutrition and hygiene. At the end of the experiment, tests were made on the blood of the two groups (plasmic protein, hematocrit, hemoglobin) to determine if there had

NUTRITIVE VALUE OF WSB-SKIM MILK MIXTURES FOR INFANTS

been a significance after receiving the Fortesan formula for 9 months. These experiments were concluded only recently and the data obtained are now being processed. A preliminary analysis of the data indicates that the results were very satisfactory. The details of the full experimental studies will be published in the near future.

NOTE

This study was supported by Grant U.S./A.I.D./csd-3646.
Rhode Island Agricultural Experiment Station Contribution #1578

REFERENCES

Campbell, J.A. 1957. *In* FAO Committee on Protein Requirements. Food and Agriculture Organization of the United Nations, Rome. Vol. 16, Nutrition Studies.

Miller, D.S. and A.E. Bender. 1955. The determination of the nutritional utilization of protein by a shortened method. Brit. J. Nutr. 9:382.

Monckeberg, F. 1967. Efecto de la desnutricion en el organismo en desanollo. Medicina (Buenos Aires, Argentina) 27:401.

Yanez, E., D. Ballester, A. Maccioni, R. Spada, I. Barja, N. Pak, C.O. Chichester, G. Donoso and F. Monckeberg. 1969. Fish protein concentrate and sunflower presscake meal as protein sources for human consumption. Amer. J. Clin. Nutr. 22:878.

19

WHEY PROTEINS FOR FOOD AND FEED SUPPLEMENT

Elisabeth Forsum

Institute of Nutrition
University of Uppsala
Uppsala, Sweden

GENERAL ASPECTS ON WHEY AND WHEY PRODUCTION

During recent years the interest in the utilization of whey has markedly increased due to several reasons. Important aspects on the special problems associated with the handling of whey are presented in the Proceedings of the Whey Utilization Conference (1971) and of the Whey Product Conference (1973). The reader is referred to these Proceedings to obtain more detailed information on special aspects of whey and whey products. This paper will deal with special aspects on the whey proteins which represent only a small fraction of total whey solids.

Whey is the liquid residual of casein and cheese manufacture. Its composition is shown in Table 1. It is seen that the protein content of whey is very low, approximately 0.6 percent while the lactose content is nearly 5 percent. Many of the problems associated with whey utilization and processing are due to the fact that whey is more than 90 percent water. Liquid whey is a bulky material, very inconvenient to handle and difficult to transport since it easily deteriorates. Owing to the high water content the drying costs in preparing whey powder are high. Furthermore, lactose constitutes approximately 75 percent of the whey solids and protein only 10-15 percent. The high lactose:protein ratio complicates the utilization

TABLE 1

Approximate Composition of Liquid Whey[a]

Component	Approximate composition % (w/v)
Total solids	6.5
Lactose	4.4
Crude protein	0.8
True protein nitrogen	0.10
Non-protein nitrogen	0.03
Ash	0.6
Water	94

[a]Modified after McDonough (1971).

of whey in different ways. Firstly, low lactose activity with consequent sensitivity to a high dietary lactose content is a feature of nearly all adult mammals and often rendering whey less suitable in human as well as in animal diets. Secondly, since lactose is a reducing sugar, it might react with the amino acid lysine in the whey proteins during processes involving heat and make this amino acid biologically unavailable (the so-called Maillard reaction) which might diminish the nutritive value of the protein.

The properties of whey vary depending upon which type of cheese manufacture it is derived from. Generally it is customary to distinguish between "sweet" and "acid" whey. These latter terms are extensively used although their definitions are not always clearcut. Nielsen (1974) defines sweet whey as "the whey resulting from the manufacture of cheese made from milk coagulated primarily with rennet at relatively low acidity" and acid whey as "the whey resulting from the manufacture of cheese or casein made from milk coagulated primarily with acid." In general, rennet whey is derived from the manufacture of hard cheese such as Cheddar, Swiss, etc., while acid whey is obtained during the production of cottage cheese (coagulated by lactic fermentation) or casein (precipitated by the addition of hydrochloric acid).

The world's production of whey is considerable. As seen in Table 2, the annual world production of liquid whey was 57 million tons in 1966 and 71 million tons in 1973 (FAO, 1974), which coresponds to an increase of 25 percent. The main producers are the United States and the countries in the common market. It may be noted that about one-third of the total world production of whey is produced in developing countries which is of interest in discussions on the world food supply.

This increase in whey production, together with the development of the cheese industry, has given rise to serious pollution problems. Formerly cheese was manufactured in small plants situated near the farms supplying the cheese milk. Fluid whey was returned to the farms and utilized for the feeding of animals. However, fluid whey can only be transported short distances if high costs and deterioration of the whey are to be avoided and thus, as the dairy industry developed larger plants, returning of fluid whey to the producers became uneconomical. Owing to this structural rationalization of the dairy industry, the cheese-making factory often produced more whey than could be utilized and in this situation whey presented a pure disposal problem. Furthermore, milk production and consequently the production of cheese and whey varies greatly with the seasons, being highest in early summer, which makes the disposal problem even more complicated. This has led to development of other disposal routes, e.g., through municipal sewage systems or land disposal practices. Such alternatives could give rise to serious water pollution problems, since whey is a powerful pollutant with a high biological oxygen demand.

Statistical data on the utilization of whey in feeds and food is scarce, which precludes an adequate calculation of the amounts of whey wasted. It is estimated that in many developed countries at least 50 percent of the total production of whey has been disposed of as waste in recent years. The proportion wasted seems to be

TABLE 2

Estimated World Whey Production from Cheese and Cottage Cheese[a]

Producer	Source of whey	1966	1971	1972	1973 preliminary
			Thousands of tons		
U.S.A.	cheese	6,728	8,608	9,449	9,621
	cottage cheese	1,890	2,275	2,355	2,215
	total	8,618	10,883	11,804	11,836
Canada	cheese	704	888	904	810
	cottage cheese	70	110	115	125
	total	774	998	1,019	935
Belgium--Luxembourg	cheese	232	200	192	150
	cottage cheese	50	90	90	80
	total	282	290	282	230
Denmark	total	1,000	960	1,048	1,024
France	cheese	4,328	4,728	5,040	5,176
	cottage cheese	550	875	920	960
	total	4,878	5,603	5,960	6,136
Germany, Federal Republic	cheese	1,472	1,840	1,992	2,008
	cottage cheese	1,040	1,445	1.490	1,560
	total	2,512	3,283	3,482	3,568

WHEY PROTEINS FOR FOOD AND FEED SUPPLEMENT

Ireland	total	136	264	364	328
Italy	total	3,912	3,840	3,880	3,960
Netherlands	total	1,864	2,424	2,504	2,616
United Kingdom	total	872	1,296	1,469	1,447
Total EEC	total	15,456	17,962	18,989	19,309
Other western Europe	total	4,649	5,083	5,200	5,232
Total western Europe	total	20,105	23,045	24,189	24,541
Australasia	total	1,352	1,440	1,502	1,512
Other developed countries	total	492	768	800	832
Total developed countries	total	31,345	37,134	39,314	39,656
U.S.S.R.	cheese	3,456	3,624	3,808	4,328
Eastern Europe	total	4,968	6,088	6,090	6,300
Developing countries	total	17,344	19,344	19,736	20,723
Total world	total	57,113	66,190	63,948	71,007[a]

[a]Data obtained from FAO (1974). Estimated on the basis of 8 and 5 kg of whey per kg of cheese and cottage cheese, respectively. In addition to whey from cheese and cottage cheese making, over 3 million tons of whey were derived from casein production in 1973, with New Zealand, Australia, Ireland, France, Federal Republic of Germany, Argentina, Poland, and the U.S.S.R. being the main producers.

lowest in North America, Scandinavia, and the Netherlands, while in France, the Federal Republic of Germany, and Italy, waste probably accounts for well over half of the total supplies.

However, since it has gradually been recognized that whey is a serious pollutant, disposal of whey through the sewage system has been prohibited in many countries. This fact together with the increasing costs of dried skim milk has contributed to the strong interest in utilization of whey solids in foods and feeds which has become evident in recent years. As a result of this interest new processes for recovery of whey solids have been developed and it could be anticipated that this technology will continue to develop in the near future.

Concentration by evaporation followed by roller drying or spray-drying for production of whey powder is one method by which recovery of total whey solids is possible. Partly due to improved manufacturing techniques, and partly to increasing demands for whey powder, this method represents the most economical way of whey utilization. Whey powder is extensively used in animal feeds, and its use in the food industry is increasing, especially in the United States.

Manufacture of lactose represents partial utilization of whey solids. As a by-product of lactose manufacture a solution rich in whey proteins which could be used as a food ingredient is obtained (Nickerson, 1970). However, this by-product is mostly used as an animal feed.

The low protein content of whey has complicated the production of whey proteins. Older methods for preparation of whey proteins often involved acid precipitation of heat denatured whey proteins. Such products, generally called lactalbumin, contained proteins of high nutritional quality but without functional properties which limited their use in the food industry (Wingerd, 1971).

Recently, methods for production of undenatured whey protein concentrates have been developed, i.e., gel filtration, ultrafiltration, and reverse osmoses. The base of these methods has been dealt with extensively by O'Sullivan (1971) and McDonough (1971).

WHEY PROTEINS FOR FOOD AND FEED SUPPLEMENT

Using these methods, products with a high protein content and
reduced lactose and mineral contents could be produced. These
concentrates possess not only an excellent protein nutritive quality
but also interesting functional properties which will probably make
them very useful in industrial food applications. Treatment with
lactase has also been tried in an attempt to reduce the lactose
content of whey (Guy et al., 1974; Wierzbicki et al., 1974).

UTILIZATION OF WHEY AND WHEY PROTEINS

In Human Nutrition

There are several traditional means of utilizing whey in human
foods, e.g., in whey beverages and whey cheeses. Among the former,
both alcoholic and non-alcoholic examples are numerous, and are
produced by a large number of processes (Holsinger et al., 1974;
Mann, 1972). However, whey is often only one component of the
product. One of the most successful whey beverages appears to be
the Swiss drink "Rivella," a carbonated soft drink made from deproteinized whey. This usage of whey represents only a small proportion of the whey available and generally these beverages do not
contribute significantly to human protein nutrition. In Scandinavian
countries, for a long time whey has been converted into the whey
cheese "Mesost" by prolonged boiling. Although this is now made on
an industrial scale, it corresponds to only a small fraction of the
whey produced. Another example of whey cheese is the Italian
Ricotta cheese which is manufactured from whey by heat coagulation
of the whey proteins.

During recent years, the use of various whey preparations in
the food industry has increased (Mann, 1974). Whey is extensively
used at present in baked goods, fruit drinks, sherbets, and candies,
particularly in the United States (Jacobsen, 1974). However, the
overall contribution of whey proteins to the quantity and quality
of human food protein is negligible. It is probable that the earlier
mentioned development of new whey protein products will increase the

use of these proteins in the food industry and consequently in human nutrition. However, such products will probably be marketed mainly in industrialized countries where protein nutrition does not present any problems.

Of special interest is the use of whey proteins in so-called adapted milk formulas or "humanized" infant foods. It is a well-known fact that human milk contains relatively little casein as compared with cow's milk. The ratio of casein to whey protein in human milk is generally claimed to be 2:3 as compared with 4:1 in cow's milk. Tomarelli and Bernhart (1962) reported a high nutritive value of bovine casein and whey proteins mixed according to the human milk protein composition. These findings have found application in the preparation of breast milk substitutes where the protein composition often is adjusted to simulate that of human milk. However, utilization of whey constituents in such products represents only a small fraction of the total whey production.

In conclusion, traditional uses of whey and whey proteins in human nutrition contribute only marginally to the protein nutrition of man and it is unlikely that their importance with respect to protein nutrition will increase significantly in the near future. However, in a few applications the whey proteins might make a significant contribution to human protein nutrition, i.e., in protein-rich weaning foods and in emergency food mixtures. It is possible that whey proteins might also be valuable in dietetic foods and in further developed infant food formulas. These applications will be discussed later.

In Animal Nutrition

Use of whey in animal nutrition represents one of its major pathways of utilization. Feeding fresh liquid whey to livestock, especially pigs, but also calves, is one of the dominating traditional ways of utilization which is still of importance even in highly industrialized countries (Lettner, 1972). However, this form of use is declining although recent increases in energy costs for drying whey might slow down this decline. Gradually, during recent years, the use of whey powders has gained more importance and both in the United States and Europe.Skim milk protein as well as fish meal and oilcake protein are being replaced by whey powder (FAO, 1974). Varying degrees of success have been reported regarding the use of dried whey in animal nutrition; for calves (Cottyn et al., 1969; Morrill, 1973; Bouchard et al., 1973); for pigs (Hanrahan, 1971a, b; Noland et al., 1969); and poultry (Amon, 1972; Damron et al., 1971). Less successful trials might well, at least partly, be due to the fact that whey powders seem to show large quality variations (Nielsen, 1972) which greatly influence their value as feed ingredients. Many positive observations on the use of whey powder in animal nutrition can be found in the literature, however (Oborn, 1968). Nevertheless, the contribution of whey protein from whey powder to the protein nutrition of the animal is comparatively small, since the crude protein content of dried whey is only about 12%. Furthermore, a significant amount (20-25%) of the nitrogen in whey powder is present as non-protein nitrogen. However, the whey proteins per se are known to be of high nutritive quality (Forsum, 1974). Roy (1964), for example, showed that casein was of lower quality than skim milk protein in the feeding of calves, which he explained by the presence of undenatured whey proteins in skim milk. Furthermore, whey proteins in whey protein concentrates are of high value as supplements to vegetable proteins (Forsum, 1975a). Whey proteins in whey powder are, owing to the latter's low content of true protein, relatively high contents of non-protein nitrogen, and high content of lactose, less effective as supplementary proteins than concentrated whey proteins. However, they have a small but definite effect as a supplement to other feed proteins. This is illustrated in Figures 1-4. Figure 1 shows protein and lactose contents as well as lysine and sulfur-containing amino acid concentrations in mixtures of defatted soy flour and whey powder. It is seen that high levels of dried whey are needed to improve the concentrations of these amino acids in this mixture. Nevertheless,

441

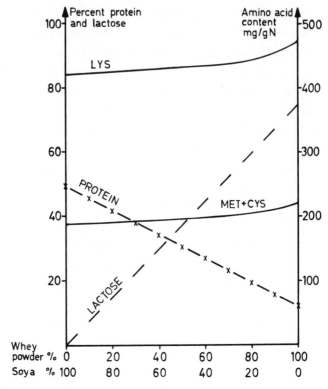

FIG. 1. Protein and lactose contents (in percent) as well as levels of lysine and methionine plus cystine (in mg amino acid per g total nitrogen) in mixtures of defatted soy flour and dried whey powder.

several authors reported success with the use of soy-whey mixtures in animal feeds. Morrill et al. (1971), for instance, described the successful use of a soy-enriched whey in the feeding of calves. Similarly, Miller et al. (1973) reported good results from the use of partly delactosed whey in corn-soybean meal rations for early weaned pigs. This was, at least partly, due to the increased levels of lysine, sulfur-containing amino acids, tryptophan, and threonine obtained when the whey product was added. Volcani et al. (1974) claimed that a soy-enriched whey, without any additives, could be used as a milk replacer for calves.

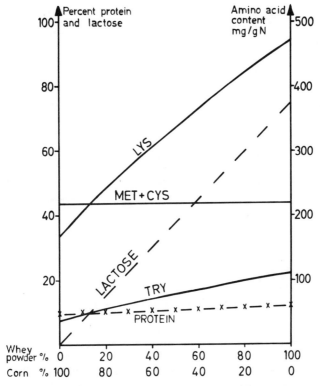

FIG. 2. Protein and lactose contents (in percent) as well as levels of lysine, tryptophan, and methionine plus cystine (in mg amino acid per g total nitrogen) in mixtures of corn and dried whey powder.

Cheeke et al. (1973) reported that corn and barley give a better performance together with whey powder than does wheat. Figures 2-4 show the protein and lactose contents as well as the concentrations of certain important amino acids in mixtures of whey powders with these three cereals. It is seen that all these three types of protein mixture benefit from incorporation of whey powder protein. However, as pointed out earlier, this effect is small and cannot be expected to give any marked improvements in dietary protein quality. Similar conclusions were drawn from corresponding calculations of the supplementary effect of whey powder protein when added

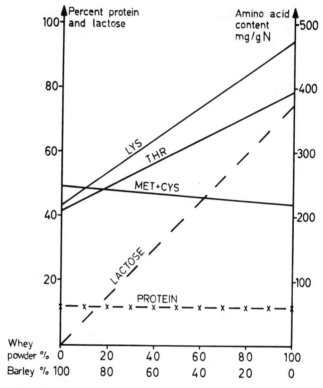

FIG. 3. Protein and lactose contents (in percent) as well as levels of lysine, threonine, and methionine plus cystine (in mg amino acid per g total nitrogen) in mixtures of barley and dried whey powder.

to other feed proteins. This conclusion is in agreement with the results of Morrill (1973) who found no profound effects of whey products in whey-grain blends for dairy calves.

There are several reports on the use of whey proteins as a substitute for skim milk proteins in calf feeds (Toullec et al., 1969, 1971; Bech, 1970; Raven, 1972; Stewart et al., 1974). Generally, the results are satisfactory although Toullec et al. (1969) found that the rate of stomach emptying was higher when whey proteins rather than skim milk proteins were fed. Adams (1974) commented on the utilization of whey in animal feeds and pointed

WHEY PROTEINS FOR FOOD AND FEED SUPPLEMENT

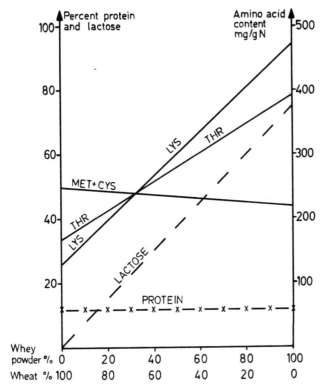

FIG. 4. Protein and lactose contents (in percent) as well as levels of lysine, threonine, and methionine plus cystine (in mg amino acid per g total nitrogen) in mixtures of wheat and dried whey powder.

out that dried whey as a milk replacer for dairy calves must be of good quality and supplemented by protein.

In conclusion, whey protein from whey powder or liquid whey makes a small but definite contribution to the protein nutrition of many domestic animals. However, its value for improving the total protein quality of various feed mixtures is limited.

PROPERTIES OF WHEY PROTEINS

The chemical properties of milk proteins have been extensively dealt with by several authors, e.g., in a book on milk proteins

445

edited by McKenzie (1970, 1971) and in an article by Lyster (1972) who provide detailed information upon this subject. Here only the biological and nutritional properties of these proteins will be briefly commented on.

The approximate content of different whey proteins in fluid whey is shown in Table 3. It is seen that the main protein is β-lactoglobulin, which contributes to about 50% of total whey proteins. This protein is known to be a specific milk protein, i.e., it is synthesized by the mammary gland and is not found in blood serum. The exact biological function of this protein is unknown. It is of interest that this protein has not been detected in human milk (Bell and McKenzie, 1964). α-Lactalbumin, another specific milk protein, is present in whey from cow's milk in comparatively low amounts. This protein is a component of the enzyme lactose synthetase and its concentration in the milk of different mammals is generally correlated to the milk lactose content. Consequently, since human milk is rich in lactose, the content of this protein in human milk is high (Forsum, 1975c).

Immunoglobulins and bovine serum albumin represent proteins derived from blood serum. Protection from infections in the calf is mediated to a large extent by immunoglobulins, mainly of the IgG class, in the milk. They are especially high in colostrum and it is generally claimed that they are able to pass through the intestinal mucosa of the calf during the first days of life. The serum albumin of the whey is reported to be identical to blood serum albumin.

These proteins are quantitatively the most important of bovine whey, but several other proteins are present in small amounts. Among these, the casein residues vary depending on the type of cheese manufacture from which the whey is derived. In rennet whey, where casein is precipitated by the addition of rennin, a casein derived peptide, called the macropeptide, is present. The macropeptide is part of the casein subunit, κ-casein, which stabilizes the casein micelle. When rennin acts on casein, the macropeptide is split off, the stabilizing property of κ-casein is lost, and

WHEY PROTEINS FOR FOOD AND FEED SUPPLEMENT

TABLE 3

Approximate Concentration of Major Whey Proteins in
Liquid Whey and Their Respective Percentage of Total Whey Proteins

Protein	Approximate concentration (% w/v)	Approximate percent of total whey protein
β-Lactoglobulin	0.3	50
α-Lactalbumin	0.07	12
Immunoglobulins	0.06	10
Bovine serum albumin	0.03	5
Other proteins (including residual casein)	0.14	23

consequently casein is precipitated. Finally, there are several other proteins which are present in small quantities in the whey, i.e., lactoferrin, lactollin, transferrin, glycoproteins, and various enzymes.

In connection with the nomenclature of the whey proteins a few points should be noted. In older literature the terms lactalbumin and lactoglobulin are often used. These terms refer to different whey protein fractions obtained by salt fractionation (McKenzie, 1971) and should be avoided as the whey proteins have now been characterized more exactly with the use of modern biochemical methods. Furthermore, the term lactalbumin often refers to commercial whey protein products of ill-defined protein composition. Rose et al. (1970) have made an excellent review of the modern nomenclature of milk proteins and the reader is referred to this article for further details.

Most probably, one important biological function of the whey proteins is their contribution of amino acids to the suckling, i.e., their nutritive function. The milk protein casein is a unique protein since it carries large amounts of calcium and phosphorus which are important for the bone development of the offspring. However, the amino acid composition of casein is not optimal from the nutritional point of view and one important function of the whey proteins is probably to improve the overall amino acid pattern of the milk protein. The nutritive value of the whey proteins has long been known to be superior to that of casein. Henry (1957) thus found that lactalbumin had higher protein efficiency ratio (PER) and biological value (BV) values than casein, and this observation has been extensively confirmed in recent years (Lindquist and Williams, 1973; Wingerd et al., 1970; Wingerd, 1971).

The amino acid compositions of two whey protein concentrates (WPC) produced by large-scale gel filtration and ultrafiltration are shown in Table 4 (Forsum et al., 1974). These concentrates contain essentially all proteins present in whey, but not the free amino acids and small peptides which are present in small quantities in liquid whey. It is seen that the contents of essential amino acids are high and of special interest are the high contents of lysine, threonine, tryptophan, and cystine. However, the contents of phenyl-alanine and tyrosine are comparatively low. The low content of phenylalanine could be utilized in the dietary treatment of phenyl-ketonuria (PKU). This inherent metabolic disorder is due to an impaired ability to metabolize the amino acid phenylalanine to tyrosine, and instead toxic metabolites, so called phenylketons, are formed. These compounds are fatal to mental development and their occurrence in the patient's blood has to be avoided if a normal mental development is to be achieved. Most food proteins contain comparatively high amounts of phenylalanine and thus a child with phenylketonuria cannot tolerate a normal diet. This necessitates the use of special formulas, generally consisting of mixtures of synthetic amino acids without phenylalanine, or protein hydrolysates from which phenylalanine has been removed. However, since phenyl-alanine is an essential amino acid, it is necessary to some extent even in the diet of phenylketonurics. Thus, their diet generally contains a natural protein source which provides the phenylalanine required plus a phenylalanine-low formula which is needed to com-pletely cover the nitrogen requirement. Since these phenylalanine-low formulas are expensive and unpalatable and since nutrition with

TABLE 4

Amino Acid Composition of Gel-Filtered and Ultrafiltered
Whey Protein Concentrate   (mg amino acid/g total nitrogen)

| Amino acid | Whey protein concentrate | |
	Ultrafiltered	Gel-Filtered
Ile	461	474
Leu	708	709
Lys	617	630
Met	147	124
Cys	166	169
Phe	213	218
Tyr	201	210
Thr	516	512
Trp	160	147
Val	423	435
Arg	171	172
His	122	131
Ala	336	335
Asp	741	743
Glu	1,217	1,206
Gly	124	126
Pro	441	451
Ser	391	381

intact protein might be advantageous to nutrition with free amino
acids (Holdsworth, 1972), it is desirable that the natural protein
source used should have a low phenylalanine content but otherwise a
well-balanced amino acid composition. A lower percentage of the
nitrogen requirement of the child then has to be covered by special
phenylalanine-low formulas. Hambraeus et al. (1970, 1974) reported
on the use of whey protein containing formulas in the dietary treatment of PKU. In one test, on a girl with hyperphenylalaninemia, a
formula based on a gel-filtered WPC was used as the sole source of

nitrogen (Hambraeus et al., 1974). This resulted in a higher nitrogen retention but a lower level of phenylalanine in the blood than with the conventional treatment. These findings are not only of interest in connection with phenylketonuria but also show that the whey proteins are of high nutritive quality for humans also.

Whey proteins in whey protein concentrates prepared by comparatively gentle methods and consequently containing proteins which to a large extent are undenatured, show a very high nutritional value. However, most whey proteins consumed by man or animals are derived from whey which to some extent has been processed under less gentle conditions. For example, dried whey for foods and feeds are often preconcentrated before drying, at a comparatively high temperature. The whey cheese mentioned earlier is subjected to heat treatment in the presence of lactose for a considerable time during manufacture. A preliminary study by Forsum indicates that the biological value as well as the digestibility remain high even in products exposed to considerable heat treatment. This is possibly due to the high lysine content of the whey proteins since the Maillard reaction has to be very extensive if sufficient lysine is to be damaged to make this the limiting amino acid. Furthermore, this study indicates that denaturation of the whey proteins per se does not seem to impair their nutritional quality. However, it should be noted that although heat treatment does not seem to affect the nutritive value of whey proteins if the damage is not serious enough to make lysine the limiting amino acid, it could affect their value as supplements to proteins with low lysine content.

Although it has long been known that the nutritive value of total whey proteins is high, few investigations have been made on the nutritive quality of the separate whey proteins. The bovine whey proteins β-lactoglobulin and α-lactalbumin have interesting amino acid compositions, but owing to difficulties in preparing sufficient amounts of pure proteins for nutritional studies conventional evaluation of the nutritive value using growing rats has not until recently been performed with these proteins. In studies on growing mice, Bosshardt et al. (1961) found the nutritive value of crystalline β-lactoglobulin to be inferior to that of casein.

During recent years, however, methods for large-scale fractionation of proteins have been developed. For example, the Sephadex gel filtration process could be applied for preparation of the individual whey proteins in sufficient amounts for nutritional studies. Large-scale fractionation by whey proteins could also be accomplished by other methods as, for example, by fractionated precipitation by carboxymethyl cellulose (CMC) (Hidalgo and Hansen, 1971). Forsum et al. (1974) described large-scale fractionation of two different whey protein concentrates, using preparatory gel filtration, one prepared by gel filtration and one by ultrafiltration. A prototype of a stacked column, KS 450 Pharmacia Fine Chemicals, Sweden, with a total volume of 124 l and packed with Sephadex[R] G-75 was utilized.

As shown in Figure 5, three protein fractions were obtained from both types of concentrates (fractions one, two, three). This figure also shows the recovery of sample nitrogen in the different fractions. It is seen that the nitrogen recovery in fractions one and three was similar in the two types of concentrates. However, in the second fraction of gel-filtered WPC, only 29% of the sample nitrogen was recovered, while the corresponding figure for ultrafiltered WPC was 48%. In the case of gel-filtered WPC, 22% of the sample nitrogen was collected as a precipitate before application of the sample, while the corresponding figure for ultrafiltered WPC was only 0.4%. In the production of this particular gel-filtered WPC a certain amount of heat treatment is used during concentration and it seems likely that β-lactoglobulin, the protein obtained in this second fraction (Table 5), is to some extent denatured and made insoluble during this heat treatment.

The protein fractions were characterized by means of starch-gel electrophoresis, immunoelectrophoresis, and amino acid analysis. The casein contents of the different fractions were estimated by acid precipitation at pH 4.6. The first fraction was found to contain high molecular weight proteins, i.e., bovine serum albumin

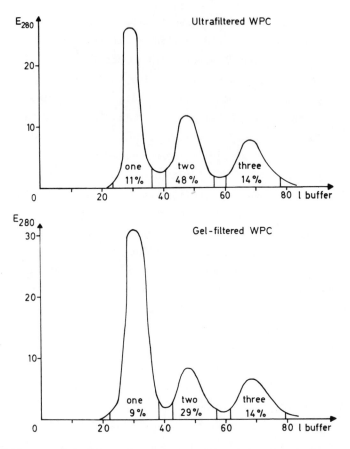

FIG. 5.   Gel filtration of ultrafiltered and gel-filtered whey protein concentrates on Sephadex[R] G-75.   Recovery of sample nitrogen in the different fractions is indicated.   Column: five segments each measuring 45 x 15 cm.   Buffer: 0.1 M phosphate, pH 613, 0.02% NaN$_3$.   Flow rate: 10 1/h.

and casein, while the second and third fractions contained β-lacto-globulin and α-lactalbumin, respectively (Table 5).   Furthermore, analyses showed that the β-lactoglobulin present in the second fraction was comparatively pure, while the main protein in fraction three, α-lactalbumin, was contaminated by some β-lactoglobulin.   It was concluded, however, that large-scale gel filtration offers a possibility of preparing large amounts of the main whey proteins with a fairly high degree of purity.

TABLE 5

Nutritive Values of Gel-Filtered and Ultrafiltered
Whey Protein Concentrates (WPC) and the Respective Whey
Protein Fractions; and the Major Protein Components of the Fractions

Item	Major components	PER[a]	NPU[b]
Gel-Filtered WPC			
Total		4.0	94
Fraction one	Bovine serum albumin, casein	--	82
Fraction two	β-Lactoglobulin	3.0	87
Fraction three	α-Lactalbumin	4.2	87
Ultrafiltered WPC			
Total		4.3	85
Fraction one	Bovine serum albumin, casein	--	75
Fraction two	β-Lactoglobulin	3.5	87
Fraction three	α-Lactalbumin	4.0	90
Reference casein		3.3	79

[a]Protein efficiency ratio.
[b]Net protein utilization.

Nutritional evaluation of ultrafiltered and gel-filtered WPC as
well as of their respective fractions prepared by large-scale gel
filtration was carried out and the results are shown in Table 5
(Forsum, 1974). The nutritive values of the two whey protein concentrates were high and similar, as indicated by the protein
efficiency ratio and net protein utilization values. Likewise,
the biological estimations showed the nutritive value of the
fractions to be high. However, the PER estimations indicated that
the nutritive value of the second fraction (β-lactoglobulin) was
lower than that of the third fraction (α-lactalbumin) which is of
interest since α-lactalbumin is a major protein in human whey.

As mentioned earlier, whey proteins are utilized at present in
so-called "humanized" breast milk substitutes where the ratio of

casein to whey protein is adjusted to simulate that of human milk. However, the amino acid composition of such formulas differs from that of human milk in several respects, e.g., they have high contents of methionine which might be undesirable since the enzyme for transformation of methionine into cystine is not developed during early life (Sturman et al., 1970). Several reasons for the discrepancies can be found. Firstly, bovine whey has a high content of β-lactoglobulin; secondly, the statement that breast milk protein consists of 40% casein and 60% whey protein is uncertain (Lönnerdal et al., 1975); and thirdly, it is reported that about 20% or even more of the nitrogen in human milk is non-protein nitrogen (Macy et al., 1931; Lönnerdal et al., 1975).

Large-scale fractionation of whey proteins offers a possibility of making breast milk substitutes more similar to human milk. Figure 6 shows the amino acid composition of a hypothetical breast milk substitute in percent of the amino acid composition of human milk (Forsum, 1974). In this breast milk substitute 40% of the nitrogen is derived from bovine casein, 40% from fraction three of ultra-filtered WPC (which is rich in α-lactalbumin), and 20% from non-protein nitrogen. In this figure, the amino acid composition of a commercial Swedish breast milk substitute is also given for comparison. The amino acid composition of the hypothetical protein mixture is more similar to that of human milk than is the commercial breast milk substitute. Furthermore, it is probable that further improvement could be achieved if the protein composition of human milk was known with greater accuracy. These considerations indicate that fractionated whey proteins might be utilized for improving infant formulas. However, whether this will be of any importance in the future is dependent upon the cost of production and fractionation of whey proteins. Furthermore, the possible nutritional advantage of such formulas should be evaluated in clinical trials.

Another application of large-scale gel filtration of whey proteins has been reported by Forsum and Hambraeus (1972). Using this technique a whey protein fraction with a phenylalanine content still

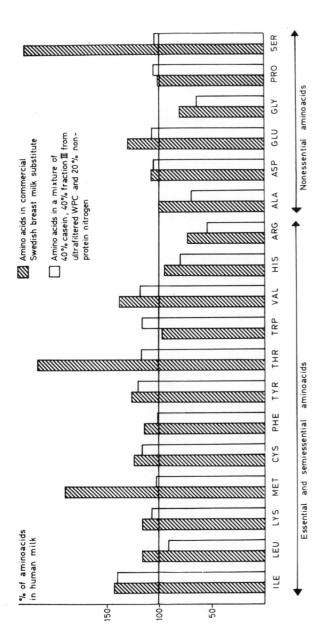

FIG. 6. The amino acid composition of a protein mixture consisting of 40% casein, 40% fraction three from ultrafiltered whey protein concentrate (WPC), and 20% non-protein nitrogen, and of a commercial breast milk substitute, shown in percent of the amino acid contents of human milk. Reproduced with permission of the American Dairy Science Association and the Journal of Dairy Science.

lower than that of total whey protein was obtained. This fraction was shown to have a high nutritive value when used in combination with a special phenylalanine-free formula of free amino acids when measured on growing rats.

SUPPLEMENTARY VALUE OF WHEY PROTEINS

As mentioned earlier, the contents of essential amino acids in whey proteins are high. This indicates that whey proteins could be of value as supplements to proteins of low nutritional quality. The contents of essential amino acids expressed in percent of amino acids of FAO amino acid reference pattern (1973) for a whey protein concentrate (WPC) produced by gel filtration as well as for wheat, corn, and rice protein are shown in Figure 7. It is seen from this figure that wheat is deficient in lysine and threonine and corn in lysine and tryptophan, while rice protein is low in lysine and iso-leucine. Because of these inadequacies in amino acid composition, much work has been devoted to the improvement of the quality of cereal protein. In the case of wheat, lysine supplementation has been much discussed, while the development of "high lysine corn" represents an effort to improve the quality of corn protein. Since WPC contains large amounts of amino acids low in cereal proteins, the supplementary effect of WPC protein on wheat, corn, and rice protein was studied.

In the case of wheat protein, the supplementary effect of WPC was compared with that of a fish protein concentrate (FPC), dried skim milk (DSM), and lysine (Forsum et al., 1973).

Wheat flour was supplemented by WPC, FPC, DSM, and lysine, respectively, to obtain the same lysine score (Table 6). To obtain this, less supplementary protein had to be incorporated into the WPC-wheat mixture than into wheat-DSM or wheat-FPC. In spite of this, the chemical scores, using egg protein as reference, were similar for wheat-WPC, wheat-DSM, and wheat-FPC (Table 6). Further-more, the PER value of the wheat-WPC mixture was higher than that of wheat-FPC, and approximately the same as that of wheat-DSM (Table 6).

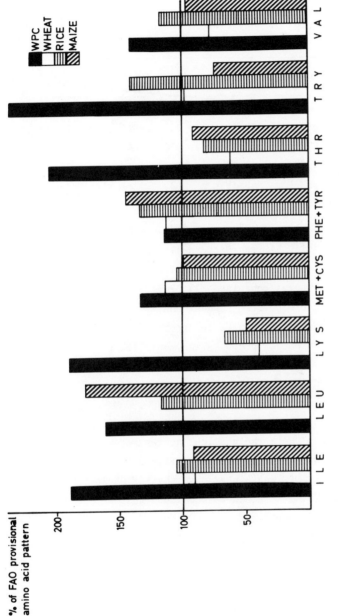

FIG. 7. Essential amino acid contents of a whey protein concentrate, wheat, corn, and rice, expressed in percent of the FAO provisional amino acid reference pattern (1973).

TABLE 6

Nutritive Value of Wheat Protein when
Supplemented by Whey Protein Concentrate (WPC),
Dried Skim Milk (DSM), Fish Protein Concentrate (FPC), and Lysine

Mixture	Protein ratio	Lysine score	Chemical score[a]	PER
Wheat + lysine	--	82	53 (Thr)	0.8
71% Wheat + 29% DSM	39:61	82	69 (Met + Cys)	2.4
89% Wheat + 11% FPC	47:53	82	67 (Ile)	2.4
92% Wheat + 8% WPC	65:35	82	70 (Phe + Tyr)	2.5
85% Wheat + 15% DSM	65:35	64	64 (Lys)	1.8
93% Wheat + 7% FPC	65:35	70	64 (Ile)	1.8
Reference casein	--	129	58 (Met + Cys)	2.5

[a]Estimated using FAO egg protein 1965 as reference.

However, these mixtures contained 11% FPC, 29% DSM, and 8% WPC,
respectively. In products for human consumption, to avoid gritti-
ness, no more than 7% FPC can be incorporated and if the wheat
mixture is to be used for bread baking, only 16% DSM can be added
if the dough-forming qualities of the mixture are to be satisfactory.
Eight percent WPC can be added to wheat without any of these problems.

In addition, mixtures of wheat with WPC, DSM, and FPC, respectively, containing the same amount of supplementary protein, namely
35%, were studied. Here the chemical scores for wheat-WPC were
higher than for wheat-FPC or wheat-DSM (Table 6). Likewise, the
PER value of wheat-WPC was higher than that of wheat-DSM or wheat-
FPC (Table 6). Thus, it could be concluded that WPC is more useful
as a wheat protein supplement than FPC or DSM.

Wheat supplemented by lysine had a PER value of only 0.8
(Table 6), while the PER of unsupplemented wheat is 0.5 (Abrahamsson
et al., 1974a). The value of lysine fortification of wheat has been
much discussed and the results of this study indicate that it may be
of limited value.

In the case of corn and rice protein, the supplementary effect of WPC was compared with that of DSM (Forsum, 1975a). In addition, corn supplemented by lysine and tryptophan was studied. Biological tests of protein quality were performed on raw (PER) as well as on boiled (NPU) protein mixtures. In both rice diets and corn diets supplemented by DSM or WPC, cereal protein constituted approximately half of the dietary protein, the rest being supplementary protein (WPC or DSM) (Table 7).

Calculation of chemical scores, using the FAO provisional amino acid pattern (1973) as reference, showed that both rice-WPC and corn-WPC had scores above 100, while the scores of rice-DSM and corn-DSM were below 100 (Table 7). The PER values of WPC-supplemented cereals were higher than those of DSM-supplemented cereals. Likewise, the NPU values were higher when WPC was used as the supplementary protein than when DSM was used (Table 7). Since the NPU estimations were performed on boiled protein sources, it was concluded that the WPC-cereal mixtures still had a high protein quality even after moderate heat treatment. The protein of corn supplemented by lysine and tryptophan was of moderate quality (Table 7).

TABLE 7

Nutritive Values of Corn and Rice Protein when Supplemented by Whey Protein Concentrate (WPC) and Dried Skim Milk (DSM)

Diet	Protein ratio	Chemical score[a]	PER	NPU
Corn + lysine + tryptophan	--	91 (Thr)	2.4	60
Corn + DSM	48:52	89 (Ile)	3.6	71
Corn + WPC	48:52	>100	4.1	76
Reference casein	--	91 (Met + Cys)	3.4	77
Rice + DSM	47:53	95 (Thr)	3.8	65
Rice + WPC	47:53	>100	4.1	71
Reference casein	--	91 (Met + Cys)	2.9	79

[a]Calculated using FAO provisional pattern 1973 as reference.

Thus, both chemical and biological evaluation indicated that WPC is a more efficient supplement to corn and rice protein than is DSM. However, DSM as well as WPC were found to be efficient cereal supplements. PER of WPC and of DSM are approximately 4.0 and 3.6, respectively. When these proteins were mixed with about 50% of poor cereal protein, the PER values were not reduced.

In conclusion, the results of these studies showed that supplementation of wheat, corn, and rice by WPC is an efficient way of utilizing this concentrate. These findings are in agreement with those of Womack and Vaughan (1972), who compared the value of DSM and a whey product produced by reverse osmosis as cereal supplements. They concluded that the supplementary value of "reverse osmosis whey" and DSM were similar. However, it can be calculated from their data that cereals supplemented by "reverse osmosis whey" had PER values significantly higher than had cereals supplemented with DSM. By measuring PER of malnourished or stunted rats, these authors have also shown that "reverse osmosis whey" and DSM were equally effective as protein supplements to corn diets (Womack and Vaughan, 1974). Furthermore, Al-Ani et al. (1973) found that the protein quality of diets based on wheat was markedly improved by adding dried partially delactosed whey. However, Al-Ani et al. (1972) studied the supplementation of wheat by dried whey and found that dried whey appeared to be more useful as such a supplement when fed in combination with milk than by itself. This was explained by the low lysine and methionine contents and the high lactose content of their dried whey product. These findings also agree with those aspects earlier mentioned in this paper that dried whey is of limited value as cereal protein supplement due to its low protein content and high contents of lactose and non-protein nitrogen. Thus, it can be concluded that when fortification of cereal and cereal products is discussed, WPC should be taken into consideration.

During his studies on the nutritional value of protein for man, Kofranyi (1973) found a mixture of egg and potato protein to have a nutritional value superior to that of all other proteins. However,

WHEY PROTEINS FOR FOOD AND FEED SUPPLEMENT

Jekat (1971) found a mixture of 31% lactalbumin and 69% potato protein to be of nearly the same nutritional quality. The whey proteins are subjected to milder treatment in the production of gel-filtered WPC than in the production of lactalbumin. Thus, it is possible that the nutritional quality of whey proteins is higher in a gel-filtered WPC than in lactalbumin. The nutritive value of the lactalbumin-potato mixture of Jekat was compared with that of a mixture where WPC was used instead of lactalbumin (Forsum, 1975a). The NPU value of this potato-WPC mixture was 56, as compared with 31 for Jekat's potato-lactalbumin mixture, this difference being significant $(0.001 < p < 0.01)$. These findings indicate that a nutritional evaluation of a potato-WPC mixture in human nutrition would be of interest.

The above results suggest that use of whey proteins as supplements to protein of poor quality represents an effective and economical way of utilizing them. Thus, the use of a gel-filtered WPC in protein-rich weaning foods (Forsum, 1973) and emergency food mixtures (Abrahamsson, 1974a, b) has been tested.

So-called protein-rich weaning foods usually contain mainly vegetable protein sources. According to the Protein Advisory Group (PAG) they should contain at least 5% from an animal source, generally dried skim milk. This should ensure that the protein quality of the product is adequate. However, during recent years the production of DSM has been decreasing, and thus the effect of replacement of DSM by WPC on the protein quality in protein-rich weaning foods was investigated.

When the essential amino acid compositions of WPC and DSM were compared with that of the essential amino acid contents of human milk (Figure 8), it was found that the surplus of several essential amino acids, especially lysine, threonine, and tryptophan, was greater in WPC than in DSM. Since vegetable proteins often are limited by these amino acids, this suggests that WPC would be more useful than DSM as an animal protein source in protein-rich weaning foods.

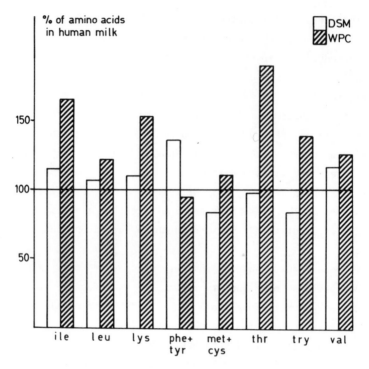

FIG. 8. Essential amino acid contents of dried skim milk (DSM) and whey protein concentrate (WPC) expressed in percent of the FAO human milk amino acid reference pattern 1973.

The effect on the protein quality of three protein-rich weaning foods, CSM (corn soy milk), Faffa, and Superamine, when protein from DSM was replaced by protein from WPC, was studied. CSM is manufactured by the Lanhoff Grain Company, Danville, Illinois, and its composition in g/100 g is: precooked corn flour, 64; defatted soy flour, 24; DSM, 5; soy oil, 5; vitamins and minerals, 2. Faffa is manufactured by the Ethiopian Nutrition Institute, Addis Ababa, Ethiopia, and its composition in g/100 g is: wheat flour, 57; defatted soy flour, 18; chick pea flour, 10; DSM, 5; sugar, 8; minerals and vitamins, 2. Superamine is manufactured by S N Sempac, Alger, Algeria, and its composition in g/100 g is: chick pea flour, 38; durum wheat flour, 28; lentil flour, 18; dried skim milk, 10; sugar, 5; vitamins and minerals, 1. In these formulas protein from

DSM constitutes 9-18% of the total protein. The protein quality was evaluated by chemical and biological methods. Theoretically, this change of animal protein source increased the chemical scores of CSM, Faffa, and Superamine by 4-5 units.

As shown in Table 8, considerable improvements in PER and NPU were obtained when DSM was replaced by WPC in Superamine and CSM. In Superamine, the PER value was increased by 43% and the NPU value by 14% while the NPU of CSM was increased by 17% as a result of this change in animal protein source. Only a slight improvement in the quality of Faffa protein was observed when DSM protein was replaced by WPC protein, the increase in PER as well as NPU being 7%. It should be noted that recently a dry 29% whey protein concentrate has been approved as an optional ingredient in CSM.

Utilization of whey protein concentrate in emergency food mixtures based on Swedish ingredients has also been studied. The mixtures contained mainly wheat which was supplemented by protein sources to satisfy the recommendations of PAG for protein-rich weaning foods. Chemical and biological testing of mixtures containing 5-10% WPC showed the whey proteins to be of value for the protein quality of the mixture (Abrahamsson et al., 1974a). When these mixtures were used for preparation of bread or porridge, the

TABLE 8

Nutritive Value of Some Protein-Rich Weaning Foods,
when Animal Protein is Supplied by
Dried Skim Milk (DSM) or Whey Protein Concentrate (WPC)

Diet	PER	NPU
Corn soy milk with DSM	--	71
Corn soy milk with WPC	--	83
Faffa with DSM	2.8	59
Faffa with WPC	3.0	63
Superamine with DSM	2.3	59
Superamine with WPC	3.3	67
Reference casein	3.2	61

presence of WPC was not found to impair the appearance or palatability of the product. Furthermore, field testing of emergency
foods, containing WPC, in Afghanistan and West Africa, showed that
the product was well accepted and tolerated (Abrahamsson et al.,
1974b). Similar results were obtained by Rodier et al. (1974) in
the field testing of a soy-whey beverage which showed that such a
beverage will probably be acceptable in preschool feeding programs
in most parts of the developing world.

Interesting aspects of the utilization of whey proteins in
human nutrition have been published by Hutton (1974). His paper
deals with technological, environmental, and nutritional as well as
agricultural and economic viewpoints on whey protein utilization,
and the outstanding ability of the whey proteins to boost the food
value of cereal proteins is stressed.

GENERAL ASPECTS ON THE UTILIZATION OF WHEY AS A SOURCE OF NUTRIENTS

It can be calculated that all the whey produced during 1973
contained 426 thousand tons of protein and 3,195 thousand tons of
lactose equivalent to 60,830 million k Joule. If it is assumed that
the daily energy requirement of a human being is 10,500 k Joule and
that the world population is 6 billion people, it can be estimated
that the energy value of the whey produced in 1973 corresponded to
about 2.5% of the energy needs of the human population. This calculation illustrates the enormous wastage and inefficient utilization of whey.

It is sometimes pointed out that whey powders contain the main
proportion of the skim milk nutrients, practically all the lactose
and vitamins present in the milk, and a significant part of the
minerals and proteins (Cox, 1973; Anon., 1974). However, as mentioned earlier, it is the unbalanced relative proportion of these
nutrients in the whey solids, from a nutritional point of view, that
complicates the use of dried whey products in human and animal
nutrition. The high mineral content is a problem when whey is
utilized in baby foods, and the low protein content is a problem

WHEY PROTEINS FOR FOOD AND FEED SUPPLEMENT

in the manufacture of whey protein products. Most of the difficulties, however, are due to the high lactose content of the whey.
As mentioned earlier, a low lactase activity and a reduced ability
to tolerate lactose are widespread among the world's population.
Although lactose occasionally could be valuable as a component in
whey powders for different uses, e.g., bread baking (Guy, 1973),
its level in dried whey is often higher than desirable. However,
the importance of low lactase activity has sometimes been over-
emphasized and it should be stressed that most people, even those
with a low intestinal lactase activity, are able to tolerate a
limited amount of lactose. Furthermore, studies on rats, of an age
when the intestinal lactase activity is low, have shown that limited
levels of lactose in the diet might be beneficial to the biological
value of proteins (Eggum, 1973; Forsum, 1975b). Thus, it should be
noted that although the lactose level in whey powders often is too
high, it is seldom necessary to completely remove the lactose to
obtain a valuable and useful food.

The following conclusions can thus be drawn. Firstly, although
whey contains valuable nutrients, its use in foods and feeds is complicated for several reasons. Secondly, the most valuable components
among the whey solids are the whey proteins which have interesting
nutritional qualities that could probably be utilized in a nutritionally meaningful way. Finally, the future use of whey and whey
proteins in foods and feeds will be dependent upon economic factors
which today are difficult to predict.

ACKNOWLEDGMENTS

These studies were supported by grants from the Swedish Inter-
national Development Authority (SIDA), the Swedish Nutrition Founda-
tion, the Semper Fund for Nutritional Research, Mjölkcentralen,
Stockholm Sweden, Swedish Medical Research Council, the Bank of
Sweden Tercentenary Fund, and from the Faculty of Medicine,
University of Uppsala.

Mrs. Maivor Sjöstrand is acknowledged for preparing the drawings.

REFERENCES

Abrahamsson, L., E. Forsum and L. Hambraeus. 1974a. Nutritional evaluation of emergency food mixtures based on wheat supplemented by different protein concentrates. Nutr. Rep. Int. 9:169.

Abrahamsson, L., L. Hambraeus and B. Vahlquist. 1974b. An ongoing applied nutrition research program. PAG Bull. IV, 4:26.

Adams, R.S. 1974. Whey too nutritious to be wasted. Dairy Herd Manag. 11, 9:24.

Al-Ani, M.R., H.E. Clark and J.M. Howe. 1972. Evaluation of whey as a protein supplement for wheat flour. Nutr. Rep. Int. 5:111.

Al-Ani, M.R., H.E. Clark and J.M. Howe. 1973. Effect of adding varying levels of lysine or delactosed demineralized whey to wheat flour on growth and body composition of young rats. J. Nutr. 103:515.

Amon, E. 1972. Einsatz von Süssmolkenpulver in der Geflügelmast. Die Bodenkultur 23:384.

Anonymous. 1974. An expanding future for whey as a source of human protein. Milk Ind. 75, 4:23.

Bech, H.V. 1970. Anvendelse af valle og valleprodukter til foderbrug. Melkeritidende 83:579.

Bell, K. and H.A. McKenzie. 1964. β-Lactoglobulins. Nature 204:1275.

Bosshardt, D.K., E. Brand and R.H. Barnes. 1961. Nutritional equivalence of β-lactoglobulin and its corresponding amino acids. Proc. Soc. Exp. Biol. Med. 107:979.

Bouchard, R., G.J. Brisson and J.P. Julien. 1973. Nutritive value of bacterial sludge and whey powders for protein in calf milk replacers and on chromic oxide as indicator of digestibility. J. Dairy Sci. 56:1445.

Cheeke, P.R., T.P. Davison, R.O. Myer and D.E. Stangel. 1973. Utilization of dried whey by growing-finishing swine. Feedstuffs 45, 30:25.

Cottyn, B.G., M.R. Casteels and F.X. Buysse. 1969. Le remplacement de la poudre de lait écrémé par de la poudre de sérum de lait et de la levure S.A.V. dans les rations pour veaux de boucherie. Rev. L'agr. 22:83.

Cox, A.C. 1973. Whey powder. Food Process. Ind. 42, 505:49.

Damron, B.L., D.P. Eberst and R.H. Harms. 1971. The influence of partially delactosed whey, fish meal and supplemental biotin in broiler diets. Poultry Sci. 50:1768.

Eggum, B.O. 1973. The influence of lactose on protein utilization. A study of certain factors influencing protein utilization in rats and pigs. Landhusholdningsselskabets forlag, Copenhagen. p. 120.

WHEY PROTEINS FOR FOOD AND FEED SUPPLEMENT

FAO Nutritional Meetings Report Series No. 52. WHO Technical Report Series No. 522. 1973. Energy and protein requirements. Rome, Italy.

FAO Commodity Note. 1974. Whey--an important potential protein source. Monthly Bull. Agr. Econ. Stat. 23, 4:12.

Forsum, E. 1973. The use of a whey protein concentrate as animal protein source in protein-rich weaning foods. Envir. Chld. Hlth. 19:333.

Forsum, E. 1974. Nutritional evaluation of whey protein concentrates and their fractions. J. Dairy Sci. 57:665.

Forsum, E. 1975a. Use of a whey protein concentrate as a supplement to maize, rice and potatoes: a chemical and biological evaluation using growing rats. J. Nutr. 105:147.

Forsum, E. 1975b. Effect of dietary lactose on nitrogen utilization of a whey protein concentrate and its corresponding amino acid mixture. Nutr. Rep. Int. (In press).

Forsum, E. 1975c. Determination of α-lactalbumin in human milk. (To be published).

Forsum, E. and L. Hambraeus. 1972. Biological evaluation of a whey protein fraction with special reference to its use as a phenylalanine-low protein source in the dietary treatment of PKU. Nutr. Metabol. 14:48.

Forsum, E., L. Hambraeus and I.H. Siddiqi. 1973. Fortification of wheat by whey protein concentrate, dried skim milk, fish protein concentrate and lysine monohydrochloride. Nutr. Rep. Int. 8:39.

Forsum, E., L. Hambraeus and I.H. Siddiqi. 1974. Large-scale fractionation of whey protein concentrates. J. Dairy Sci. 57:659.

Guy, E.J. 1973. Use of whey in baking. *In* Proceedings of Whey Product Conference (June 14-15, 1972). Agricultural Research Service, USDA. p. 34.

Guy, E.J., A. Tamsma, A. Kontson and V.H. Holsinger. 1974. Lactase-treated milk provides base to develop products for lactose-intolerant populations. Food Prod. Dev. 8, 8:50.

Hambraeus, L., L. Wranne and R. Lorentsson. 1970. Whey protein formulas in the treatment of phenylketonuria in infants. Nutr. Metabol. 12:151.

Hambraeus, L., L.I. Hardell, E. Forsum and R. Lorentsson. 1974. Use of a formula based on a whey protein concentrate in the feeding of an infant with hyperphenylalaninemia. Nutr. Metabol. 17:84.

Hanrahan, T.J. 1971a. Whey solids in the diet of growing-finishing pigs. 1. Dried whey as a feed for pigs. Ir. J. Agr. Res. 10:1.

Hanrahan, T.J. 1971b. Whey solids in the diet of growing-finishing pigs. 2. Concentrated whey as a feed for pigs. Ir. J. Agr. Res. 10:9.

Henry, K.M. 1957. Dairy Sci. Abstr. 19:603.

Hidalgo, J. and P.M.T. Hansen. 1971. Selective precipitation of whey proteins with carboxy methyl cellulose. J. Dairy Sci. 54:1270.

Holdsworth, C.D. 1972. Absorption of protein, amino acids and peptides--a review. In W.L. Burland and P.D. Samuel (Eds.) Transport Across the Intestine. Churchill, Livingstone, Edinburgh. p. 136.

Holsinger, V.H., L.P. Posati and E.D. DeVilbiss. 1974. Whey beverages: a review. J. Dairy Sci. 57:849.

Hutton, J.T. 1974. Whey protein. Activities Report 26:102.

Jacobsen, D.H. 1974. Use of modified whey products and lactose in the food industry. Amer. Dairy Rev. 36:34.

Jekat, F. 1971. Studien auf dem Stickstoffgebiet und ihr Bezug zur Ernährung. Ernährungs-Umschau 18:252.

Kofranyi, E. 1973. Evaluation of traditional hypothesis on the biological value of proteins. Nutr. Rep. Int. 7:45.

Lettner, F. 1972. Schweinemast mit flüssiger Molke. Gute Rat in Futterungsfragen 11, 3:6.

Lindquist, L.O. and K.W. Williams. 1973. Aspects of whey processing by gel filtration. Dairy Ind. 38:459.

Lönnerdal, B., E. Forsum and L. Hambraeus. 1975. The protein content of human milk. I. A transversal study of Swedish normal material. (To be published).

Lyster, R.L.J. 1972. Reviews of the progress of dairy science. Section C. Chemistry of milk proteins. J. Dairy Res. 39:279.

Macy, I.G., B. Nims, M. Brown and H.A. Hunscher. 1931. Human milk studies. VII. Chemical analyses of milk representative of the entire first and last halves of the nursing period. Amer. J. Dis. Children 42:569.

Mann, E.J. 1972. Whey beverages. Dairy Ind. 37:153.

Mann, E.J. 1974. Whey utilization--parts 1 and 2. Dairy Ind. 39:303, 343.

McDonough, F.E. 1971. Concentration and fractionation of whey by reverse osmosis. In Proceedings of Whey Utilization Conference (June 2-3, 1970). Agricultural Research Service, USDA. p. 36.

McKenzie, H.A. (Ed.). 1970, 1971. Milk Proteins: Chemistry and Molecular Biology. Academic Press, New York.

Miller, E.R., D.E. Orr, P. Tummasang, J.P. Hitchcock and D.E. Ullrey. 1973. Use of dried whey product in early weaning rations. Res. Rep. 232:51.

Morrill, J.L., S.L. Melton and A.D. Dayton. 1971. Evaluation of milk replacers containing a soy protein concentrate and high whey. J. Dairy Sci. 54:1060.

Morrill, J.L. 1973. Utilization of whey-grain blends by calves. *In* Proceedings of Whey Product Conference (June 14-15, 1972). Agricultural Research Service, USDA. p. 74.

Nickerson, T.A. 1970. Lactose. *In* B.H. Webb and E.O. Whittier (Eds.) By-products from Milk. Avi Publishing Co., Westport, Connecticut. p. 356.

Nielsen, V.H. 1972. New uses for whey. Amer. Dairy Rev. 34, 8:42.

Nielsen, V.H. 1974. What exactly is whey. Amer. Dairy Rev. 36, 9:68.

Noland, P.R., C.A. Baugus, R.M. Sharp and E.M. Funderburg. 1969. Economical rations for early-weaned pigs. Arkansas Farm Res. 18, 2:9.

Oborn, J. 1968. A review of methods available for whey utilization in Australia. Australian J. Dairy Tech. 23:131.

O'Sullivan, A.C. 1971. Whey processing by reverse osmosis ultra-filtration and gel filtration. Dairy Ind. 36:636, 691.

Proceedings of Whey Utilization Conference (June 2-3, 1970). 1971. Agricultural Research Service, USDA.

Proceedings of Whey Product Conference (June 14-15, 1972). 1973. Agricultural Research Service, USDA.

Raven, A.M. 1972. Nutritional effects of including different levels and sources of protein in milk replacers for calves. J. Sci. Food Agr. 23:517.

Rodier, W.I., W.C. Wetsel, H.L. Jacobs, R.C. Graeber, H.R. Moskowitz, T.J.E. Reed and D. Waterman. 1974. The acceptability of whey-soy mix as a supplementary food for preschool children in developing countries. Technical Report for U.S. Agency for International Development.

Rose, D., J.R. Brunner, E.B. Kalan, B.L. Larson, P. Melnychyn and H.E. Swaisgood. 1970. Nomenclature of the proteins of cow's milk: third revision. J. Dairy Sci. 53:1.

Roy, J.H.B. 1964. The nutrition of intensively-reared calves. Vet. Rec. 76:511.

Stewart, J.A., L.L. Muller and A.T. Griffin. 1974. Use of whey solids in calf feeding. Australian J. Dairy Tech. 29:53.

Sturman, J.A., G. Gaull and N.C.R. Raiha. 1970. Absence of cysta-thionase in human fetal liver: is cystine essential? Science 169:74.

Tomarelli, R.M. and F.W. Bernhart. 1962. Biological assay of milk and whey protein compositions for infant feeding. J. Nutr. 78:44.

Toullec, R., C.M. Mathieu, L. Vassal and R. Pion. 1969. Utilisation digestive des protéines du lactoserum par le veau préruminant a l'engrais. Ann. Biol. anim. Bioch. Biophys. 9:661.

Toullec, R., P. Thivend and C.M. Mathieu. 1971. Utilisation des protéines du lactosérum par le veau préruminant a l'engrais. Ann. Biol. anim. Bioch. Biophys. 11:435.

Volcani, R., Z. Holzer and A. Ben-Asher. 1974. Soy-enriched whey as a milk replacer for pail-fed calves. Feedstuffs 46, 17:37.

Wierzbicki, L.E., V.H. Edwards and F.V. Kosikowski. 1974. Hydrolysis of lactose in acid whey by lactase bound to porous glass particles in tubular reacters. J. Food Sci. 39:374.

Wingerd, W.H. 1971. Lactalbumin as a food ingredient. J. Dairy Sci. 54:1234.

Wingerd, W.H., S. Saperstein and L. Lutwak. 1970. Bland soluble whey protein concentrate has excellent nutritional properties. Food Technol. 24:758.

Womack, M. and D.A. Vaughan. 1972. Whey and whey products as cereal supplements. J. Dairy Sci. 55:1080.

Womack, M. and D.A. Vaughan. 1974. Evaluation of whey products as supplements for maize by using protein-calorie malnourished or stunted rats. Nutr. Rep. Int. 9:241.

20

THE NUTRITIVE QUALITY OF POTATO PROTEIN

P. Markakis

Department of Food Science and Human Nutrition
Michigan State University
East Lansing, Michigan

INTRODUCTION

The potato tuber, henceforth referred to as potato(es), contains on the average 2.1% crude or total protein (%N x 6.25) on a fresh weight basis. This protein represents 10.4% of the total solids of the potato, a percentage lying between those for wheat flour (13.4%) and white rice (7.6%) (USDA Agr. Handbook No. 8, 1963). A hectare (2.47 acres) produces 226 kg of potato protein as a world average; this is a yield greater than that in wheat grain protein (200 kg/ha) or rice grain protein (168 kg/ha), but lower than that in soybean protein (470 kg/ha) (FAO Production Yearbook, 1972). Potatoes provide the world with 6 million metric tons of protein, wheat with seven times, and rice with four times as much. Both the protein content of the potato and the protein yield per hectare cultivated with potatoes vary widely under the influence of genetic and environmental factors, including cultivation practices.

Of Andean origin, the potato is now a worldwide crop and a particularly important staple in Europe and the USSR--together they grow 75% of the world production. The nutritive value of its protein has become the subject of numerous studies, in which amino acid analysis, animal feeding, and human feeding tests were used. These studies, as well as those pertaining to the effect of processing on the quality of potato protein, will be briefly discussed here.

THE AMINO ACIDS OF THE POTATO TUBER

A diet must provide the essential amino acids, which the body cannot synthesize, and the nitrogen of the non-essential amino acids, which is also necessary for the synthesis of body protein and other nitrogen-containing compounds. It is possible for a certain amount of a food, e.g., milk, to satisfy the human requirements in essential amino acids, but not the requirements in total utilizable nitrogen (Snyderman et al., 1962). The entire "nitrogen profile" of a food is therefore significant nutritionally. The total or crude protein content of potatoes, conventionally considered to be the Kjeldahl %N x 6.25, may be broken down as in Table 1, which was compiled by Schreiber (1961) on the basis of many analyses by various authors. It is interesting that the factor 7.5 has been recently proposed for converting Kjeldahl N to total protein in potatoes (Desborough and Weiser, 1974). The true protein fraction has been further subdivided into tuberin (a globulin, 76.4%), globulin II (1.4%), tuberinin (an albumen, 4.0%), glutelin (5.5%), prolamin (1.8%), and an uncharacterized subfraction (10.9%) (Lindner et al., 1960). Gel electrophoresis and electrofocusing have shown that these subfractions do not represent single molecular species (Macko and Stegeman, 1969).

The amino acid composition of potatoes is shown in Table 2. Of the many amino acid analyses of potatoes, those by FAO (1970) and Orr and Watt (1957) are most frequently quoted, although the latter is incomplete. In the analysis by Kaldy and Markakis (1972), the S-containing amino acids were determined after performic acid oxidation, a treatment resulting in greater accuracy in the determination of these amino acids, especially when carbohydrates are present during hydrolysis.

An idea of the variability among values for the same amino acid is provided by %CV, which was calculated on the basis of the FAO data

THE NUTRITIVE QUALITY OF POTATO PROTEIN

TABLE 1

Nitrogen Containing Compounds (Crude Protein) of the Potato[a]

N-fraction	% of total N
True protein N	50
Nonprotein N	50
Inorganic N	
Nitrate N	1
Nitrite N	trace
Ammonia N	3[b]
Amide N	
Asparagine N	13
Glutamine N	10
Remaining N	
Free amino acid N	15
Basic N	8[c]

[a]From Schreiber (1961).

[b]It is doubtful that there is so much free NH_3 in potatoes; probably part of it is formed from the easily hydrolyzable glutamine during analysis.

[c]Alkaloids, certain vitamins, purines, pyrimidines, quaternary ammonium compounds, etc.

alone. The FAO report (1970) also cites the ranges for individual amino acid concentrations. For methionine and cystine, which as a group are limiting the nutritive value of potato protein, these concentrations vary from 54 to 125 (methionine) and 4 to 81 (cystine) mg amino acid per g total N. Assuming equal accuracy in securing these various values, the large ranges indicate that (a) the nutritional value of the potato nitrogen may vary considerably among cultivars (Schuphan and Postel, 1957) and (b) the possibilities for genetic improvement of the potato protein quality are good, as they are for the genetic improvement of the potato protein quantity (Desborough and Weiser, 1972).

A number of procedures have been proposed for estimating the nutritive value of either pure proteins or the mixture of proteins,

TABLE 2

Amino Acid Composition of Potatoes (mg per g total N)[a]

Amino acid (AA)	FAO (1970) CC	M	Orr and Watt (1957) (method unspecified)	Schwerdtfeger (1969) CC	Kaldy and Markakis (1972) CC	Average	% CV
Essential AA							
Isoleucine	236	303	275	206	262	257	27.6
Leucine	377	361	312	381	375	362	30.2
Lysine	299	351	334	338	387	342	43.5
Methionine	81	106	78	94	100	92	27.9
Cystine	37	67	59	33	81	55	77.2
Phenylalanine	251	293	275	300	281	280	24.8
Tyrosine	171	171	113	175	231	172	38.6
Threonine	235	204	247	238	238	233	24.3
Tryptophan	--	103	66	75	94	85	(33.4M)
Valine	292	331	334	300	356	323	22.0

Nonessential AA

Arginine	311	345	309	250	306	305	14.9
Histidine	94	96	91	94	143	103	29.1
Alanine	287	375	404	225	194	297	20.5
Aspartic acid	775	682	--	1550	1531	1138	29.4
Glutamic acid	639	463	625	938	968	729	28.7
Glycine	237	188	--	238	188	214	18.6
Proline	235	188	209	194	238	213	16.1
Serine	259	163	250	231	275	236	14.8
Protein score		70	61	55	70		
MEAA index		73	66	66	72		

[a]Notations: CC = chemical method

M = microbiological method

MEAA = modified essential amino acid (index)

$$\% \; CV = \text{percent coefficient of variation} = \frac{\text{standard deviation}}{\text{mean}} \times 100, \text{ on CC data by FAO}$$

peptides, and free amino acids present in diets, on the basis of their content of essential amino acids (Sheffner, 1967). The protein score procedure was developed by an FAO/WHO Expert Group (1965) and is based on the concept of the limiting amino acid(s), with whole egg protein as the 100% standard. This procedure applied to the four analyses presented in Table 2 gave protein scores 70, 61, 55, and 70, respectively. The low scores obtained from Schwerdtfeger's data and from those by Orr and Watt are mainly due to the small concentrations of S-containing amino acids in their reports. The higher scores should be viewed as more representative of the nutritive value of potato protein because the S-containing amino acids are often underestimated when chemical methods are used for their determination. For comparison with other foods the following protein scores are given: beef 80, fish 75, soyflour 70, milk 60, wheat flour 50, and navy bean 42.

The essential amino acid index, as developed by Oser and modified by Mitchell (Sheffner, 1967), is based on the geometric mean of the egg ratios. This procedure was applied to the four analyses of Table 2 and gave the indices 73, 66, 66, and 72, respectively. The MEAA indices of some other proteins are: casein 90, soyflour 81, and white flour 64.

Complete amino acid analyses of pure potato proteins are scarce. Hughes (1958) analyzed the heat-coagulable fraction of potato nitrogen and reported the following results in g amino acid/16 g total N: arginine 5.5, histidine 2.4, isoleucine 6.8, leucine 11.1, lysine 8.3, phenylalanine 6.2, methionine 2.8, cystine 1.6, threonine 5.7, tryptophan 1.8, valine 8.0, alanine 4.7, aspartic acid 13.0, glutamin acid 11.3, glycine 4.9, proline 5.1, serine 5.8, tyrosine 6.1, γ-amino butyric acid 0, and ammonia 1.7. A protein score of 70 and a MEAA index of 98 can be calculated for this protein. What is more remarkable than the extremely high MEAA index of this protein is that it is a better source than whole egg protein of every essential amino acid except the S-containing amino acids, in g/16 g total N. The excellent amino acid composition of this protein is in accord with the results

obtained from human potato-feeding experiments which will be
described later.

Because of the high content of free amino acids in potatoes,
and the possibility for these amino acids to be leached out during
cooking and hence lost (it is recommended to discard the water in
which unpeeled potatoes have been boiled as solanine may be concentrated in it), or to react with sugars during chipping and cause
browning, a number of analyses have been carried out on these amino
acids. While the amino acid composition of the potato proteins is
constant for the same cultivar (genetic control), the composition
of the free amino acid fraction of the tuber is affected by storage,
nutrition of the plant, climatic conditions, and treatment with
chemicals such as ethylene chlorohydrin (Mulder and Bakema, 1956;
Schwimmer and Burr, 1967). The natural variability of the free
amino acid composition of the potato tuber and the variety of
methods used in extracting and separating them from the proteins
(e.g., by dialysis, 70% ethanol extraction, protein precipitation
by heat or picric acid or trichloroacetic acid) have resulted in
widely differing results. Table 3 lists the figures obtained by
several different investigators. An interesting observation regarding the distribution of amino nitrogen in the potato tuber is that
the outer layers (cortex) have a much higher concentration of
essential amino acids than the inner layers (Schuphan, 1970).
Plant breeders may find it feasible to increase the cortical area
of the tuber. The periderm (the brown skin) does not seem to have
any protein value (Thompson, 1975).

ANIMAL FEEDING EXPERIMENTS

In contrast to the human feeding experiments, which will be
described later, animal feeding tests have not been consistent in
the evaluation of the protein quality of potatoes. In early experiments (McCollum et al., 1918 and 1921), diets containing 7-8% crude
potato protein hardly increased the weight of young rats. Growth
was no better when cereal proteins were fed alone at the same level.

TABLE 3

Free Amino Acid Composition of Potatoes (mg per g nonprotein N)

Amino acid	Chick and Slack (1949)	Thompson and Steward (1952)	Mulder and Bakema (1956)	Hughes[a] (1958)	Kaldy (1971)
Isoleucine	--	} 84	} 137	31	206
Leucine	--			0	106
Lysine	119	51	trace	169	275
Methionine	50	67	63	31	131
Cystine	75	--	19	38	trace
Phenylalanine	256	112	81	106	244
Tyrosine	--	98	81	100	206
Threonine	69	82	38	106	--
Tryptophan	--	--	--	44	--
Valine	206	196	106	106	419
Arginine	163	288	300	256	631
Histidine	69	--	38	88	181
Alanine	--	107	38	69	150
Aspartic acid	--	86	319	1775[a]	806
Glutamic acid	--	144	644	1944[a]	1106
Glycine	--	22	trace	13	19
Proline	--	trace	trace	19	69
Serine	--	53	38	69	--

[a]These results pertain to cooked potato; the values for aspartic and glutamic acid include amounts derived from asparagine and glutamine.

However, when cereals and potatoes were mixed, and the total protein in the diet was raised to 9%, growth was much better and reproduction occurred. This is understandable in view of the high lysine content of potatoes and the low lysine content of wheat and other cereals. Use of the amino acid complementarity between potatoes and cereals was made in preparing a chip-type product (Markakis et al., 1962). Mitchell (1924) put the biological value of potato nitrogen for growth and maintenance of young rats at 68.5 when the diet contained 5% protein and at 66.7 when it contained 10% protein. Hartwell (1925, 1927) found that potatoes providing all of the 7.6% crude protein of a diet supported very poor growth in rats and were insufficient for lactation. Kon (1928) tested tuberin, the chief protein of potatoes, and found its biological value to be 71 compared to 68 for casein(ogen). Jones and Nelson (1931) obtained poor growth with rats fed a 9% potato protein diet. The potato protein was fed as a concentrate containing 90% of the original N. A supplement of tryptophan, or tyrosine and cystine did not improve matters. Almost contemporarily, however, Beadles et al. (1930) showed that cystine did accelerate the growth of rats when added to a potato diet containing 8-9% crude protein. Chick and Cutting (1943) demonstrated that the value of potato nitrogen in supporting the growth and maintenance of young rats was greater than that of whole wheat but lower than that of milk.

Schiftan (1933) conducted N-balance experiments with pigs and calculated a biological value of 73.2 for a diet containing 13% potato protein; the value for fishmeal protein was about the same, but those for milk nitrogen and casein were superior. On the other hand, Hutchison et al. (1943) found that the biological value of potato nitrogen was inferior to that of barley for growing pigs.

Joseph et al. (1963) determined the protein efficiency ratios (PER) of three potato cultivars and reported rather widely differing values: 1.99 for President, 1.23 for Great Scott, and 0.95 for Up-to-Date.

Iriarte et al. (1972) used the meadow vole as an experimental animal in growth studies and found broad differences in PER values among the six potato cultivars they tested in the form of flakes. At the 5.28% protein level in the diet the PER for casein was 1.7, for Russet Burbank potatoes 0.6, and for the experimental cultivar No. 58 it was 1.3; the other four experimental cultivars had PER values lying between these two extremes. Addition of methionine increased the PER values of the potato diets considerably.

HUMAN FEEDING EXPERIMENTS

As early as 1913, Hindhede maintained nitrogen equilibrium in three men on a diet in which practically all nitrogen was supplied by potatoes. Rose and Cooper (1917) successfully repeated Hindhede's experiment with a young woman; in her case, N-balance was achieved by an average daily intake of 0.096 g N/per kg body weight (bw); 99.9% of this N was of potato origin--about 1500 g potatoes daily for seven days. Kon and Klein (1928) kept a man and a woman in nitrogen equilibrium and good health for 167 days on a diet in which all the nitrogen required was supplied by potatoes. The daily need for potato protein was found to be 35.6 g for the man and 23.8 g for the woman on a 70 kg bw basis.

Rather surprising are the results obtained by Kofranyi and Jekat (1965, 1967) at the Max-Planck Institute for Nutritional Physiology. In carefully conducted experiments, these authors fed healthy college students with protein present in either single foods or in pairs of foods mixed at definite protein ratios and determined the smallest amount of protein from each diet that was necessary for nitrogen balance maintenance. Two subjects needed less potato protein than (whole) egg protein to maintain nitrogen balance: one subject needed 0.469 g potato protein vs. 0.575g egg protein daily per and the other 0.569 g potato protein versus 0.575 g egg protein per kg bw. A third subject needed more potato protein, 0.597 g, than egg protein, 0.469 g. The average of the three subjects was 0.545 g/kg bw for the potato protein and 0.505 g/kg bw for the egg protein. The authors further found that, in terms of quantities required to maintain nitrogen balance in adult humans, and with the exception of egg protein, the protein of potatoes had better nutritive quality than the protein of any other single food they tested: beef, tuna fish, wheat flour, soybean, rice, corn, beans, and seaweeds. Even more interesting are their protein-protein supplementation experiments. When the subject who needed 0.469 g potato protein or 0.472 g egg protein per kg bw to reach nitrogen balance was fed a diet in which 75% of the protein originated from eggs and 25% from potatoes, the equilibrium protein requirement was reduced to 0.424 g; for a mixture of 50% egg protein and 50% potato protein, the requirement was 0.365 g; for 35% egg protein and 65% potato protein, the requirement was 0.346 g; and for 25% egg protein and 75% potato protein, the requirement was 0.387 g. The 35:65 egg:potato mixture of proteins resulted in a minimum protein requirement for a second subject, too. Many other pairs of proteins were similarly tested, but none was found to result in as low a minimum total protein requirement as the 35:65 egg:potato mixture of protein (Figure 1). Only a case of amino acid supplementation extremely favorable to meeting the nutritional requirements of human adults might explain this lowering of adequate protein need. It is a thought-provoking situation.

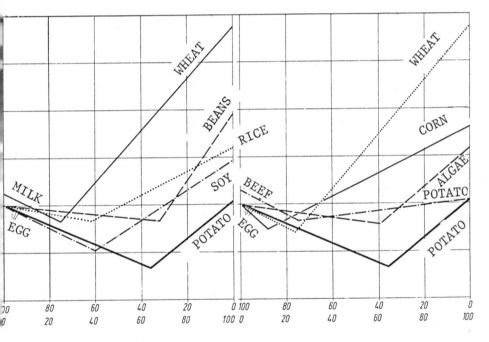

FIG. 1. Minimum quantities of protein in g/kg body weight/day required for maintaining nitrogen balance in human adults (from Kofranyi and Jekat, 1967).
A: Protein of milk, whole eggs, or beef as percentage of the mixture.
B: Protein of potatoes, soybeans, rice, beans, wheat, corn, or algae as percentage of the mixture.

EFFECT OF STORAGE AND PROCESSING ON POTATO PROTEIN

Habib and Brown (1957) reported that storage of potato tubers for a month at 40°F resulted in slight or no change in the free amino acid composition of four cultivars, Katahdin, Red Kote, Red Pontiac, and Russet Rural; but reconditioning at 75°F resulted in a marked decrease in total free amino acids and complete loss of arginine, histidine, and lysine. Fitzpatrick and Porter (1966), however, found considerable increase in the free amino acid content and no change in the total nitrogen content of Kennebec potatoes stored at 36°F for 5-10 months and reconditioned at room temperature; they assumed that metabolic hydrolysis of the proteins occurred, especially during reconditioning. Desborough and Weiser (1974) stored 12 genotypes from October to January at 38-40°F and found an average loss of 3% in total protein.

The effect of chipping on the nitrogenous compounds of potatoes was studied by Fitzpatrick and Porter (1966). They found that the greater the accumulation of reducing sugars in stored potatoes, the greater the loss of free amino acids after chipping; in one case, 88.4% of the free amino acids and 88.7% of the sugars could not be recovered from the chips, presumably as a result of the Maillard browning reaction. But even when the reducing sugars were not abundant considerable quantities of free amino acids were lost during chipping.

Jaswal (1973) also studied the effect of chipping on the amino acid content of potatoes. His results are summarized in Figure 2. The losses of bound and free amino acids in low specific gravity potatoes after chipping amounted to 36.9% and 44.8%, respectively. The corresponding losses in high specific gravity potatoes were 20.2% (bound AA) and 33.2% (free AA). From these figures the conclusion may be drawn that chipping causes considerable damage to the protein value of potatoes, as 1/4 to 1/3 of the amino acids of raw potatoes cannot be recovered in the chips. The same author calculated the losses of amino acids occurring during canning, drum drying, and french frying of potatoes. Canning caused almost as much destruction

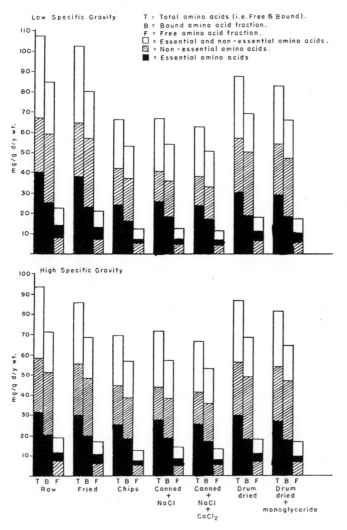

FIG. 2. Amino acid contents of low and high specific gravity potatoes and their products (from Jaswal, 1973).

to amino acids (essential and nonessential) as did chipping. Interestingly, drum drying resulted in much less damage to amino acids and french frying resulted in an almost insignificant loss of amino acids.

Hughes (1958) determined 19 amino acids in prepeeled boiled potatoes. His results are of particular interest because they illustrate the discordance among at least two methods of evaluating protein on the basis of amino acid analysis. He reported his results in g amino acid/16 g total N as follows: arginine 4.6, histidine 1.8, isoleucine 2.4, leucine 3.7, lysine 4.8, phenylalanine 3.4, tyrosine 3.3, methionine 1.3, cystine 1.0, threonine 3.2, tryptophan 1.1, valine 4.1, alanine 2.4, aspartic acid 22.7, glutamin acid 23.8, glycine 1.9, proline 2.1, serine 2.8, γ-amino butyric acid 1.6, and ammonia 4.6. From these data a protein score of 75 can be calculated, but a MEAA Index of only 57. The reason is that the deficit in S-containing amino acids among essential amino acids is not very great; when, however, the concentrations of all the essential amino acids on a total N basis is considered the protein quality index drops, as there is a large proportion of nonessential nitrogen in the boiled potato ($\frac{EAA}{Total\ AA}$ x 100 is 37 for the average potato of Table 2, and 31 for the boiled potato). By calculation, Hughes also arrived at an estimate of the composition of the non-protein nitrogen in boiled potatoes; per 16 g N this fraction contained 28.4 g aspartic acid, 31.1 g glutamine acid, and 19.9 g of all the other amino acids, put together. He concluded that the amino acid composition of boiled potato is not very different from that of raw potato. In contrast to this conclusion, Desborough and Weiser (1974) reported a 50% loss of total protein for 12 genotypes after boiling for 30 minutes. It appears that additional studies on the changes in protein quantity and quality of potatoes during boiling are desirable. Kies and Fox (J.Fd.Sci.37:378,1972) showed that protein quality of potato flakes can be improved by adding L-methionine to the diet of human adults.

CONCLUSION

Potatoes contribute substantial quantities of proteinaceous nitrogen to the human diet. Only 50% of this nitrogen is true protein, the remaining consisting mostly of free amino acids (15% of total N), and asparagine plus glutamine (23% of total N). Amino acid analysis of the heat-coagulable protein of potatoes suggests a very high nutritive quality for it. The protein score and the modified essential amino acid index of the totality of nitrogen substances indicate a potato protein quality close to 70% that of whole egg

THE NUTRITIVE QUALITY OF POTATO PROTEIN

protein. The S-containing amino acids limit the nutritive value of potato protein. Animal feeding experiments do not all agree on the nutritive evaluation of potato nitrogen. But human feeding experiments attribute extraordinarily high quality to the protein of this commodity. Chipping and canning may result in considerable damage to the quality of potato protein, but it is doubtful that similar damage is caused by boiling. French frying does not appear to change appreciably the quality of potato protein. This protein is rich in lysine and an excellent supplement for lysine-poor proteins, such as those of cereals. This supplementarity is attested by the historical fact that bread and potatoes have sustained peoples through adverse nutritional circumstances.

REFERENCES

Beadles, J.R., W.W. Braman and H.H. Mitchell. 1930. The cystine deficiency of the proteins of garden peas and potatoes. J. Biol. Chem. 88:615.

Chick, H. and M.E. Cutting. 1943. Nutritive value of the nitrogenous substances in the potato. Lancet 245:667.

Chick, H. and E.B. Slack. 1949. Distribution and nutritional value of the nitrogenous substances in the potato. Biochem. J. 45:211.

Desborough, S.L. and C.J. Weiser. 1972. Protein comparisons in selected Phureja-Haploid Tuberosum families. Amer. Potato J. 49:227.

Desborough, S.L. and C.J. Weiser. 1974. Improving potato protein. I. Evaluation of selection techniques. Amer. Potato J. 51:185.

FAO. 1970. Amino Acid Content of Foods and Biological Data on Proteins. Rome, Italy.

FAO. 1972. Production Yearbook. Rome, Italy.

FAO/WHO Expert Group. 1965. Protein requirements. Geneva, Switzerland.

Fitzpatrick, T.J. and W.L. Porter. 1966. Changes in the sugars and amino acids in chips made from fresh, stored and reconditioned potatoes. Amer. Potato J. 43:238.

Habib, A.T. and H.D. Brown. 1957. Role of reducing sugars and amino acids in the browning of potato chips. Food Technol. 11:85.

Hartwell, G.A. 1925. A possible correlation between dietary protein and loss of fur in young growing rats. Biochem. J. 19:75.

Hartwell, G.A. 1927. The dietary value of potato protein. Biochem. J. 21:282.

Hindhede, M. 1913. Studies on protein minimum. Skand. Arch. Physiol. 30:97 (in German).

Hughes, B.P. 1958. The amino acid composition of potato protein and of cooked potato. Brit. J. Nutr. 12:188.

Hutchison, J.C.D., J.S.D. Bacom, T.F. Macrae and A.N. Worden. 1943. The nutritive value of potato protein for the pig. Biochem. J. 37:550.

Iriarte, R.J.R., N.R. Thompson and C.L. Bedford. 1972. Protein in potato flakes: evaluation by the meadow vole (*Microtus pennsylvanius*). Amer. Potato J. 49:255.

Jaswal, A.F. 1973. Effect of various processing methods on free and bound amino acid content of potatoes. Amer. Potato J. 50:186.

Jones, D.B. and E.M. Nelson. 1931. Nutritive value of potato protein and of gelatin. J. Biol. Chem. 91:705.

Joseph, A.A., R.N.R. Choudhuri, K. Indiramma, M.N. Rao, M. Swaminathan A. Sreenivasan and V. Subrahmanyan. 1963. Food Science (Mysore) 12:255.

Kaldy, M.S. 1971. Evaluation of potato protein by amino acid analysis and dye-binding. Ph.D. Thesis, Michigan State University, East Lansing, Michigan.

Kaldy, M.S. and P. Markakis. 1972. Amino acid composition of selected potato varieties. J. Food Sci. 37:375.

Kofranyi, E. and F. Jekat. 1965. The biological value of potato proteins. Forschber. Landes NRhein-Westf. No. 1582 (in German).

Kofranyi, E. and F. Jekat. 1967. The biological value of food proteins. Hoppe-Seyler's Z. physiol. Chem. 34884 (in German).

Kon, S.K. 1928. The nutritional value of tuberin, the globulin of potato. Biochem. J. 22:261.

Kon, S.K. and A. Klein. 1928. The value of whole potato in human nutrition. Biochem. J. 22:258.

Lindner, K., S. Jaschik and I. Korpaczy. 1960. Amino acid composition and biological value of potato protein fractions. Qual. Plant. Mater. Veg. 7:289 (in German).

Macko, V. and H. Stegeman. 1969. Mapping of potato proteins by combined electrofocusing and electrophoresis. Hoppe-Zeyler's Zeitschr. f. Physiol. Chem. 350:917.

Markakis, P., T.M. Freeman and W.H. Harte. 1962. Method of producing a chip-type product. U.S. Patent 3,027,258.

McCollum, E.V. 1921. The supplementary dietary relations between proteins of cereal grains and the potato. J. Biol. Chem. 47:175.

McCollum, E.V., N. Simmonds and H.T. Parsons. 1918. The dietary properties of the potato. J. Biol. Chem. 36:197.

THE NUTRITIVE QUALITY OF POTATO PROTEIN

Mitchell, H.H. 1924. Biological values of proteins at different levels of intake. J. Biol. Chem. 58:905.

Mulder, E.G. and K. Bakema. 1956. Effect of N, P, K and Mg nutrition of potato plants on the content of free amino acids and on the amino acid composition of the protein of the tubers. Plant and Soil 7:135.

Orr, M.C. and B.K. Watt. 1957. Amino acid composition of foods. Home Econ. Res. Report 4. USDA, Washington, D.C.

Rose, M.S. and L.F. Cooper. 1917. The biological efficiency of potato nitrogen. J. Biol. Chem. 30:201.

Schiftan, H. 1933. Arch. Tierernaehr. Tierz. 8:212. Cited by Hutchison et al. (1943).

Schreiber, K. 1961. Chemistry and biochemistry. *In* R. Schick and M. Klinkowski (Eds.) The Potato. VEB Deutscher Landwirtshafts-verlag, Berlin (in German).

Schuphan, W. 1970. Control of plant proteins: the influence of genetics and ecology on food plants. *In* R.A. Lawrie (Ed.) Proteins as Human Foods. Avi Publishing Co., Westport, Conn.

Schuphan, W. and W. Postel. 1957. The biological value of potato protein. Naturwissenschaften 44:40 (in German).

Schwerdtfeger, E. 1969. Effect of home preparation on valuable constituents of potatoes. Part 3. Proteins and amino acids. Qual. Plant. Mater. Veg. 17:191.

Schwimmer, S. and H.K. Burr. 1967. Structure and chemical composition of the potato tuber. *In* W.F. Talburt and O. Smith (Eds.) Potato Processing. Avi Publishing Co., Westport, Conn.

Sheffner, L. 1967. In vitro protein evaluation. *In* A.A. Albanese (Ed.) Newer Methods of Nutritional Biochemistry. Academic Press, New York. Vol. III.

Snyderman, S.E., L.E. Holt, J. Danois, E. Roitman, A. Boyer and M.E. Balis. 1962. "Unessential" nitrogen: a limiting factor for human growth. J. Nutr. 78:57.

Thompson, J.F. and F.C. Steward. 1952. The analysis of the alcohol-insoluble nitrogen of plants by quantitative procedures based on paper chromatography. II. The composition of the alcohol-soluble and insoluble fractions of the potato tuber. J. Exp. Bot. 3:170.

Thompson, N.R. 1975. Personal communication.

Talley, E.A., F.L. Carter and W.L. Porter. 1958. Determination of end points in extraction of amino acids from potatoes. J. Agr. Food Chem. 6:608.

USDA Agr. Handbook No. 8. 1963. Composition of Foods. Agricultural Research Service, USDA, Washington, D.C.

21

EFFECTS OF ENZYMES ON NUTRITIONAL QUALITY AND AVAILABILITY OF PROTEINS

S. Schwimmer

Western Regional Research Center
Agricultural Research Service
U.S. Department of Agriculture
Berkeley, California

INTRODUCTION

We shall examine the following general areas: (1) enzymatic transformations of toxicants, antinutrients, and other undesirable substances; (2) how to prevent enzyme action in the food when this action renders an otherwise good source of protein unavailable or unacceptable for human consumption although there may be no direct interaction with the protein; (3) the effect and use of proteolytic enzymes added to food on the availability (extractability, solubility) and nutritional and chemical parameters associated with protein quality; (4) autolytic processes in which the endogenous proteinases modify the protein; (5) addition of other non-proteolytic enzymes to improve availability *via* enhanced extractability of the protein; (6) non-proteolytic enzyme action in the food resulting in undesirable modification of the protein.

It may be worthwhile as an aid in delineating the range of the ensuing discussion to list related topics which will not be covered or at best, discussed peripherally in conjunction with main topics: the use of enzymes to manufacture proteinaceous food ingredients, which are not used primarily for their nutritional value; i.e., flavoring ingredients cloudifiers, stabilizers, and other substances which affect textural and functional properties; the enzymes of protein-consuming subjects--how they are affected and how their synthesis is controlled by the protein that is being consumed; enzyme action arising as the result of natural or deliberate microbial fermentation; the role of enzyme action in the production of such conventional products as cheese and bread; antinutritional effects of inhibitors of the consumers own enzymes including antitrypsin inhibitors and other toxins and antinutrients (see Liener, this volume).

ENZYMATIC REMOVAL OF TOXIC SUBSTANCES FROM HIGH-PROTEIN FOODS

As shown in Table 1, we discuss in this section the exploitation of enzyme action for the removal of unwanted, mostly toxic, substances from foods and high protein feeds which have potential for human consumption. By far the greatest research effort has been put into the removal of lactose from dairy foods by addition of external sources of lactase (β-galactosidase, E.C. 3.2.1.23). The attention paid to the use of this enzyme derives from increasing evidence that large segments of the adult population of various ethnic groups are lactase deficient. A good review is that of Kretchmer (1972).

In general, the lactase preparations proposed to remove lactose from milk are derived from three microorganisms or close variants thereof: primarily a yeast, *Saccharomyces lactis*; a fungus, *Aspergillus niger*; and a bacterium, *Bacillus subtilis*. Of course, active exploration for other sources continues unabatedly (Borglum and Sternberg, 1972; Wierbicki and Koisikowski, 1973; Blanchon and Wells, 1974).

Investigations on the effectiveness and safety of adding preparations of lactase directly to milk have been underway for at least 10 years. In the Netherlands lactase from *S. lactis* as a commercial preparation (Maxilact) which was used to prepare powder from both skim milk (Lactalac V) and from whole milk (Lactalac M).

EFFECTS OF ENZYMES ON PROTEIN QUALITY

TABLE 1

Removal of Unwanted Substances by Enzymes

Substance(s)	Food	Toxicity	Enzyme, Action	Source
Lactose	Milk	Intestinal upset	β-Galactosidase	O
Oligo-galacto-saccharides	Beans	Flatulence	α-Galactosidase	O, I
Nucleic acid	Single cell protein	Gout	Ribonuclease Plastein synthesis	O, I O
Lignan glycoside	Safflower seed	Catharsis	β-Glucosidase	O
Phytic acid	Beans, Wheat	Mineral deficiency	Phytase (phosphatase)	O, I
Trypsin inhibitor	Soybean	Protein utilized	Urease-NH_3 production	I
Ricin	Castor bean	Paralysis of resp. and vasomotor system	Proteinase	I

O = External source of enzyme; I = Potentiation of foods' own enzyme, enzyme autolysis. See also, Montgomery, 1969; Leopold and Ardrey, 1972.

According to Olling (1972), both were acceptable to lactase deficient infants and adults. A similar, if not identical enzyme preparation was used in the U.S. to remove lactose from milk (Kosikowski and Wierbicki, 1973). On the other hand, Rand and Linklater (1973) preferred a fungal lactase added to milk intended primarily for persons deficient in intestinal lactase. The reason they used fungal instead of yeast lactase was the superior heat stability of the former which enabled them to add the fungal enzyme during pasteurization. This eliminated the cost of interposing an extra step in the processing procedure.

Various schemes have been tried and proposed for the incorporation of an immobilized enzyme system to remove lactose from dairy
products and waste streams. Only limited studies are available on
the actual application of immobilized lactase to remove lactose
from milk. Woychick (1974) feels that the problem of the rich
medium for the growth of microorganisms provided by milk remains
a major obstacle to commercial adaptation of immobilized lactase.
On the other hand, Pastore et al. (1974) report no external contamination of milk passing through a column of lactase entrapped in
cellulose triacetate. They were able to hydrolyze 75% of the
lactose in milk in 4 hr at 50°C.

The action of α-galactosidases in removing unassimilable
oligosaccharides is discussed by Olson (this volume).

The high purine content of single cell protein (SCP) is
due to the high nucleic acid content which plays a role in the
etiology of gout. Nucleic acid can be removed by non-enzymatic
methods such as that of Hedenskog and Mogren (1973) in which
protein is separated from nucleic acid by precipitating the latter
in hot strong alkali. One would expect a lowering of nutritional
value of the protein by such drastic treatment. A milder alternative, adopted by a group of investigators at MIT (Ohta et al.,
1971) is to potentiate the nucleases of the unicellular organism.
Thus the yeast *Candida utilis* was subject to a heat shock at pH
4.0 at 68° for one to three seconds. This treatment probably
damages the internal membranes of the yeast cells so that the
ribonuclease has unlimited access to the RNA. Subsequent pro-
grammed incubation for somewhat longer periods at somewhat lower
temperatures results in the degradation of the RNA to 3'-nucleo-
tides. At first the latter accumulate in the cell, but the nucleo-
tides diffuse out of the cell without a concomitant loss of protein.
In this vein, Chao et al. (1974) have been granted a patent in
which it is claimed that the nucleic acid content of SCP material
is reduced to acceptable level in food products by "physiological

conditioning", followed by the action of endogenous ribonuclease.

In a subsequent study the MIT group developed an alternative enzyme treatment (Castro et al., 1971). Pancreatic ribonuclease was added to heat-shocked yeast cells (80° for 30 sec) thus allowing the added enzyme (enzyme:cell = 1:10,000) access to the nucleic acid.

The plastein reaction discussed below, has been applied to SCP (Fujimaki et al., 1973). The reduced fluorescence and UV absorbance of the plastein as compared with the starting SCP suggests that nucleic acid level was reduced.

Phytic acid, *myo*-inositol hexaphosphate, ubiquitously distributed throughout the plant kingdom, has been implicated as an antinutrient in beans and grains (Liener, 1969; Liener, this volume). Historically, phytic acid was pinpointed as the putative culprit of calcium deficient disease increase among children during World War II. In an attempt to upgrade the nutritional protein quality of bread, bran enriched whole wheat bread was used instead of white bread. Bran is very rich in phytic acid. Since then, more carefully controlled investigations suggest that phytic acid, under certain conditions, limits the availability of certain metals especially zinc, and also calcium and perhaps iron. Furthermore its phosphorus may be unavailable as a nutrient. The phytic acid is almost always accompanied by phytase(s) which hydrolyze it to inorganic orthophosphate and inositol. As expected, autolytic conditions for the hydrolysis of oligosaccharides in bean slurries also result in the augmentation of inorganic orthophosphate and increase of inositol (Becker et al., 1974) and decreases in the phytic acid (Chang, 1975). The latter investigator presented direct evidence for the decrease of phytic acid in whole beans even when the only source of added water comes from the atmosphere. The key to successful degradation of phytic acid is the use of temperatures (50-60°C) which destroy viability (*via* damage to intracellular membranes) without destroying the enzymes. The phytase activity in soybeans is low and heat-sensitive as compared with that of

a food such as wheat (Ranhotra, 1973; Chang, 1975). It is probable
that phytase action, as well as other autolytic enzyme action,
occurs during the various fermentations of soy bean to produce
tempeh, miso, tofu, etc.

Safflower seed *(Catharmus tinctorus)* has been proposed as yet
another untapped source of protein-rich human food (Anon, 1967).
In addition to the problem caused by difficultly removable hulls,
the oil-free protein-rich meal contains compounds known as lignan
glycosides. One of these is bitter and the other (2-hydroxyarctiin)
is cathartic (Palter et al., 1972). The bitter and cathartic
effects may be eliminated by removing the sugars with β-glucosidase
used by Palter et al., for their structural studies.

The leaves and other green parts of the tomato plant are a
potential source of protein which cannot be used for feed or food
because of the presence of the bitter and toxic alkaloid tomatine.
Ripe tomatoes, which of course do not contain tomatine, do possess
an enzyme system for degrading tomatine (Heftmann and Schwimmer,
1972). According to Darzins (1960) autolytic processes in castor
bean can remove the extremely toxic protein ricin.

Although enzyme action is usually not used to remove the
antinutrient trypsin inhibitor from soybean, potentiation of the
soybean's urease by adding urea has been used for this purpose.
According to a patent by Rambaud (1975), spraying urea on unex-
tracted soybean (crushed to allow endogenous urease action to
occur) results in the liberation of ammonia which destroys the
trypsin inhibitor when followed by rolling, flaking, and cooking
in steam.

Glucose is an unwanted substance interfering with the use of
a rich protein source, eggs, when the latter is stabilized by
drying. Glucose interacts with proteins at low water activities
during and after dehydration to form non-enzymatic browning products. This reaction may also decrease the nutritive value of the
eggs. Glucose can be removed with glucose oxidase (Vadehra and
Nath, 1973).

EFFECTS OF ENZYMES ON PROTEIN QUALITY

PREVENTION OF NON-PROTEIN LINKED UNDESIRABLE ENZYME ACTION

Under this heading we include those enzyme reactions which make an otherwise good source of protein unfit to eat. These products may be toxic or esthetically or sensorily objectionable. Stratagems have to be devised to prevent their action or to remove reaction products.

Perhaps the most well-known enzyme, in relation to protein foods, is lipoxygenase. In addition to its possible involvement with the proteins it is now definitely established that its stable end-products possess many of the objectional flavors associated with soybean meal (Kalbrenner et al., 1974). The presence of soy flour can be detected organoleptically after a 750-fold dilution with wheat flour (Moser et al., 1967). Heating soybean meal destroys lipoxygenase activity. However, it is necessary, at times to keep the proteins in their native state as in the preparation of protein isolates. Debittering methods include attempts to extract the substrates of lipoxygenase with organic solvents or to use the latter to inactivate the enzyme, in combination with heat or pH denaturation (Baker and Mustakas, 1973). The use of proteinase action will be discussed later.

Common beans also possess lipoxygenase activity whose end-products are readily detected when bean meal is slurried in water. This is one reason why whole beans are soaked overnight, then cooked. In the subsequent cooking the cells do not separate and it has been suggested that this could lead to a decrease in the availability of protein. Kon et al. (1974) showed that blending the beans in acid prevented lipoxygenase-produced off-flavor and also improved starch digestibility. The Protein Efficiency Ratio (PER) method for acid treated pinto beans cooked for 15 min was 1.04 as compared with a value of 0.77 for beans cooked whole. Lipoxygenase in rice bran was allowed to self destruct by reaction inactivation before being added to lipid-containing high protein products (Wheeler and Wallace, 1973).

Activity of lipase in a high protein fortified flour blend produced off-flavor upon prolonged storage. This could be prevented by simply depriving the lipase of reaction medium, water, by lowering the moisture content of the flour from 13 to 10% and keeping it low by proper packaging (Bean et al., 1974).

Three varieties of crucifer seeds have been investigated as sources of protein. These are white mustard (*Sinapis alba*), Crambe seed (*Crambe abyssinia*), and rapeseed (*Brassica compestris, B. napus*). The first is in present use as a condiment and the latter two seeds are used for oil production, especially erucic acid used in nylon synthesis. They all contain glucosinolates (mustard oil glucosides, thioglucosides) and enzymes attacking them (glucosinolases, thioglucosidases, myrosin, E.C.3.2.3.1).

$$\underset{\text{R-C-NOSO}_3^-}{\overset{\text{S-Glucosyl}}{|}} + H_2O \longrightarrow \underset{\text{R-C-NH-OSO}_3^-}{\overset{S}{\|}} + \text{Glucose}$$

A variety of end products can be formed from this active primary product of the enzyme action, a thiohydroxamic O-sulfonate; depending on the aglycone of the substrate and conditions of the enzyme reaction, these can be isothiocyanates, thiocyanates, nitriles, and oxazolidinethiones. The former compounds impart objectionable flavors and the latter are highly goitrogenic (Schwimmer, 1960, 1961; Schwimmer and Friedman, 1972; Van Etten, 1969; Van Etten et al., 1969).

One can distinguish five general approaches to prevent the formation of this class of antinutrient; one or more in combination have been proposed (Table 2).

With regard to the last approach, Table 2, the Scandinavian countries have launched a breeding program whose aim is to lower the glucosinolates, especially the progoitrin component, of rapeseed (Josefsson and Munck, 1972). That they have succeeded is attested to by the finding of only 0.1 mg of each of the products of glucosinolase reaction, oxazolidinethione and isothiocyanate, per

EFFECTS OF ENZYMES ON PROTEIN QUALITY

. TABLE 2

Preventing Glucosinolase Action in Crucifer Seeds

Method	Reference
Potentiate enzyme, Remove products	Goering (1961)
Inactivate enzyme	Eapen et al. (1973); Hill-Cucurella (1971)
Leach out substrate	Kozlowska et al. (1972); Eapen et al. (1973)
Destroy substrate chemically (Ferrous salts)	Kirk et al. (1971)
Breed out substrate	Josefsson and Munck (1972)

g of dry weight of the seed of *Bronowski* cultivar bred for the purpose of removing the glucosinolates. This is to be compared with values of 11.2 and 3.7 mg per g for a non-bred variety. The latter, as expected, was highly toxic to mice. They died within eight days after the start of the diet. Unfortunately, these authors found that the low-glucosinolate variety, while not so toxic, did appear to contain high-molecular weight compounds which exerted a detrimental effect on the nutritional value of the rapeseed meal. McLaughlan et al. (1975) attribute antinutritional effects of rapeseed and mustard protein concentrates to zinc deficiency occasioned by high phytic acid levels.

There are instances in which a step in food processing designed to stop undesirable enzyme action can result in a net decrease in the protein nutritional value of the food. It is well known that the processing step known as blanching can, especially if hot water rather than steam is used, result in the leaching out of nutrients including protein and its nutritional equivalent, amino acids. To cite an example especially significant for protein nutrition is shrimp processing in India and Pakistan. Haq et al. (1969) found

that the blanch water disposed of as the result of shrimp canning
in Pakistan contained 16.6% extracted protein. This amounted to a
loss of about 30,000 lb of protein in an 8-hr shift. Shrimp
account for nearly 20% of the sea food catch in India (Srinivas
et al., 1974). They found that the blanching step in an improved
method for stabilizing shrimp using low doses of ionizing radia-
tion resulted in a decrease in protein from 89% to 82% (dry basis).
Although better than other methods, they found some loss of available lysine upon prolonged storage but no loss in digestibility.
On the other hand, in processing of turnip greens, Meredith et
al. (1974) found very little, if any, loss of lysine as a result
of blanching, *per se* especially as compared with losses occurring
in the draining steps. Recent innovations in blanching technology,
designed primarily to solve pollution and energy problems, also
improve the retention of nutritional value of the food including
that of the protein (Bomben et al., 1973; Lazar and Lund, 1974).

ADDITION OF PROTEOLYTIC ENZYMES

Some of the health-associated reasons for adding proteolytic
enzymes to foods are as follows: (1) to increase extractability
of proteins in foods; (2) to improve the digestibility of the
food's protein; (3) to solubilize protein denatured in the course
of processing of the food; (4) to maintain protein solubility in
acid media so that the proteins (or the products of their partial
degradation) can be incorporated into carbonated beverages; (5) to
manufacture of soy milk; (6) to prepare hydrolyzates for parenteral nutrition (intravenous feeding); (7) to avoid alkali extraction of proteins which renders some essential amino acids such as
lysine (as lysino-alanine) and methionine nutritionally unavailable
(DeGroot and Slump, 1969); (8) to partially hydrolyze proteins in
foods and feedstuffs as a preliminary to acid hydrolysis in the
quantitative determinations of the amino acids in the protein (cf.
Gehrke and Neuner, 1974); (9) to assess the digestibility of food

protein as a guide or as an indicator of its *in vivo* digestibility;
(10) to improve the nutritional quality of the animal feeds by the
addition of commercial preparations of proteolytic enzymes;
(11) to use protein hydrolysate as a synergist with phenolic anti-
oxidants (Bishov and Henick, 1975); (12) to aid in the removal of
unwanted substances such as those posessing noxious odors and
tastes which associate with the intact but not with partially
hydrolyzed protein. The release of these flavors was the primary
objective of Fujimaki co-workers at the Department of Agricultural
Chemistry of the University of Tokyo when they published the first
of a series of remarkable papers (Fujimaki et al., 1968). The
results through 1971 were summarized by Fujimaki et al., (1971).

They succeeded in removing the objectionable substances responsible for the bitter taste and odor associated with purified
soybean protein by the use of commercial and pure endopeptidases
(proteinases). However, the peptides produced were bitter. Since
it appeared that bitterness seemed to be associated with peptides
bearing C-leucine as their carboxyl termini, the carboxypeptidases
should, and indeed did, debitter these hydrolysates. Especially
effective was a commercial enzyme preparation, Molsin, which contains an *Aspergillus* acid carboxypeptidase.

The alternative approach was to abolish these C-termini
through synthesizing new peptide bonds by incorporating these
peptides into resynthesized protein-like molecules *via* the plastein
reaction. The Tokyo group showed that the key to successful
plastein synthesis was dependent on a substrate concentration of at
least 20% oligopeptides, *ca* 0.2 M (optimum around 30%) and an
optimum degree of hydrolysis amounting to the splitting of 70 to
90% of the available peptide bonds. The first step in the plastein
synthesis catalyzed by chymotrypsin appears to be the formation of
a peptidylchymotrypsin through serine-195. This is followed by a
general base catalyzed nucleophilic attack (assisted by histidine-
57 of the enzyme) of this complex by another peptide resulting in
the aminolysis or iminolysis and thus a new peptide bond.

Finley and co-workers (1975) have succeeded in synthesizing plastein by passing caseinolytic peptides through a column of papain immobilized on chitin.

Whatever occurs in the formation of plastein, we know now that it leads to a product which is at least nutritionally wholesome as the soybean protein from which it came (Yamashita et al., 1970). Thus, the chemical score with respect to sulfur containing amino acids and leucine were, respectively, 94.3% and 102.5% of the untreated protein. *In vitro* digestibilities were about the same (100%) and true digestibility of the plastein fed to rats was 90.3%. Biological Value was 66.8, comparing favorably with the starting material. After supplementation with essential amino acids to give an amino acid pattern similar to that of casein, the ration yielded rates of growth equal to 96% of that of rats fed casein.

The Tokyo group have applied the plastein reaction to enrich soybean protein with methionine supplement incorporated directly into the protein (Yamashita et al., 1970; Yamashita et al., 1972; Arai et al., 1974). This first enrichment was accomplished by either providing the proteolytic enzymes, as substrate for plastein synthesis, a mixture of soy protein hydrolysates and hydrolysates from methionine-rich protein such as ovalbumin or by supplementing the soybean protein hydrolysates with L-methionine derivatives. By such means they were able to raise the level of soybean protein 7-fold. The advantage of incorporating methionine rather than adding it as a free amino acid is that it may be lost during processing *via* several routes. These include oxidation to the sulfoxide or to methional *via* the Strecker degradation. As pointed out by Schwimmer and Friedman (1972), such degradations would not only destroy an essential amino acid, but would also give rise to undesirable flavors.

On the other hand, too high a level of methionine, at least when fed in the free form can, be deleterious nutritionally (Scrimshaw and Altschul, 1971). At any rate, such high methionine-containing proteins can be diluted with proteins which are deficient

500

in this amino acid. Furthermore, evidence available suggests that intestinal absorption of dietary nitrogen in the form of peptides or partially digested proteins may be preferable to absorption of free amino acids. Imondi and Stradely (1974) found that soybean partially hydrolyzed by proteinase (and supplemented with essential amino acids) was much more fully and efficiently utilized by rats with pancreatic insufficiency that was a mixture of essential amino acids or unhydrolyzed protein.

A study of the proteolysis of soy protein which appears to be nutritionally significant is of Kirchgessner and Steenhart (1974) on the distribution of amino acids peptide cores remaining after partial hydrolysis with pepsin. They found that the essential amino acids threonine, valine, isovaline, leucine, and phenylalinine are present in the undigested core. This suggests that these amino acids might be less readily available than one would predict from a total amino acid analysis. In relation to question of the availability of methionine incorporated into protein *via* plastein synthesis one would expect that this amino acid would be more readily available since it is attached to the end of peptide chains and not the core. Similarly, some twenty years ago, Birk and Bondi (1955) reported that after the *in vitro* action of proteolytic enzymes of the gastro-intestinal tract on proteins present in a variety of plant feeds (soy, peanuts, wheat maize, etc.), a trichloracetic acid-precipitable "core" about 20 to 30 amino acids long was obtained. Such a core was never found when animal proteins were subjected to the same enzyme action.

Enzyme-chemical treatment of coconut meal by Molina and Lachance (1973), was found to be superior to treatment with either enzyme alkali or alone. They were able to extract 80-90% of the protein on a pilot-plant scale. The nutritive value of this extracted protein was much higher than that of the original coconut meal (Lachance and Molina, 1974). Part of this superiority, in addition to removal of fiber, was due to a relatively favorable distribution of essential amino acids, especially lysine. The

PER values (corrected) of the original coconut meal, the enzyme-
chemical treated extract, the extract supplemented with fiber and
of casein were respectively 2.32, 2.72, 2.55, and 2.50. The corresponding values for the net protein retention were 3.8, 4.5, 3.9
and 3.7. These papers also provide a summary of previous literature.

Using a heat-denatured protein fraction prepared from defatted
cottonseed meal so as to have as much insoluble protein as possible,
Arzu et al. (1972) were able to solubilize 40-60% of the protein
at optimal experimental conditions of 45° in five hr. Out of ten
commercial proteases tried, two from bacteria and bromelain from
pineapple proved to be the most active.

Childs (1975) was able to extract more than 50% of the protein
from screw-expressed commercial cottonseed meal by the use of an
enzyme-chemical method adapted from that used by Molina and Lachance
(1973), for coconut meal. Neither of these cottonseed studies presented any criteria of the nutritional value of the preparations.
Martinez et al., 1970.

Enzyme processing of a variety of seed proteins - defatted
sesame and peanut meals and four varieties of bean species, chick-
peas, green gram, black gram and field bean--resulted in increased
solubility and nutritive value according to Sreekantiah et al.
(1969). Some of their results, shown in Table 3 demonstrate increased extractability and lysine content of sesame and chickpeas.
However, the methionine appeared to be quite sensitive to their
treatment; incubation of 10% cooked suspensions of the meals with
commercial fungal protease preparations of Japanese origin for 5
hr at 45°C. According to the authors suitable blending of the
hydrolysates should yield a protein rich food with a reasonably
balanced amino acid composition. The values they obtained are
comparable to those for microbially fermented or predigested
oriental foods such as tempeh and miso.

Sunflower seed is another source of potentially valuable protein. Saint-Rat (1971) points out that the biological value of the

EFFECTS OF ENZYMES ON PROTEIN QUALITY

defatted seed cake is about the same as soybean meal. However, its
digestibility is inferior due to the presence of difficultly removable hulls. As an alternative to the complex and expensive process
of mechanical decortication, he incubated sunflower cake for short
periods with a commercial enzyme preparation possessing proteinase,
amylase, polygalacturonase, and cellulase activity. The protein
content of the resulting extract was 63.75% as compared with 42.5%
for enzyme-treated defatted soymeal and 26% for similarly treated
coconut and meal. However, the sunflower is very poor in lysine.
For similar reasons of difficulties with intractable husks, it
might be worthwhile to apply such proteolytic enzyme processing
to safflower seed (Anon, 1967a).

Proteolytic enzymes have been applied to leaf protein. In one
process (Edwards and Edwards, 1974), alfalfa or clover is first
treated with alkali, then neutralized and digested with a mixture
of pancreatin and bile and the high-protein-containing extract -
then separated. The presence of bile in conjunction with pancreatin suggests concomitant action of both lipase and proteinases.

TRANSFORMATION OF FISH PROTEIN BY PROTEINASES

Utilization of proteolytic action to transform the protein of
fish and other marine creatures has been reviewed by Finch (1970)
and Hale (1974). Mackie (1974) provides a short review on the
recovery of protein from waste fish by proteolytic enzymes. These
enzymes may be derived from microorganisms growing in fish fermentations, enzymes may be added, or the fishes' own enzymes can effect
such transformations (autolysis). Undoubtedly autolytic process
act in concert with added proteolytic enzymes. Thus, Mackie (1974)
stated that at least in one process raw fish were digested more
rapidly than were cooked fish after the addition of enzyme. In
some fish foods, especially in the fish sauces of Southeast Asia,
all three processes may be operative (VanVeen, 1965).

503

TABLE 3

Enzyme Processing of Seed Proteins

| Measurement | Seed Meal[a] | | | |
| | Sesame | | Chick Pea | |
	Control	Processed	Control	Processed
Soluble protein, %	4.63	31.31	7.38	19.00
Amino - N, %	0.29	4.50	0.29	3.68
Lysine mg/g	14.9	18.5	26.0	17.1
Methionine, mg/g	10.3	6.2	2.8	2.8
Total protein solubilized, %	--	64.14	--	86.12

[a]From the data of Sreekantiah et al. (1969).

In a statement by the Protein Advisory Committee (Anon, 1972), it was suggested that enzyme processing, although at that time less developed than alternative processing methods for the production of fish protein concentrate (FPC) could eventually result in the production of inexpensive milk analogues. This statement briefly describes three such processes. One process was proposed for the production of FPC in the United States. In this process, said to be at that time at the plant planning stage, hake protein is first subjected to partial hydrolysis by enzymes followed by solvent extraction as an alternative to removal of the fat by centrifugation. The resulting product is said to be completely water soluble and has a slight meaty flavor.

A second process, then at the pilot plant stage, involved enzyme digestion of the whole fish, fish meal or press cake followed by oil separation to yield a product free of fish odor and has been used so far as an animal feed. In the third method, pilot plant studies of which have been carried out in Chili, the PAG statement outlines a procedure in which eviscerated deboned fish are subjected to a "mild" enzyme treatment. This treatment is followed by addition of stabilized fat. The mixture is then pasteurized and spray dried to yield a light colored powder with no fish flavor which is readily dispersible in water.

In contrast to all of the above described methods, which apparently have not advanced beyond the pilot plant stage, according to Mackie (1974) the French are successfully engaged in a combined fishing-processing operation involving the addition of proteolytic enzymes. In this operation, fish waste and even whole fish treated with proteinase are converted directly into hydrolysate aboard ship. After being held at 0°C on board until the ship returns to port, the hydrolysate is separated into oil and liquid. The latter is dried to be used as FPC.

Two problems which arise in conjunction with proteinase action are loss of protein owing to excessive enzyme action and microbial contamination. Archer et al. (1973) solved the latter problem by conducting the hydrolysis at 50° and pH 8.8 using BASAP, *B. subtilis* alkaline protease (Monozyme). When pepsin is used in acid medium, quite a bit of salt can accumulate upon subsequent neutralization concentration. The same investigators used ammonia which is evaporated off during the drying step. Of course this would expose the protein in conditions in which there is a loss in nutritive value. Tarky et al. (1973) solved this problem passing the dilute hydrolysate through tubular ultrafiltration membranes. One of the advantages of FPC preparations derived from processes in which proteinase action has occurred is elimination of gristly textural characteristics of FPC made by non-enzymatic processes.

In this connection, fish protein hydrolysates as milk replacers is satisfactory, as measured by PER, if not more than 40% of the casein is replaced when used for such purposes (Toullec et al., 1973).

As with other hydrolysates, fish digests can be quite bitter due to the formation of bitter peptides (Mackie, 1974). Fujimaki et al. (1973), while testing various enzyme preparations, found that Pronase produced an acidic oligopeptide which had a desirable brothy flavor with a strong aftertaste. Neither glutamic nor aspartic acid was present. The plastein reaction was applied to recovery of protein from fish waste (Onue and Riddle, 1973).

With regard to the nutritional value, Hale (1974) has commented on the loss of essential amino acids, especially isoleucine and phenylalanine from the hydrolysis of hake protein. Again BASAP came to the rescue. When hydrolyzed at a pH equal or greater than 8.5, the resulting fish protein concentrate (FPC) gave the best balance of amino acids. The PER of the totally soluble FPC from alewives was found to be equal to that of casein. Tarky et al. (1973) found that FPC from waste fish has a low PER of 1.65 owing to a deficiency of tryptophan. After supplementation of the rations with an equal weight of casein, which has an excess of tryptophan, the PER was raised to 3.39 as compared to a value of 3.33 of casein alone. (See also, Linson, 1968; Lum, 1969;McBride et al., 1961).

PROTEIN HYDROLYSIS *VIA* AUTOLYTIC PROCESSES

Autolysis is an alternative to adding enzyme to solubilize proteins or otherwise transform the food in which they are present. Its application is, of course, limited to those foods in which the proteolytic activity is sufficiently high to effect the desired changes. The food cannot be heated or otherwise treated to inactivate the proteinases prior to autolysis. During autolysis provision has to be made for protection against microbial contamination. Furthermore, one must anticipate that autolytic processes other than those due to endogenous proteinases will go on simultaneously. Reference to such non-proteinase action will be discussed later.

Fish are the principle food in which gross quantitative autolysis of the protein has played a major role. This is because fish have abundant proteolytic activity and because the native fish proteins (in contrast to plant proteins) are highly susceptible to proteolysis.

Some of the resulting food, such as nauc-mam sauce of Viet-Nam, are treasured for their sensory attributes rather than as a source of protein nutrition. Also, it should be realized that in these foods we seldom can separate pure autolysis from concomitant microbial protease action (ensilage).

Very little has been published concerning the effect of auto-lysis on the nutritive value of the protein of fish. According to Tomiyama (1968), the nutritional value of FPC prepared from auto-lyzed protein is similar to that of isolate fish protein. Autolytic proteinase action occurs during the marinating of herring according to Sicho et al. (1972). They found that marinating too long leads to losses of valuable amino acids into the marinade.

Autolysis of plants as means of releasing and making available proteins goes back to at least 1936 in a patent on the production of yeast protein autolysate for feed and food use (Weizmann, 1936). In subsequent patents the yeast proteinase was supplemented by papain and that from seeds such as soybean (Weizmann, 1939).

Since soybeans possess proteolytic activity (Circle, 1950; Anon, 1967b, Rackis, 1972) it should be possible to transform some of the soy protein *via* autolysis.

From point of view of utilizing autolysis it is of interest to note that the soy proteinases are maximally active below neutra-lity where the main lipoxidase of soybean is practically inactive (Whitaker, 1972).

Although autolysis as a distinct procedure or process has not been reported for the extraction and solubilization of soybean pro-tein, it probably occurs in many processes. As in the case of some fish protein isolation procedures it may occur when it is not wanted. On the other hand, it appears to play an important role in soy milk preparation. Lo et al. (1968) reports a ten-fold increase in non-protein nitrogen during a 24-hour soak, a step in the preparation of soy milk. During the preparation of unheated soybean meal for extraction or for extrusion, temperatures of 50-60°C, in the range of activity of soybean proteases, are used.

A promising high protein food source which does have relatively high proteolytic activity is the peanut. Mosley and Ory (1973) showed that autolysates prepared from 10% suspensions of peanut cotyledon after 12 hr at 37° were hazy in appearance but remained essentially clear when refrigerated for a long time and should be suitable as a beverage supplement. As expected, there was a progressive increase in low molecular weight components.

IMPROVEMENT OF PROTEIN NUTRITION BY THE ACTION OF NON-PROTEOLYTIC ENZYMES

One advantage in using non-proteolytic enzymes is that it is possible to obtain the protein in a undegraded form. Another is that it may not be necessary to denature the proteins so that they become more susceptible to the proteinases. Therefore, the food does not have to be heated or cooked during processing.

Polysaccharidase application is not always successful. Commercial cellulases were not effective in liberating protein in cottonseed meal (Molina and Lachance, 1973) nor did a hemicellulase preparation help extract protein from coconut meal (Arzu et al., 1972). On the other hand, Saunders et al. (1972) was able to increase the *in vitro* digestibility of the high quality protein locked in the protein bodies of wheat bran by as much as 35% as the result of the action of the cellulases present in the commercial enzyme Pectinol 41P. Rats fed treated bran grew 25% faster than control rats. Microscopic studies showed that the bran wall was the primary substrate for these enzymes.

Partially purified fungal cellulases from *Trichoderma viridae* and as well as from *Aspergillus* and *Rhizopus* were effective in extracting 20 to 35% of the protein from sun-dried khesari (*Lathyrus sativum*) and from gram and soybean in a three hour treatment at 40°C (Ghose et al., 1970). Several groups of Japanese investigators have been engaged in studies on applying the action of microbial "macerating" enzymes, probably a mixture of enzymes, which hydrolyze cellulose, hemi-celluloses and pectin. This action produces single cell suspensions and helps to liberate nutrients from the tissues and cells of vegetables (Kawai et al., 1972; Toyama, 1969). Instead of microbial enzymes, Bock et al. (1971) advocated the use of polysaccharide-degrading enzyme complex of tomato and avocado as "Macerase" to convert vegetables to stable single-cell suspensions. This presumably results in improved protein availability. According to Yamatsu et al. (1966) the combined action of the polymer-degrading enzymes from *Trametes sanguina* on yeast and soybean meal results in the solubilization of almost 80% of the total nitrogen at pH 3. No antisepsis is necessary.

Many patents have been issued on the use of "macerase" cellulytic enzymes in recovery of protein. Thus, Blanchon (1966) claimed to separate the nutritive constituents contained in the cortical layer and envelope of cereal grains. Silberman (1971) claimed to convert food by-products such as grass, leaves, roots, seeds, stems, etc., to an end product as which can be used in soft drinks. With a commercial enzyme (Cellulase-36, Rohm and Haas). Hang et al. (1970) increased the nitrogen extracted from mung bean from 10 to 60% and that from peas 30 to 60%. A more grandiose role of cellulase in the production of SCP has been proposed (Mandels et al., 1974). In this scheme, waste cellulose would be converted into glucose which would then serve as food nutrient for the production of SCP.

A powerful non-cellulolytic enzyme from *Pestalotiopsis westerdijkii* improved the extractability of protein in soybeans from 74 to 95% as a step in the preparation of soy milk which was used for infant feeding (Abdo and King, 1967).

In some instances the polysaccharidases are used to provide more food value per unit weight of the food by converting insoluble polysaccharides to utilizable sugars. Thus, Uhlig and Grampp (1972) treated soy meal with pectinolytic enzymes alone or in combination with cellulase and/or hemicellulase in order to make available more soluble carbohydrate and thus improve the nutritional value. Digestibility of pea flour in milk replacers is improved by addition of amylase whose action provides the sugar required to replace milk lactose (Bell et al., 1974).

Finally, brief mention should be made of enzymes which do not degrade polymers, in relation to their effect of their action on the nutritive value of proteins. Naguib (1972) reports that treatment of milk with catalase (after hydrogen peroxide sterilization) does not affect the nutritional value of the milk protein. One can improve the protein content of fish simply by removing the fat. This can be accomplished by exposing the fish to lipase action (Burkholder et al., 1968).

IMPAIRMENT OF PROTEIN QUALITY BY ENZYME ACTION

This section explores the nutritional consequences of the action of endogenous food enzymes which results in deleterious modifications of the protein. Endogenous proteolytic action can, under some circumstances, lead to losses in yield and availability. This is an example of direct action of the enzyme on the protein. Another mode of modification, not always readily distinguishable from the first mode, is interaction of the protein with highly reactive intermediates or end-products of the enzyme action. A case in point is the interaction with proteins of polyphenol oxidases, PPO (Mason and Peterson, 1965).

Insight into the nature of what happens to proteins is afforded by work of Pierpont (1969) on the interaction of PPO-generated o-quinones with amino acids, peptides, and proteins. Pierpont found that such quinones can interact with sulfhydryl and free amino groups, amino acids, peptides, and proteins. The o-quinones react with descending preference with sulfhydryl groups of cysteine, free epsilon-amino groups of lysine and N-terminal amino acids. About half of the lysine of bovine serum albumin reacted in 30 min at 30°, pH 5.5. Thus, the nutritional quality may be impaired due to the unavailability of lysine and to some of the sulfur amino acids, especially if the protein is methionine-deficient.

The most direct evidence that impairment of the nutritional value of the protein does indeed occur is afforded by the experiments of Horigome and Kandatsu (1968). The nutritional implication of PPO systems on protein quality is especially relevant to forage plants and presumably to future use of these plants as high-protein human foods. As shown in Table 4, casein recovered from solutions in which PPO was oxidizing caffeic acid, isochlorogenic acid or the phenolic compounds of red clover leaves lost a significant amount of its nutritive quality.

TABLE 4

Nutritional Value of Casein Exposed to Polyphenol Oxidase Action

Substrate	Enzyme Source	Nutritional Parameters[b]			
		Biol. value	Available lysine	Digesti-bility	Color
Caffeic acid	None	97.3	99.8	99.7	White
Caffeic acid	Orchard Grass	89.4	87.3	96.3	Brown
i-Chlorogenic Acid	Orchard Grass	87.3	90.7	96.7	Green-Brown
Red Clover	Red Clover	85.9	95.3	95.3	Brown

[a]Adapted from the data of Horigome and Kandatsu (1968).

[b]Casein alone = 100.

In contrast to the above studies it appears that the interaction of some phenolic compounds with protein without subsequent enzymatic oxidation is attended by an increase in the nutritive value of the protein. Thus Drieger and Hatfield (1972) found that daily weight gains, feed efficiency, and nitrogen balance were all significantly greater (P< 0.05) in lambs fed soybean meal plus 10% tara tannins than lambs receiving soybean meal alone. Hrdlicka and Janicek (1972) observed a protective effect of tannins on the digestibility of egg albumin exposed to non-enzymatic browning by glucose.

Another enzyme we have previously discussed whose action may alter or modify protein molecules is lipoxygenase (lipoxidase). The primary action of this enzyme is to add oxygen to a double bond of a fatty acid with a *cis,cis* pentadiene configuration ($-CH=CH-CH_2-CH$ $=CH-$) to form a lipid peroxide which probably exists, at least momentarily, as a highly reactive hydroperoxy free radical. This free radical, in both enzymatic oxidation and non-enzymatic autooxidation can self-propogate and interact with a variety of substances, including protein. For instance, peroxidized lipids interact with proteins to form, or induce the formation of insoluble crosslinked complexes involving protein-protein interactions (Roubal and Tappel, 1966). Such hydroperoxides can destroy many essential amino acids in proteins, especially methionine, as well as lysine and, to some extent, phenyl alanine, threonine and also cysteine (Gamage et al., 1973).

St. Angelo and Ory (1975) present evidence for a lipoxygenase-generated lipoperoxide-protein interaction in stored peanuts. Indirect nutritional evidence of hydroperoxide damage to proteins is afforded by observations that anti-oxidant treated herring meals protected the protein therein from deterioration of nutritional properties (S.El-Lakany and B.E. March, J. Fd. Sci. 25:899, 1974).

There are undoubtedly many more enzyme reactions in foods which can give rise to highly reactive intermediates which in turn might damage the protein. For example, the enzymes responsible for the

EFFECTS OF ENZYMES ON PROTEIN QUALITY

formation of the flavor of onion and crucifers form highly reactive
primary products (Schwimmer and Friedman, 1972). Since in many
foods the enzymes are no longer acting as parts of integrated systems
(Schwimmer, 1972) non-physiological end-products may accumulate; or
ordinarily readily-converted substances such as hydrogen peroxide
may have the opportunity of reacting with protein. Perhaps the
most damaging of all of such uncontrolled reactions would be that
leading to the formation of the radical, $OH\cdot$, which can arise, in
the absence of superoxide dismutase (E.C. 1.15.1.1) from the following reaction (Fridovich, 1974, 1975).

$$O_2^- + H_2O_2 \longrightarrow OH^- + OH\cdot + O_2$$

The reactants in this equation are generated by flavoprotein oxidase-
mediated enzyme reactions. Normally this reaction in the living
cell is prevented by catalase, by peroxidases, and especially by
superoxide dismutases which catalyze the dismutation of superoxide
anion, O_2^-, to hydrogen peroxide and water.

$$O_2^- + O_2^- + 2H^+ \longrightarrow H_2O_2 + O_2$$

A more detailed treatment of the subject will appear in a future
publication.

REFERENCES

Abdo, K. M. and A. King. 1967. Enzymatic modification of the
    extractability of protein from soybeans, *Glycine max*. J. Agr.
    Food Chem. 15:83.

Anon. 1967. Nutritional value of safflower meal. Nutr. Rev. 25:
    29.

Anon. 1972. The potential of fish protein concentrate for devel-
    oping countries. PAG. Bulletin 2:24.

Arai, S., K. Aso, M. Yamashita, and M. Fujimaki. 1974. Note on
    an enlarged-scale method for processing a methionine-enriched

plastein.from soybean protein. Cereal Chem. 51:143.

Archer, M. C., J. O. Ragnarsson, S. R. Tannenbaum, and I. C. Wong. 1973. Enzymatic solubilization of an insoluble substrate, fish protein concentrate: Process and kinetic considerations. Biotech. Bioeng. 15:181.

Arzu, A., H. Mayorga, J. Gonzalez, and C. Rolz. 1972. Enzymatic hydrolysis of cottonseed protein. J. Agr. Food Chem. 20:805.

Baker, E. C. and G. G. Mustakas. 1973. Heat inactivation of trypsin inhibitor and urease in soybeans: Effect of acid and base. J. Amer. Oil Chem. Soc. 50:137.

Bean, M., D. K. Mecham, M. M. Hanamoto, and D. A. Fellers. 1974. Status of high-protein bread flours for government purchase. Baker's Dig. 48(4):34.

Becker, R. et al. 1974. Conditions for the autolysis of alpha-galactosidases and phytic acid in California small white beans. J. Fd. Sci. 39:766.

Bell, J. M., G. F. Royan, and C. G. Youngs. 1974. Digestibility of pea protein concentrates and enzyme-treated pea flour in milk replacers for calves. Can. J. Anim. Sci. 54:355.

Birk, Y. and A. Bondi. 1955. The action of proteolytic enzymes on protein feeds. Intermediary products precipitated by trichloroacetic acid and phosphotungstic acid from peptic digests and pancreatic digests. J. Sci. Food Agric. 6:549.

Bishov, S. J. and A. S. Henick. 1975. Antioxidant effect of protein hydrolyzates in freeze-dried model systems. J. Food Sci. 40:345.

Blanchon, E. 1966. Process for separating the enzymes and nutritive constituents contained in the envelope and cortical layer of cereal grains. U.S. Patent 3,255,015. June 7.

Bock, W., M. Krause, and G. Dongowski. 1971. Method of manufacture of vegetable macerates. (German) DAR Patent 84,317.

Bomben, J. L. et al. 1973. Pilot plant evaluation of individual quick blanching (IQB) for vegetable. J. Food Sci. 38:590.

Borglum, G. B. and M. Z. Sternberg. 1972. Properties of a fungal lactase. J. Food Sci. 37:619.

Burkholder, L. et al. 1968. Fish fermentations. Food Technol. 22:1278.

Castro, A. C., A. J. Sinskey, and S. R. Tannenbaum. 1971. Reduction of nucleic acid content in Candida yeast cells by pancreatic ribonuclease treatment. Appl. Microbiol. 22:422.

Chang, H. 1975. Removal of phytic acid from beans by potentiation of *in situ* phytase. Dissertation Abst. In press.

EFFECTS OF ENZYMES ON PROTEIN QUALITY

Chao, K. C. 1974. Enzymatic degradation of nucleic acids. U.S. Patent 3,809,776. May 7.

Childs, E. A. 1975. An enzymatic-chemical method for extraction of cottonseed protein. J. Food Sci. 40:78.

Circle, S. J. 1950. Proteins and other nitrogenous constituents. In "Soybeans and Soybean Products," Vol. 1. K. S. Markley (Editor). John Wiley and Sons, New York, N.Y.

Darzins, E. 1969. Edible castor cake product and method of producing same. U.S. Patent 2,929,963. January 12.

DeGroot, A. P. and P. Slump. 1969. Effects of severe alkali treatment on amino acid composition and nutritive value. J. Nutr. 98:45.

Driedger, A. and E. E. Hatfield. 1972. Influence of tannins on the nutritive value of soybean meal for ruminants. J. Anim. Sci. 34:465.

Eapen, K. E., N. W. Tape, and R. P. A. Simm. 1973. Oilseed flour. U.S. Patent 3,732,108. May 15.

Edwards, G. W. and A. W. Edwards. 1974. Alfalfa extracts. U.S. Patent 3,833,738. September 10.

Finch, R. 1970. Fish protein for human food. Crit. Rev. Food Technol. 1:519.

Finley, J. W. 1975. Personal Communication. Albany, CA.

Fridovich, I. 1974. Superoxide dismutase. Adv. Enzymol. 41:35.

Fridovich, I. 1975. Oxygen: Boon and bane. Amer. Sci. 63:54.

Fujimaki, M., H. Kato, S. Arai, and E. Tamaki. 1968. Applying proteolytic enzymes on soybeans. I. Proteolytic enzyme treatment of soybean protein and its effect on flavor. Food Technol. 22:889.

Fujimaki, M., H. Kato, S. Arai, and M. Yamashita. 1971. Applications of microbial proteases to soybean and other material to improve acceptibility especially through the formation of plastein. J. Appl. Bact. 39:119.

Fujimaki, M., K. Utaka, M. Yamashita, and S. Arai. 1973. Production of higher-quality plastein from a crude single cell protein. Agr. Biol. Chem. 37:2303.

Fujimaki, M. et al. 1973. Taste peptide fractionation from fish protein hydrolysate. Agr. Biol. Chem. 37:2891.

Gamage, P. T., and S. Matsushita. 1973. Interactions of autooxidized products of linoleic acid with enzyme proteins. Agr. Biol. Chem. 37:1.

Gehrke, C., and T. E. Neuner. 1974. Automated chemical determination of methionine. J. Assoc. Off. Anal. Chem. 57:682.

Ghose, K. C., and P. Haldar. 1970. Application of cellulase. III. Extraction of protein from khesar and gram plants with fungal cellulases. J. Food Sci. Technol. 2:160.

Goering, K. J. 1961. Process of obtaining the proteinaceous material from mustard seed, rape seed, and similar seeds. U.S. Patent 2,987,399. June 6.

Hale, M. B. 1974. Using enzymes to make fish protein concentrate. Marine Fisheries Review 36:15.

Hang, Y. D. et al. 1970. Enzymatic modifications of nitrogenous constituents of pea beans. J. Agr. Food Chem. 18:1083.

Haq, S. et al. 1969. Blanched water, a waste product of the shrimp-canning industry. Pak. J. Sci. Ind. Res. 12:49.

Hedenskog, G. and H. Mogren. 1973. Some methods for processing of single-cell protein. Biotec. and Bioeng. 15:1755.

Heftmann, E. and S. Schwimmer. 1972. Degradation to tomatine to 3-beta-5-alpha-pregn-16-en-20-one by ripe tomatoes. Phytochem. 11:2783.

Hill Cucurella, J. 1971. Isothiocyanate and 5-vinyl-2-oxazolidine-2-thione content in rape seed and rape seed meal made in five Chilean oil factories (Spanish). Oli, Grassi, Deriv. 7:2.

Horigome, T., and M. Kandatsu. 1968. Biological value of protein allowed to react with phenolic compounds in the presence of o-diphenolic oxidase. Agr. Biol. Chem. 32:1093.

Hrdlicka, J., and G. Janicek. 1972. Study of changes in the course of thermal and hydrothermal processes. XXIII. Digestibility determination of model mixtures containing egg albumin, glucose, and tannin after thermic treatment. Sbornik Vysoke Skoly Chemicko-Technologicke v Praze E, No. 35, 67 (Czechosl.).

Imondi, A. R. and R. P. Stradley. 1974. Utilization of enzymatically hydrolyzed soybean protein and crystalline amino acid diets by rats with exocrine pancreatic insufficiency. J. Nutr. 104:793.

Josefsson, E. and L. Munck. 1972. Influence of glucosinolates and a tentative high-molecular detrimental factor on the nutritional value of rape seed meal. J. Sci. Food Agr. 23:861.

Kalbrennar, J. E., K. Warner, and A. C. Eldridge. 1974. Flavors derived from linoleic and linolenic acid peroxides. Cereal Chem. 51:406.

Kawai, M. 1972. Maceration of plant tissues by crude enzyme preparations. III. Fractionation of crude enzyme preparations. J. Ferment. Technol. 50:698.

Kirchgessner, M. and H. Steinhart. 1974. Distribution of amino acids of molecular weights after pepsin *in vitro* digestion of soybean protein. Z. Tierphysiol. Tierenaehr. Futtermittelkd. 32:240.

Kirk, L. D., G. C. Mustakas, E. L. Griffin, Jr., and A. N. Booth. 1971. Crambe seed processing: Decomposition of glucosinolates. J. Amer. Oil Chem. Soc. 48:845.

Kon, S., J. R. Wagner, and A. N. Booth. 1974. Legume powders: Preparation and some nutritional and physicochemical properties. J. Food Sci. 39:897.

Kosikowski, F. V. and L. E. Wierbicki. 1973. Lactose hydrolysis of raw and pasteurized milk by *Saccharomyces lactis* lactase. J. Dairy Sci. 56:146.

Kozlowska, H., F. W. Sosulski, and C. G. Youngs. 1972. Extraction of flucosinolates from rape seed. Can. Inst. Food Sci. 5:149.

Kretchmer, N. 1972. Lactose and lactase. Sci. Amer. 227(4):70.

Lachance, P. A. and M. R. Molina. 1974. Nutritive value of a fiber-free coconut protein extract obtained by an enzymic-chemical method. J. Food Sci. 39:581.

Lazar, M. E. and D. B. Lund. 1974. Deactivation of inner core enzymes by retained blanching heat. U.S. Patent 3,794,500. February 26.

Leopold, A. and R. Ardrey. 1972. Toxic substances in plants and food habits of early man. Science 176:512.

Liener, I. E. (Editor). 1969. Toxic Constituents of Plant-Foodstuffs. Academic Press, New York, N. Y.

Linson, E. V. 1968. Edible marine protein concentrate. S. African Patent 6,705,900.

Lipmann, F. 1941. Metabolic generation and utilization of phosphate bond energy. Advan. Enzymol. 1:99.

Lo, Y. Y. et al. 1968. Soaking soybeans before extraction as it affects chemical composition and yield of soymilk. Food Technol. 22:1188.

Lonnerdal, B. and J. C. Janson. 1973. Studies on myrosinase. II. Purification and characterization of myrosinase from rape seed. Biochem. Biophys. Acta 315:421.

Lum, K. C. J. 1969. Fish concentrate. Brit. Patent 1,157,415. July 9.

McBride, J. R., D. R. Idler, and R. A. Macleod. 1961. The liquefaction of British Columbia herring by ensilage, proteolytic enzymes and acid hydrolysis. J. Fisheries Res. Board Canada 18:93.

McCabe, E. M. 1973. Soy protein fraction. U.S. Patent 3,733,207. May 15.

Mackie, I. M. 1974. Proteolytic enzymes in the recovery of proteins from fish waste. Proc. Biochem. 9:12.

Mandels, M., L. Hontz, and J. Nystrom. 1974. Enzymatic hydrolysis of waste cellulose. Biotechnol. Bioengin. 16:1471.

Mason, H. S. and E. W. Peterson. 1965. Melanoproteins. I. Reactions between enzyme-generated quinones and amino acids. Biochim. Biophys. Acta 111:134.

Martinez, W. H., L. C. Berardi, and L. A. Goldblatt. 1970. Cottonseed protein products-composition and functionality. J. Agr. Food Chem. 18:961.

Meinke, W. W. and K. F. Mattil. 1973. Autolysis as a factor in the production of protein isolates from whole fish. J. Food Sci. 38:864.

Meredith, F. I., M. H. Gaskins, and G. G. Dull. 1974. Amino acid losses in turnip greens (*Brassica L.*) during handling and processing. J. Food Sci. 39:689.

McLaughlan, J. M., J. D. Jones, B. G. Shak, and J. L. Beare-Rogers. 1975. Reproduction in rats fed protein concentrate from mustard or rapeseed. Nutr. Rep. Int. 15:325.

Molina, M. R. and P. A. Lachance. 1973. Studies on the utilization of coconut meal. A new enzymic-chemical method for fiber-free protein extraction of defatted coconut flour. J. Food Sci. 38:607.

Montgomery, R. D. 1969. Cyanogens. *In* "Toxic Constituents of Food Plantstuffs." I. E. Liener (Editor). Academic Press, New York, N.Y. and London, England.

Mosely, M. H. and R. L. Ory. 1973. Purification, characterization, and utilization of a proteolytic enzyme in peanuts. Abst. Amer. Chem. Soc. 165:AGDF 82.

Moser, H. A. et al. 1967. Sensory evaluation of soy flour. Cereal Sci. Today 12:296.

Naguib, K. 1972. The effect of hydrogen peroxide treatments on the bacteriological quality and nutritive value of milk. Milchwiss. 27:748.

Ohta, S., S. Maul, A. J. Sinskey, and S. R. Tannenbaum. 1971. Characterization of a heat shock process for reduction of the nucleic acid content of *Candida utilis*. Appl. Microbiol. 22:415.

Olling, C. C. J. 1972. Lactase-treatment in the dairy industry. Ann. Technol. Agr. 21:243.

Onue, Y. and V. M. Riddle. 1973. Use of the plastein reaction in recovering protein from fish waste. J. Fish. Res. Board Canada 30:1745.

Palter, R., R. E. Lundin, and W. F. Haddon. 1972. A cathartic glycoside isolated from Catharmus tinctorus. Phytochem. 11: 2871.

Pastore, M., F. Morisi, and A. Viglia. 1974. Reduction of lactose of milk by entrapped beta-galactosidase. II. Conditions for an industrial continuous process. J. Dairy Sci. 57:269.

Pierpont, W. S. 1969. o-Quinones formed in plant extracts. Their reaction with bovine serum albumin. Biochem. J. 112:619.

Rackis, J. J. 1972. Biologically active components. In "Soybeans." Chemistry and Technology. A. K. Smith and S. J. Circle (Editors). Avi Publishing Co., Westport, Conn.

Rambaud, M. 1975. Antitrypsin free products. U.S. Patent 3,845,229. October 29.

Rand, A. G. and P. Linklater. 1973. Use of enzymes for the reduction of lactose levels in milk products. Aust. J. Dairy Technol. 28:63.

Ranhotra, G. S. 1973. Factors affecting hydrolysis during bread-making of phytic acid in wheat protein concentrate. Cereal Chem. 50:353.

Roubal, W. T. and A. L. Tappel. 1966. Polymerization of proteins induced by free radical peroxidation. Arch. Biochem. Biophys. 113:150.

Saint-Rat, L. Enzymatic extraction of proteins from various oilseed cakes. C. R. Acad. Agriculture de France 57:826 (French).

Saunders, R. M., M. A. Connor, R. H. Edwards, and G. O. Kohler. 1972. Enzymatic processing of wheat bran. Cereal Chem. 49:436.

Schwimmer, S. 1960. Myrosin-catalyzed formation of turbidity and hydrogen sulfide from sinigrin. Acta Chem. Scand. 14:1339.

Schwimmer, S. 1961. Spectral changes during the action of myrosinase on singrin. Acta Chem. Scand. 15:535.

Schwimmer, S. 1972. Symposium. Biochemical control systems. Cell disruption and its consequences in food processing. J. Food Sci. 37:530.

Schwimmer, S. and M. Friedman. 1972. Genesis of sulphur-containing food flavors. Flavour Ind. 3:137.

Scrimshaw, N. S. and A. M. Altschul. (Editors). 1969. Amino Acid Fortification of Foods. MIT Press, Cambridge, Massachusetts.

Sicho, V. et al. 1972. Study of proteolytic processes in fish meat in the course of marinading. Sbornik Vyoske Skoly Chemicko-Technologicke v Praze, E. No. 36, 71. (Czechosl.).

Silberman, H. C. 1971. Enzymatic by-product conversion. U.S. Patent 3,615,721. October 26.

Sreekantia, K. R., H. Ebine, T. Ohta, and M. Nakano. 1969. Enzyme processing of vegetable protein foods. Food Technol. 23:1055.

Srinivas, U. K., U. K. Vakil, and A. Sreenivasan. 1974. Nutritional and compositional changes in dehydro-irradiated shrimp. J. Food Sci. 39:807.

St. Angelo, A. J. and R. L. Ory. 1975. Effects of lipoperoxides on proteins in raw and processed peanuts. J.Ag Fd.Chem. 23:141.

Tarky, W., O. P. Argawala, and G. M. Pigott. 1973. Protein hydrolysate from fish waste. J. Food Sci. 38:917.

Tomiyama, T. 1968. Preparation of fish protein concentrates by autolysis. Zesz. Prob. Postepow. Nauk Roln. No. 80:385 (Russian).

Toullec, R. 1973. Cited by Mackie (1974).

Toyama, N. Application of cellulase in Japan. *In* "Cellulases and their Applications." Advances in Chemistry Series 95, American Chemical Society, Washington, D.C.

Uhlig, H. and E. Grampp. 1972. Soya meal treatment. U.S. Patent 3,640,723. February 8.

Vahedra, D. V. and K. R. Nath. 1973. Eggs as source of protein. Crit. Rev. Food Technol. 4:193.

Van Etten, C. H. 1969. Goitrogens. *In* "Toxic Constituents of Plant Foodstuffs," I. E. Liener (Editor). Academic Press, New York, N.Y. and London, England.

Van Etten, C. H., M. E. Daxenbichler, and I. A. Wolff. 1969. Natural glucosinolates (thioglucosides) in food and feeds. J. Agr. Food Chem. 17:483.

Van Veen, A. G. 1965. Fermented and dried seafood products in Southeast Asia. *In* "Fish and Food," Vol. III, G. Borgstrom (Editor). Academic Press, New York, N.Y.

Weizmann, C. 1936. Yeast or protein preparations. Brit. Patent 450,529. July 20.

Weizmann, C. 1939. Protein products. Brit. Patent 509,495. July 17.

Wheeler, E. L. and J. M. Wallace. 1973. Self-catalyzed destruction of lipoxygenase in wheat mill fractions. Lebensm.-Wiss. Technol. 6:205.

Whitaker, J.R. 1972. Principles of Enzymology for the Food Sciences. Marcel Dekker, New York, N.Y.

Wierzbicki, L. E. and Kosikowski, F. V. 1973. Lactase potential of various microorganisms grown in whey. J. Dairy Sci. 56:26.

Woychik, J. H., M. Wondlowski, and K. J. Dahl. 1974. Preparation and application of immobilized beta-galactosidase of *Saccharomyces lactis*. *In* "Immobilized Enzymes in Food and

Microbial Processes," A. C. Olson and C. L. Cooney (Editors). Plenum Press, New York, N.Y. and London, England.

Yamashita, M. et. al. 1970. Enzyme modification of proteins in foodstuffs. II. Nutritive properties of soy plastein and its bio-utility evaluation in rats. Agric. Biol. Chem. 34:1333.

Yamashita, M., S. Arai, K. Aso, and M. Fujimaki. 1972. Location and state of methionine in a papain synthesized plastein from a mixture of soybean protein hydrolysate and *L*-methionine ethyl ester. Agric. Biol. Chem. 36:1353.

Yamatsu, O., M. Tobari, and H. Shimazono. 1966. Studies on enzymes produced by *Trametes sanguina*. J. Ferment. Technol. 44:847.

22

EFFECTS OF ANTI-NUTRITIONAL AND TOXIC FACTORS
ON THE QUALITY AND UTILIZATION OF LEGUME PROTEINS*

Irvin E. Liener

Department of Biochemistry
College of Biological Sciences
University of Minnesota
St. Paul, Minnesota

INTRODUCTION

For reasons which scientists have yet to fathom, nature has seen fit to endow many plants with the capacity to synthesize a wide variety of chemical substances which are known to exert a deleterious effect when ingested by man or animals. Included among such plants are the many varieties of legumes** which constitute an important part of the diet of large segments of the world's population. If such toxic substances do in fact exist in plant foodstuffs commonly consumed by man, why are not their effects manifested more frequently in the polulation? It would appear that, through trial

---

*Much of the material contained in this review is taken from a similar review on this subject published elsewhere (Liener, 1973). Permission to do so has been granted by the editors of the Indian Journal of Nutrition and Dietetics.

**For the purposes of this review, the following definition proposed by Roberts (1970) has been adopted: "Food legumes include those species of the plant family Leguminosae (pea or bean family) that are consumed directly by human beings, most commonly as mature, dry seeds, but occasionally as immature, green seeds or as green pods with the immature seed enclosed. Food legumes utilized as dry seed are often referred to as pulses or grain legumes."

and error, man has not only learned to avoid those foods which produce immediate ill effects, but he has also devised ways and means of eliminating them from others. For example, cooking and other common means of preparation have, in many instances, proved to be effective in destroying many of the toxic constituents in legumes. Nevertheless, circumstances may arise whereby complete detoxification may not always take place, as, for example, the inadequate commercial processing of soybean products. Abnormal patterns of food consumption may also prove harmful as exemplified by the periodic eruption of lathyrism in certain parts of India which is associated with the consumption of certain varieties of *Lathyrus* during times of famine when cereal grains are in short supply. Then we have the well-known example of favism which affects certain individuals who consume the bean, *Vicia faba*. These few examples serve to illustrate what might be expected to become more commonplace as the shortage of protein foods becomes more acute and people are forced to become more indiscriminate in their choice of life-sustaining plant foods.

PROTEASE INHIBITORS

Historical Background

Substances which have the ability to inhibit the proteolytic activity of certain enzymes are found throughout the plant kingdom, particularly among the legumes. These protease inhibitors have attracted the attention of nutritionists because of the possible role which these substances might play in determining the nutritive value of plant proteins. It was not long after soybeans were introduced into the United States that Osborne and Mendel (1917) made the significant observation that soybeans had to be heated in order to support the normal growth of rats. Kunitz (1945) subsequently isolated from raw soybeans a protein which had the unique property of combining with trypsin to form an inactive complex. It was logical to assume at the time that the trypsin inhibitor was the substance responsible for the poor nutritive value of unheated soybeans. The hypothesis that its effect could be readily explained on the basis of its ability to inhibit intestinal proteolysis was an appealing one. The fact also that methionine exerted a marked improvement on the nutritive value of raw soybeans (Liener et al., 1949) was taken to indicate that the trypsin inhibitor somehow interfered with the availability or utilization of methionine from the raw bean.

Mode of Action in the Animal Organism

It now appears that the true explanation for the growth-inhibitory property of the trypsin inhibitor is not a simple one. Although over 25 years have elapsed since Kunitz first isolated a trypsin inhibitor, years which have witnessed literally hundreds of papers on the subject (see review by Liener and Kakade, 1969; and Liener, 1972, 1973), there is still a decided lack of certainty regarding the significance of the trypsin inhibitor and its mode of action in the intact animal. There seems to be little doubt that hypertrophy of the pancreas represents one of the primary physiological effects produced by feeding raw soybeans or the isolated inhibitor (Rackis, 1974). Booth et al. (1960) are of the opinion that pancreatic hypertrophy leads to an excessive loss of endogenous protein secreted by the pancreas. Since this protein, consisting largely of pancreatic enzymes, is quite rich in cystine, the resulting effect is a net loss of sulfur-containing amino acids from the body. This would explain why the need for methionine, which is inherently limiting in soybean protein, is rendered even more acute in diets containing raw soybeans. Evidence has recently been presented to indicate that trypsin or chymotrypsin in the intestine suppresses pancreatic enzyme secretion by feedback inhibition, and that trypsin inhibitors evoke increased enzyme secretion by counteracting the suppression produced by trypsin (Green and Lyman, 1972; Niess et al., 1972).

Trypsin inhibitors have also been found in a large number of other legumes including the peanut, navy bean, lima bean, etc.;

in fact, all legumes which have been looked at to date have been found to contain trypsin inhibitors to varying degrees (Liener and Kakade, 1969). The exact nutritional significance of these inhibitors is not clear since there does not appear to be any clear-cut correlation between the trypsin inhibitor content of various legumes and the beneficial effect which heat has on their nutritional value (Borchers and Ackerson, 1950). The presence of other growth inhibitors, which will be discussed later, no doubt tends to obscure whatever detrimental effect the trypsin inhibitors per se may have on growth.

Factors Affecting the Trypsin Inhibitor Content

Heat Treatment. The extent to which the trypsin inhibitor in legumes is destroyed by heat is a function of the temperature, duration of heating, particle size, and moisture conditions--variables which are closely controlled in the commercial processing of soybean oil meal in order to obtain a product having maximum nutritive value (Liener, 1958). In general, autoclaving in an atmosphere of steam at 15 lb/sq. in. for 15-20 min serves to inactivate almost completely the trypsin inhibitor of soybeans. If the beans are soaked overnight, then steaming at atmospheric pressure serves to inactivate the trypsin inhibitor. The extrusion cooking process developed for producing a full-fat soybean flour for village use in underdeveloped countries yields a product which is free of trypsin inhibitors and is reported to be nutritionally equivalent to good quality toasted soybean flour (Albrecht et al., 1967).

The trypsin inhibitor activity inherently present in soymilk can be effectively eliminated by proper heat treatment of the liquid product or by spray drying (Hackler et al., 1965). It is of significance to note that properly processed soybean milk has a nutritive value which is almost equivalent to that of cow's milk (Shurpalekar et al., 1961).

Germination. Although germination is known to result in improvement in the nutritive value of soybeans and a number of

legumes, this effect appears to be quite unrelated to any changes
in trypsin inhibitor activity of the germinated seeds (Liener and
Kakade, 1969). The reason for the beneficial effect of germination
on the growth-promoting property of legumes remains unknown.

Fermentation. The nutritive value of fermented soybean preparations such as *tempeh* and *natto* has been reported by some investigators to be somewhat enhanced as a result of the fermentation
process (Smith, 1963). These findings are consistent with the observation that there is no pancreatic enlargement in rats fed diets
containing tempeh (Smith et al., 1964), indicating that the trypsin
inhibitor had presumably been destroyed by the heat treatment involved in the preparation of tempeh (the beans are boiled for 30
minutes prior to the fermentation).

Soybean Isolates. More recently considerable attention has
been given to the nutritional properties of soybean isolates and
the textured meat analogues fabricated therefrom. Although the
nutritive quality of these textured food products has been reported
to be essentially equivalent to casein or beef, the protein efficiency of the original protein isolate was very low and could be
improved by heat treatment (Bressani et al., 1967). These results
would indicate the possible presence of residual growth inhibitors
in the protein isolate which were inactivated during the process of
converting the isolate into fiber. A number of these textured products have been examined for antitryptic activity, and, as the data
in Table I show, the soybean isolate and fiber are surprisingly
rich in trypsin inhibitor activity. The levels of antitryptic
activity in the processed meat analogues, however, are quite low
and of questionable significance.

Possible Significance in Animal and Human Nutrition

Not all of the growth-depressing effect of raw soybeans can be
attributed to the trypsin inhibitors (Rackis, 1965). Kakade et al.
(1973) have recently reported the results of studies designed to

TABLE 1

Trypsin Inhibitor Activities of Soybean Flour,
Isolate, Fiber, and Finished Textured Products[a]

Product	Antitrypsin activity	
	TIU/g dry solids[b] x 10^{-3}	% of soyflour
Soyflour (unheated)	86.4	100
Soybean isolate	25.5	30
Soybean fiber	12.3	14
Chicken analog	6.9	8
Ham analog	10.2	12
Beef analog	6.5	7

[a]Liener, unpublished data.

[b]Trypsin inhibitor activity determined by the method of
Kakade et al., 1969. TIU = trypsin inhibitor units as defined in
this reference.

evaluate the extent to which the trypsin inhibitors contribute to
the deleterious effects of unheated soybeans fed to rats. These
workers fed rats crude soybean extracts from which the trypsin inhibitor activity had been selectively removed by binding to Sepharose-bound trypsin. By comparison with groups of rats fed the
original extract as well as the heat-treated extract, it was concluded that approximately 40% of the growth-depressing effect of
the original unheated extract could be accounted for by the trypsin
inhibitors. The growth inhibition which persisted in the absence
of the trypsin inhibitors was attributed to the poor digestibility
of the undenatured protein.

Thus, although there seems to be little doubt that the trypsin
inhibitors play a significant role in the nutrition of experimental
animals such as the rat and chick, their significance with respect
to human nutrition may be called into question. It is important to
note that practically all of the in vitro studies with trypsin inhibitors have involved the use of bovine trypsin because of its
ready commercial availability as a crystalline preparation. More

recently, however, it has been demonstrated (Feeney et al., 1969; Travis and Roberts, 1969) that human trypsin is much less inhibited by the soybean inhibitor and ovomucoid, the egg white trypsin inhibitor, than is bovine trypsin (Figure 1). The inability of ovomucoid to inhibit human trypsin may explain perhaps why this inhibitor has virtually no effect on the nitrogen balance of human subjects (Scudamore et al., 1949). From these various lines of evidence, therefore, one is tempted to conclude that, despite the considerable body of evidence which implicates the trypsin inhibitors as a factor contributing to the poor nutritive value of improperly processed legumes in animals, their relevance to human nutrition remains uncertain.

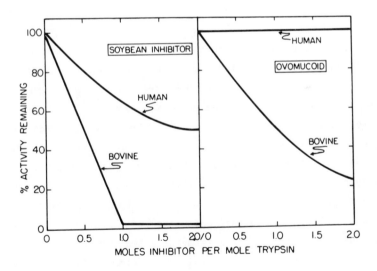

FIG. 1. Effect of soybean trypsin inhibitor and ovomucoid on the activities of human and bovine trypsins. Based on data taken from Coan and Travis, 1971.

PHYTOHEMAGGLUTININS

Another substance which appears to be universally distributed among the legumes is a protein which has the unique property of being able to agglutinate red blood cells, the so-called phyto-hemagglutinins (Lis and Sharon, 1973; Liener, 1974). In 1953 Liener isolated a phytohemagglutinin from soybeans and demonstrated its ability to inhibit growth of rats when added to a diet containing heated soybean meal at a level approximating its occurrence in the raw meal. Growth inhibition was not observed, however, when the food intake of the control diet containing the heated soybean meal was restricted to the food intake of the same diet containing the hemagglutinin. In more recent experiments (Turner and Liener, in 1975) little improvement in growth of rats was observed when the hemagglutinins were selectively removed from crude soybean extracts by adsorption to Sepharose-bound concanavalin A (Table 2). These data would suggest that the hemagglutinins must play a relatively minor role in determining the nutritive properties of soybean pro-tein.

On the other hand, the phytohemagglutinins would appear to be a significant factor contributing to the poor nutritive value of other kinds of beans which enjoy popular consumption in some of the lesser developed countries (Jaffé, 1969). In Table 3 is shown the effect of heat treatment on the nutritive value of a number of legumes which are commonly consumed in various parts of the world. It is apparent from these data that the growth-promoting properties of only the black bean and kidney bean were improved by heat treat-ment. As shown in Table 4, these same two beans were also the only ones which displayed a significant level of hemagglutinating activ-ity. The phytohemagglutinins from these two varieties of *Phaseolus vulgaris* were therefore isolated in pure form and fed at various levels to rats in a basal ration containing 10% casein. From the data presented in Table 5, it is evident that an inhibition of growth was obtained at levels as low as 0.5% of the diet, the kidney bean hemagglutinin being much more effective in this respect than

TABLE 2

Effect of Removing Soybean Hemagglutinin (SBH) on
the Growth-Promoting Activity of Raw Soybean Extracts[a]

Protein component of diet	Hemagglutinating activity units/g protein x 10^{-3}	PER[b]
Original soybean extract	324	0.91
Original soybean extract - SBH[c]	29	1.13
Original soybean extract, heated	6	2.25
Raw soy flour	330	1.01
Heated soy flour	13	2.30

[a]Turner and Liener, 1975.

[b]Protein efficiency ratio = g gain in weight per g protein consumed.

[c]SBH was removed from an aqueous extract of soybeans by passage through a column of Sepharose-bound concanavalin A.

TABLE 3

Effect of Heat on Nutritive Value of Some Legumes[a]

Source of protein	Gain in weight g/day	
	Raw[b]	Heated
Phaseolus vulgaris		
Black bean	-1.94 (4-5)	+1.61
Kidney bean	-1.04 (11-13)	+1.48
Cicer arietinum		
Bengal gram	+1.25	+1.16
Cajanus cajan		
Red gram	+1.33	+1.74
Phaseolus aureus		
Mung bean	+1.05	+1.07

[a]Data taken from Honavar et al., 1962.

[b]100% mortality observed during period (days) shown in ( ).

TABLE 4

Hemagglutinating and Antitryptic Activities

of Crude Extracts[a] of Raw Legumes[b]

Legume	Hemagglutinating activity units/ml	Antitryptic activity units/ml
Phaseolus vulgaris		
Black bean	2450	2050
Kidney bean	3560	1552
Cicer arietinum	0	220
Cajanus cajan	0	418
Phaseolus aureus	0	260

[a]A 10% suspension of the finely ground meal in 1% NaCl clarified by centrifugation.

[b]Data taken from Honavar et al., 1962.

the black bean hemagglutinin. In fact, the kidney bean hemagglutinin at a level of 0.5% caused 100% mortality after about 2 weeks, whereas 1.2% of the black bean hemagglutinin was necessary to produce a similar mortality rate. These data also show that the toxicity of these phytohemagglutinins may be destroyed by moist heat treatment. In the case of the whole bean, it is necessary to soak the beans overnight before autoclaving in order to effect complete destruction of the phytohemagglutinins (Honavar et al., 1962).

Although the toxicity of most phytohemagglutinins can be readily demonstrated by intraperitoneal injection, or, as in the case of the *P. vulgaris* legumes, by oral ingestion, there is some evidence to indicate that the toxic component may not be identical to the component responsible for hemagglutinating activity. Kakade and Evans (1965a, b), for example, have isolated fractions from the navy bean (*P. vulgaris*) which had low hemagglutinating activity but which were more toxic than fractions with higher hemagglutinating activity. Similar results were reported by Stead et al. (1966) with the Natal round yellow bean (*P. vulgaris*). Pertinent to these observations are the reports that ricin, the phytohemagglutinin of

TABLE 5

Effect of Purified Hemagglutinin Fractions
from the Black Bean and Kidney Bean on the Growth of Rats[a]

Source of hemagglutinin	Purified hemagglutinin in diet %	Average gain in weight g/day	Mortality[b] days
Black bean	0.0	+2.51	
	0.5	+1.04	
	0.5[c]	+2.37	
	0.75	+0.20	
	1.2	-0.91	15-17
	2.3	-1.61	12-14
	4.6	-1.72	5-6
Kidney bean	0.0	+2.31	
	0.5	-0.60	14.5
	0.5[c]	+2.29	
	1.0	-0.87	11-12
	1.5	-1.22	4-5

[a]Data taken from Honavar et al., 1962.

[b]100% mortality observed during period recorded here. Blank space indicates that no deaths were observed.

[c]Solution of hemagglutinin boiled for 30 minutes and dried coagulum fed at the level indicated. Hemagglutinating activity was completely destroyed by this treatment.

the castor bean (*Ricinus communis*), may be dissociated into a toxic, nonagglutinating component and a nontoxic, hemagglutinating component (Takahashi et al., 1962; Waldschmidt-Leitz and Keller, 1970). Thus far similar definitive results with the phytohemagglutinins of *P. vulgaris* have not been reported.

One of the complicating factors involved in relating hemagglutinating activity to toxicity is the fact that there are hundreds of different varieties of *P. vulgaris*. The hemagglutinins present in their seeds are known to exhibit not only different degrees of specificity towards blood cells from different species of animals, but the manifestation of activity may also depend on whether the cells have been pretreated with proteolytic enzymes or not. Jaffé and his colleagues (Brücher et al., 1969; Jaffé and Brücher, 1972; Jaffé et al., 1972) have made a systematic study of the hemaggluti-nating activity of a large number of different varieties and culti-vars of *P. vulgaris* with respect to their action on the blood cells from different animals, with and without prior trypsinization, and the toxicity of their extracts when injected into rats. They made the significant observation that only those extracts which aggluti-nated trypsinated cow cells were toxic when injected in rats (Table 6). Feeding tests confirmed the fact that those varieties which displayed agglutinating activity towards trypsinated cow cells were also toxic and inhibited growth when incorporated into the diets of rats, whereas those varieties which were nonagglutinating or agglutinated only rabbit cells were nontoxic (Jaffé and Brücher, 1972; Jaffé and Vega Lette, 1968). These results serve to emphasize the importance of testing the hemagglutinating activity of seed extracts against several species of blood cells before one is justi-fied in concluding that a particular bean is toxic or not. The use of trypsinated cow cells would appear to offer an important tool for detecting beans which are potentially toxic.

Although the toxic effects of the hemagglutinins can be generally eliminated by proper heat treatment (generally the same conditions which inactivate the protease inhibitors), it should be recognized that conditions may sometimes prevail whereby complete destruction of the phytohemagglutinins may not be achieved. For example, Korte (1972) has recently observed that in mixtures of ground beans and ground cereal prepared under the field conditions prevailing in Africa the hemagglutinin was not always destroyed, and the cooked product produced diarrhea and other signs of toxicity. A reduction in the boiling point of water in mountainous regions could also conceivably result in incomplete destruction of the hemagglu-tinins. Occasionally outbreaks of massive poisoning after the con-sumption of partially cooked bean flakes have in fact been reported from time to time (Faschingbauer and Kofler, 1929; Griebel, 1950). The marked resistance of the phytohemagglutinins to inactivation by

TABLE 6

Correlation of Specific Hemagglutinating Activity
with the Intraperitoneal Toxicity in Rats
of Extracts of Different Varieties and Cultivars of *P. vulgaris*[a]

Variety	Rabbit blood	Trypsinated cow blood	Toxicity # injected rats / # dead rats
Balin de Albenga	+	+	5/4
Merida	+	+	9/9
Negro Nicoya	+	+	5/4
Saxa	+	+	5/5
Peruvita	+	-	5/0
Palleritos	+	-	6/0
Juli	+	-	5/0
Cubagua	+	-	5/0
Porillo	-	+	5/5
Negra No. 584	-	+	5/3
Vainica Saavegra	-	+	10/6
Hallado	-	-	5/0
Madrileno	-	-	5/0
Alabaster	-	-	5/0
Triguito	-	-	6/0

[a]Data taken from Jaffé and Brücher, 1972.

dry heat (DeMuelenaere, 1964) should caution against the indiscriminate use of bean flour in foods which have been prepared by dry
heat instead of cooking, such as has been proposed for bread (Anonymous, 1948) and cakes (Marcos and Boctor, 1959).

GOITROGENS

Goitrogenic substances are most commonly found in plants of
the cabbage family which includes such common edible plants as
cabbage, turnip, cauliflower, kale, brussel sprouts, rapeseed,

535

mustard seed, etc. Among the legumes, however, only the soybeans and peanuts have been reported to produce goiterogenic effects in animals (Van Etten, 1969). Unheated soybeans, for example, cause a marked enlargement of the thyroid gland of the rat and chick, an effect which can be counteracted by the administration of iodide or partially eliminated by heat. An example of the therapeutic effectiveness of iodide in overcoming the goiterogenic effect of soymilk is shown in Figure 2. Several workers (Van Wyk et al., 1959; Hydowitz, 1960) have reported a number of cases of goiter in human infants fed soybean milk. Apparently the heat treatment employed for sterilizing these particular soybean preparations was not sufficient to destroy the goiterogenic agent. Iodine supplementation, however, alleviated this goiter condition in human infants (Van Wyk et al., 1959). The goiterogenic principle from soybeans has been recently partially purified and characterized as a low-molecular-weight oligopeptide composed of two or three amino acids or a glycopeptide consisting of one or two amino acids and a sugar (Konijn et al., 1972, 1973).

Rats fed ground nuts also develop enlarged thyroids, but in this instance the goiterogenic principle has been identified as a

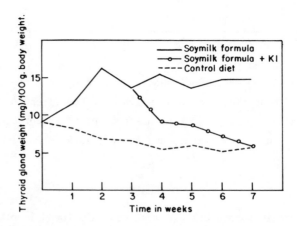

FIG. 2. Effect of a soymilk diet with and without iodine on the thyroid gland of the rat. Taken from Anderson, 1961.

phenolic glycoside which resides in the skin (Sreenivasan et al., 1957). It has been suggested that the phenolic metabolites formed from this glycoside are preferentially iodinated and thereby deprive the thyroid of available iodine. Thus the goiterogenetic effect of ground nuts is effectively counteracted by iodine supplementation but not by heat treatment.

CYANOGENS

It has been known for a long time that a wide variety of plants are potentially toxic because they contain glycosides from which HCN may be released by hydrolysis (Montgomery, 1969). It will be noted in Table 7 that the legumes predominate in terms of their cyanide-producing potential. In the years immediately following the turn of the 20th century and again during World War I lima beans imported into Europe from tropical countries (Java, Puerto Rico, and Burma) were responsible for serious outbreaks of cyanide poisoning, and

TABLE 7

Cyanide Content of Certain Plants[a]

Plant	HCN yield, mg/100 g
Lima bean (*Phaseolus lunatus*)	
Samples incriminated in fatal human poisoning	210.0-312.0
Normal levels	14.4-16.7
Sorghum	250.0
Cassava	113.0
Linseed meal	53.0
Black-eyed pea (*Vigna sinensis*)	2.1
Garden pea (*Pisum sativum*)	2.3
Kidney bean (*Phaseolus vulgaris*)	2.0
Bengal gram (*Cicer arietinum*)	0.8
Red gram (*Cajanus cajans*)	0.5

[a]Data taken from Montgomery, 1969.

cases of human intoxication from the consumption of certain varieties of lima beans are not uncommon today in some of the tropical
countries. Most of the lima beans consumed in the United States
and Europe at the present time are well below the toxic levels
implicated in fatal cases of poisoning.

Cyanide in the form of HCN is released from a glycoside
(*phaseolunatin* in the case of lima beans) through the action of
an enzyme present in the plant tissue (see Figure 3). Hydrolysis
occurs quite rapidly when the ground bean meal is cooked in water,
and most of the liberated HCN is lost by volatilization. Further
cooking also leads to the eventual destruction of the enzyme. Yet
many cases of human intoxication have occurred even with cooked
lima beans. For example, it has been reported (Gabel and Kruger,
1920) that when lima beans which had been cooked so as to destroy
the enzymes responsible for cyanide formation were fed to human
subjects, cyanide could be detected in the urine. This has led to
the supposition that perhaps enzymes secreted in the intestinal
tract, or by the microflora of the colon, may be responsible for
releasing HCN after ingestion of the cooked beans.

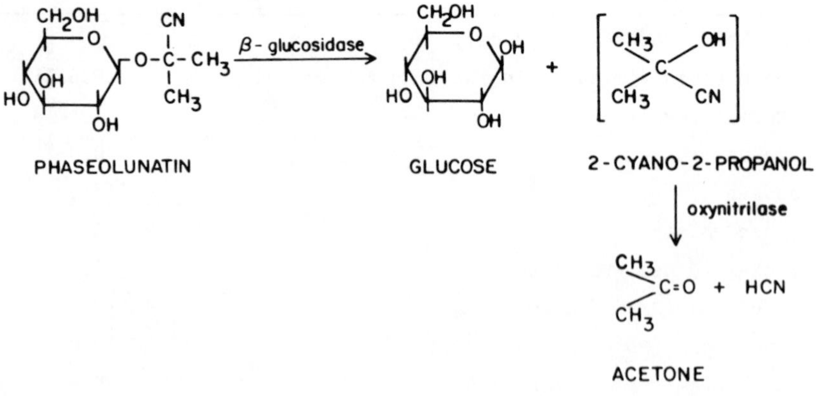

FIG. 3. Enzymatic release of HCN from phaseolunatin, the
cyanogenetic glycoside of lima beans (*Phaseolus lunatus*).

ANTI-NUTRITIONAL FACTORS OF LEGUME PROTEINS

ANTI-VITAMIN FACTORS

The inclusion of unheated soybean meal, or the protein isolated therefrom, in the diet of chicks may cause rickets unless
higher than normal levels of vitamin D_3 are added to the diet
(Carlson et al., 1964). The rachitogenic effect could be eliminated by autoclaving the soybean meal, but supplementation with
calcium or phosphorus was ineffective. Along the same lines, raw
kidney beans are believed to contain an antagonist of vitamin E as
evidenced by liver necrosis in rats and muscular dystrophy and low
levels of plasma tocopherol in chicks (Hintz and Hogue, 1964;
Desai, 1966). The anti-vitamin E effect of raw kidney beans can
be partially eliminated by heat treatment. Neither the identity
of the anti-vitamin D factor of soybeans nor of the anti-vitamin E
factor of kidney beans is known. Edelstein and Guggenheim (1970a,
b) demonstrated that unheated soyflour is deficient in vitamin B_{12}
and contains a heat-labile substance that increases the requirement
for vitamin B_{12}. The identity of this anti-vitamin B_{12} factor
remains to be established.

METAL-BINDING CONSTITUENTS

The inclusion of isolated soybean protein in animal diets has
been noted to lead to a decrease in the availability of certain
trace minerals such as zinc, manganese, copper, and iron (O'dell
and Savage, 1960). In fact, an anemia in monkeys due to a deficiency in iron may be induced in monkeys on a soybean protein diet,
an effect which may be eliminated by heat treatment or chelating
agents such as EDTA (Fitch et al., 1964). Peas (*Pisum sativum*)
have also been shown to contain a factor which interferes with the
availability of zinc for chicks (Kienholz et al., 1962). Autoclaving the peas eliminated the requirement for supplemental zinc.
Since zinc supplementation was only one-third as effective as autoclaving, the presence of an additional heat-labile growth inhibitor
in peas was postulated.

The exact mechanism whereby certain plant proteins exhibit this ability to interfere with the availability of metals is not known, although it may be related to the observation that a soy protein-phytic acid complex has a special affinity for metal ions (O'dell and Savage, 1960).

LATHYROGENS

Lathyrism is a disease associated with the consumption of certain species of peas belonging to the genus *Lathyrus*. This subject has been most recently reviewed by Rao et al. (1969) and Sarma and Padmanaban (1969). This disease is particularly prevalent in India, especially during periods of famine resulting from droughts when the crop fields become blighted and, as an alternate crop, a type of pea referred to as the chickling vetch or *L. sativus* is cultivated. *Vicia sativa* (common vetch) has also been frequently reported to be a common contaminant of *L. sativus* implicated in cases of human lathyrism. Those who eat this plant frequently suffer from an affliction of the central nervous system which causes weakness and paralysis of the leg muscles and death in extreme cases (neuro-lathyrism).

Attempts to identify the causative agent of human lathyrism have been complicated by the fact that another species of *Lathyrus*, namely *L. odoratus* or sweet pea, produces in rats a type of lathyrism (osteolathyrism) which is characterized by skeletal deformities. In contrast to this, rats thrive quite well on *L. sativus* and do not display the nervous disorder associated with the consumption of this species in man. Historically, the lathyrogen of the sweet pea was the first to be isolated and was identified as β-(N-α-glutamyl) aminopropionitrile, although β-aminopropionitrile is equally as active as an osteolathyrogen (Figure 4).

Several groups of workers in India (Adiga et al., 1962; Murti et al., 1964; Rao et al., 1964) have succeeded in isolating from *L. sativus* a compound which may very well be the causative principle of

OSTEOLATHYROGENS

C≡N
|
CH₂
|
CH₂
|
NH₂

β−aminopropionitrile
(BAPN)

Found in
L. odoratus
L. pusillus
L. hirsutus

C≡N
|
CH₂
|
CH₂
|
NH
|
C=O
|
(CH₂)₂
|
CH−NH₂
|
COOH

β−(N−γ−glutamyl)−aminopropionitrile

FIG. 4.   Structures of compounds found in certain species of *Lathyrus* which cause osteolathyrism.

human neurolathyrism.   This compound was identified as β-N-oxalyl-α,β-diaminopropionic acid (Figure 5), and its injection in young chicks, rats, and monkeys produced severe neurotoxic symptoms. Other compounds which have been isolated from other species of *Lathyrus* as well as *Vicia sativa* and which have been shown to produce neurotoxic effects when injected into animals are likewise shown in Figure 5.   Roy (1973) has recently shown that the oral administration of β-N-oxalyl-α,β-diaminopropionic acid to baby chicks can induce neurological symptoms but at a much higher dose than that required by the intraperitoneal route.

NEUROLATHYROGENS

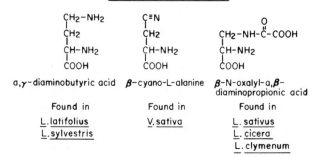

CH₂−NH₂
|
CH₂
|
CH−NH₂
|
COOH

α,γ−diaminobutyric acid

Found in
L. latifolius
L. sylvestris

C≡N
|
CH₂
|
CH−NH₂
|
COOH

β−cyano-L-alanine

Found in
V. sativa

O
‖
CH₂−NH−C−COOH
|
CH−NH₂
|
COOH

β-N-oxalyl-α,β-
diaminopropionic acid

Found in
L. sativus
L. cicera
L. clymenum

FIG. 5.   Structures of compounds found in certain species of *Lathyrus* and *Vicia* which act as neurotoxins.

Assuming that oxalyl-diaminopropionic acid is the causative factor of human lathyrism, it may come as a surprise to learn that all of the misery in the past associated with the consumption of *L. sativus* could have been avoided by a relatively simple detoxification procedure involving steeping the dehusked seeds overnight, followed by steaming for 30 minutes or roasting at 150° for 20 minutes. Amino acid analysis of the protein of *L. sativus* indicates that it is rich in lysine and is therefore potentially useful as a lysine supplement.

The breeding of species and varieties of *Lathyrus* which are genetically deficient in the neurotoxin is also a possibility. In extensive surveys of different species of *Lathyrus* and *Vicia sativa* (common vetch) a number of samples were found to have little or no oxalyl-diaminopropionic acid (Bell, 1964; Jeswani et al., 1970). Unfortunately many of these samples also contained other compounds which could be lathyrogenic, among them the compounds α, γ-diaminobutyric acid and β-cyanoalanine (Figure 5), which are also known to produce neurotoxic effects when injected into animals. It is obvious that any serious breeding program involving *Lathyrus* must take into account the possible role of these compounds as well as the pathogenesis of lathyrism.

FAVISM

Favism is a disease characterized by hemolytic anemia which affects certain individuals following the ingestion of fresh raw or cooked broad beans (*Vicia faba*). The subject of favism has been recently reviewed by Donoso et al. (1969) and Mager et al. (1969). This disease is confined largely to the inhabitants of countries surrounding the Mediterranean basin, although individuals of the same ethnic background residing in other countries frequently suffer from favism. Individual susceptibility to this disease is believed to be of genetic origin, and an attack is frequently precipitated simply by exposure to the pollen of the blossoms of this legume.

ANTI-NUTRITIONAL FACTORS OF LEGUME PROTEINS

One of the difficulties in establishing the pathogenesis of favism is the fact that it has not been possible to reproduce this disease in experimental animals. In fact, the broad bean can serve as a satisfactory source of protein in feedstuffs although it does tend to be somewhat deficient in the S-containing amino acids (Eppendorfer, 1971; Nitsan, 1971).

The red blood cells of individuals who are prone to favism exhibit a number of biochemical abnormalities, the most significant of which are diminished levels of reduced glutathione and glucose-6-phosphate dehydrogenase activity. Reduced levels of both of these factors are believed to destabilize the integrity of the cell membrane and exposure to some component of the broad bean then precipitates the hemolytic crisis.

Present evidence would suggest that the substances responsible for favism are pyrimidines which occur naturally as β-glycosides (Mager et al., 1965). These substances, known as divicine and isouramil, have the structures shown in Figure 6 and are the aglycone moieties of vicine and convicine, respectively. In vitro experiments have demonstrated that divicine and isouramil cause a rapid decrease in the glutathione content of glucose-6-phosphate dehydrogenase deficient red blood cells, an effect which could account for the hemolytic effect exerted by broad beans. Broad beans are also rich in DOPA quinone which has also been shown to catalyze the oxidation of reduced glutathione (Beutler, 1970).

It is a curious fact that divicine was first discovered in the common vetch, Vicia sativa, and the garden pea, Pisum sativum, by Schulze (1891). Divicine is also toxic when injected into experimental animals, and, because of its occurrence in Vicia sativa, was at one time thought to be the causative factor of lathyrism (Anderson et al., 1925). The fact that the occurrence of divicine is not confined to the broad bean makes it difficult to accept the idea that this compound can be responsible for a disease which, to our knowledge, can be produced only by the ingestion of this particular bean.

543

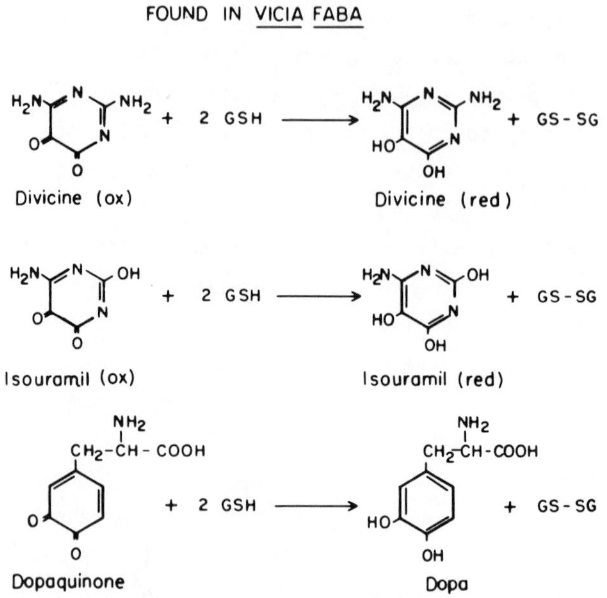

FOUND IN <u>VICIA</u> <u>FABA</u>

FIG. 6. Compounds found in *Vicia faba* which catalyze the oxidation of glutathionine (2GSH→GS-SG). The oxidative destruction of glutathione may be the underlying biochemical event responsible for favism (see text for discussion).

CONCLUSIONS

It should be apparent that, although there are numerous examples of so-called toxic constituents in legumes, they have nevertheless provided man over the centuries with a valuable source of protein. This can be attributed in part to the fact that man has learned how to detoxify them by suitable preparative measures. The varied nature of our diet also minimizes the contribution of a toxicant from any one foodstuff. Nevertheless, there is the ever present possibility that the prolonged consumption of a particular legume which may be improperly processed could bring to the surface toxic effects which would otherwise not be apparent. As the shortage of protein becomes more acute, it is not unlikely that in the future much of the population of the world will be faced with a more limited selection of protein foods, most of which will be of plant origin and hence potential carriers of toxic constituents. The nutritionist, food scientist, and plant breeder should all be at least cognizant of such a possibility and prepared to apply their knowledge and skill to meeting this challenge.

REFERENCES

Adiga, P.R., G. Padmanaban, S.L.N. Rao and P.S. Sarma. 1962. The isolation of a toxic principle from *Lathyrus sativus* seeds. J. Sci. Ind. Res. (India). 21:284.

Albrecht, W.J., G.C. Mustakas, J.E. McGhee and E.L. Griffin. 1967. A simple method for making full-fat soyflour. Cereal Sci. Today. 12:81.

Anderson, D.W. 1961. Problems in the formulation of soymilk. Proc. Conf. Soybean Products for Proteins in Human Foods, Peoria, Illinois. p. 166.

Anderson, L.A.P., A. Howard and J.L. Simonsen. 1925. Studies on lathyrism. Indian J. Med. Res. 12:613.

Anonymous. 1948. Augmenting wheat flour supplies. Chem. Ind. Eng. News. 26:2516.

Bell, E.A. 1964. Relevance of biochemical taxonomy to the problem of lathyrism. Nature. 203:378.

Beutler, E. 1970. L-Dopa and favism. Blood. 34:523.

Booth, A.N., D.J. Robbins, W.E. Ribelin and F. DeEds. 1960. Effect of raw soybean meal and amino acids on pancreatic hypertrophy in rats. Proc. Soc. Exp. Biol. Med. 104:681.

Borchers, R. and C.W. Ackerson. 1950. The nutritive value of legume seeds. X. Effect of autoclaving and the trypsin inhibitor test for 17 species. J. Nutr. 41:339.

Bressani, R., F. Viteri, L.G. Elias, S. DeZaghi, J. Alvarado and A.D. Odell. 1967. Protein quality of a soybean protein textured food in experimental animals and children. J. Nutr. 93:349.

Brücher, O., M. Wecksler, A. Levy, A. Palozza and W.G. Jaffé. 1969. Comparison of phytohemagglutinin in wild beans (*Phaseolus aborigineus*) and in common beans (*Phaseolus vulgaris*) and their inheritance. Phytochemistry. 8:1739.

Carlson, C.W., H.C. Saxena, L.S. Jensen and J. McGinnis. 1964. Rachitogenic activity of soybean fractions. J. Nutr. 82:507.

Coan, M.H. and J. Travis. 1971. Interaction of human pancreatic proteinases with naturally recurring proteinase inhibitors. *In* H. Fritz and H. Tschesche (Eds.) Proc. Int. Res. Conf. Proteinase Inhibitors. Walter de Gruyter, Berlin. p. 294.

DeMuelenaere, H.J.H. 1964. Effect of heat treatment on the hemagglutinating activity of legumes. Nature. 201:1029.

Desai, I.D. 1966. Effect of kidney beans (*Phaseolus vulgaris*) on plasma tocopherol-level and its relation to nutritional muscular dystrophy in the chick. Nature. 209:810.

Donoso, G., H. Hedayat and H. Khayatian. 1969. Favism, with special reference to Iran. WHO Bull. 40:513.

Edelstein, S. and K. Guggenheim. 1970a.Changes in the metabolism of vitamin B_{12} and methionine in rats fed unheated soya-bean flour. Brit. J. Nutr. 24:735.

Edelstein, S. and K. Guggenheim. 1970b.Causes of the increased requirement for vitamin B_{12} in rats subsisting on an unheated soybean flour diet. J. Nutr. 100:1377.

Eppendorfer, W.H. 1971. Effect of S, N, and P on amino acid composition of field beans (*Vicia faba*) and responses of the biological value of seed protein to S-amino acid content. J. Sci. Food Agr. 22:501.

Faschingbauer, H. and L. Kofler. 1929. Uber die Giftwirkung von rohen Bohnen und Bohnenkeimlingen. Wien. Klin. Wochschr. 42:1069.

Feeney, R.E., G.E. Means and J.C. Bigler. 1969. Inhibition of human trypsin, plasmin, and thrombin by naturally occurring inhibitors of proteolytic enzymes. J. Biol. Chem. 244:1957.

Fitch, C.D. W.E. Harville, J.S. Dinning and F.S. Porter. 1964. Iron deficiency in monkeys fed diets containing soybean protein. Proc. Soc. Exp. Biol. Med. 116:130.

Gabel, W. and W. Kruger. 1920. The toxic action of Rangoon beans. Muensch Med. Wochschr. 67:214.

Green, G.M. and R.L. Lyman. 1972. Feedback regulation of pancreatic enzyme secretion as a mechanism for trypsin inhibitor-induced hypersecretion in rats. Proc. Soc. Exp. Biol. Med. 140:6.

Griebel, C. 1950. Erkrankungen durch Bohnenflochen (*Phaseolus vulgaris* L.) and Platterbsen (*Lathyrus tingitanus* L.). Z. Lebensm. Unters. Forsch. 90:191.

Hackler, L.R., J.B. Van Buren, K.H. Steinkraus, I. El Rawi and D.B. Hand. 1965. Effect of heat treatment on nutritive value of soymilk protein fed to weanling rats. J. Food Sci. 30:723.

Hintz, H.F. and D.E. Hogue. 1964. Kidney beans (*Phaseolus vulgaris*) and the effectiveness of vitamin E for prevention of nutritional muscular dystrophy in the chick. J. Nutr. 84:283.

Honavar, P.M., C.V. Shih and I.E. Liener. 1962. The inhibition of the growth of rats by purified hemagglutinin isolated from *Phaseolus vulgaris*. J. Nutr. 77:109.

Hydowitz, J.D. 1960. Occurrence of goiter in an infant on soy diet. New England J. Med. 262:351.

Jaffé, W.G. 1969. Hemagglutinins. *In* I.E. Liener (Ed.) Toxic Constituents of Plant Foodstuffs. Academic Press, New York. p. 69.

Jaffé, W.G. and O. Brücher. 1972. Toxicity and specificity of different phytohemagglutinins of beans (*Phaseolus vulgaris*). Arch. Latimamer. Nutr. 22:267.

Jaffé, W.G., O. Brücher and A. Palozza. 1972. Detection of four types of specific phytohemagglutinins in different lines of beans (*Phaseolus vulgaris*). Z. Immun. Forsch. 142:439.

Jaffé, W.G. and C.L. Vega Lette. 1968. Heat-labile growth-inhibiting factors in beans (*Phaseolus vulgaris*). J. Nutr. 94:203.

Jeswani, L.M., B.M. Lal and S. Prakash. 1970. Studies on the development of low neurotoxin (β-N-oxalyl-α,β-diaminopropionic acid) lines in *Lathyrus sativus* (Khesari). Current Sci. 39:518.

Kakade, M.L., D.E. Hoffa and I.E. Liener. 1973. Contribution of trypsin inhibitors to the deleterious effects of unheated soybeans fed to rats. J. Nutr. 103:1772.

Kakade, M.L. and R.J. Evans. 1965a.Growth inhibition of rats fed navy bean fractions. J. Agr. Food Chem. 13:450.

Kakade, M.L. and R.J. Evans. 1965b.Nutritive value of navy beans (*Phaseolus vulgaris*). Brit. J. Nutr. 19:269.

Kakade, M.L., N. Simons and I.E. Liener. 1969. An evaluation of natural vs. synthetic substrates for measuring the antitryptic activity of soybean samples. Cereal Chem. 46:518.

Kienholz, E.W., L.S. Jensen and J. McGinnis. 1962. Evidence for chick growth inhibitors in several legume seeds. Poultry Sci. 41:367.

Konijn, A.M., S. Edelstein and K. Guggenheim. 1972. Separation of a thyroid-active fraction from unheated soya bean flour. J. Sci. Food Agr. 23:549.

Konijn, A.M., B. Gershon and K. Guggenheim. 1973. Further purification and mode of action of a goitrogenic material from soybean flour. J. Nutr. 103:378.

Korte, R. 1972. Heat resistance of phytohemagglutinins in weaning food mixtures containing beans (*Phaseolus vulgaris*). Ecology Food Nutr. 1:303.

Kunitz, M. 1945. Crystallization of a trypsin inhibitor from soybeans. Science. 101:668.

Liener, I.E. 1953. Soyin, a toxic protein from the soybean. I. Inhibition of rat growth. J. Nutr. 49:527.

Liener, I.E. 1958. Effect of heat on plant proteins. *In* A.M. Altschul (Ed.) Processed Protein Foodstuffs. Academic Press, New York. p. 79.

Liener, I.E. 1972. Nutritional value of food protein products. *In* A.K. Smith and S.J. Circle (Eds.) Soybeans: Chemistry and Technology. Avi Publishing Co., Westport, Connecticut. p. 203.

Liener, I.E. 1973. Toxic factors associated with legume proteins. Indian J. Nutr. Diet. 10:303.

Liener, I.E. 1974. Phytohemagglutinins: their nutritional significance. J. Agr. Food Chem. 22:17.

Liener, I.E., H.J. Deuel Jr. and H.L. Fevold. 1949. The effect of supplemental methionine on the nutritive value of diets containing concentrates of the soybean trypsin inhibitor. J. Nutr. 39:325.

Liener, I.E. and M.L. Kakade. 1969. Protease inhibitors. *In* I.E. Liener (Ed.) Toxic Constituents of Plant Foodstuffs. Academic Press, New York. p. 7.

Lis, H. and N. Sharon. 1973. The biochemistry of plant lectins. Ann. Rev. Biochem. 42:541.

Mager, J., G. Glaser, A. Razin, G. Izak, S. Bien and M. Noam. 1965. Metabolic effects of pyrimidines derived from fava bean glycosides on human erythrocyte deficient in glucose-6-phosphate dehydrogenase. Biochem. Biophys. Res. Commun. 20:235.

Mager, J., A. Razin and A. Hershko. 1969. Favism. *In* I.E. Liener (Ed.) Toxic Constituents of Plant Foodstuffs. Academic Press, New York. p. 293.

Marcos, S.R. and A.M. Boctor. 1959. The use of *Dolichos lablab* and *Lathyrus sativus* in the making of taamiah (bean cakes) in Egypt. Brit. J. Nutr. 13:163.

Montgomery, R.D. 1969. Cyanogens. *In* I.E. Liener (Ed.) Toxic Constituents of Plant Foodstuffs. Academic Press, New York. p. 143.

Murti, V.V.S., T.R. Seshadri and T.A. Venkitasubramanian. 1964. Neurotoxic compounds of the seeds of *Lathyrus sativus*. Phytochemistry. 3:73.

Nesheim, M.C., J.D. Garlich and D.T. Hopkins. 1962. Studies on the effect of raw soybean meal on fat absorption in young chicks. J. Nutr. 78:89.

Niess, E., C.A. Ivy and M.C. Nesheim. 1972. Stimulation of gallbladder emptying and pancreatic secretion in chicks by soybean whey protein. Proc. Soc. Exp. Biol. Med. 140:291.

Nitsan, Z. 1971. *Vicia faba* beans vs. soyabean meal as a source of protein. J. Sci. Food Agr. 22:252.

ANTI-NUTRITIONAL FACTORS OF LEGUME PROTEINS

O'dell, B.L. and J.E. Savage. 1960. Effect of phytic acid on zinc availability. Proc. Soc. Exp. Biol. Med. 103:304.

Osborne, T.B. and L.B. Mendel. 1917. The use of soybean as food. J. Biol. Chem. 32:369.

Rackis, J.J. 1965. Physiological properties of soybean trypsin inhibitors and their relationship to pancreatic hypertrophy and growth inhibition of rats. Fed. Proc. 24:1488.

Rackis, J.J. 1974. Biological and physiological factors in soybeans. J. Amer. Oil Chem. Soc. 51:161A.

Rao, S.L.N., P.R. Adiga and P.S. Sarma. 1964. The isolation and characterization of β-N-oxalyl-α,β-diaminopropionic acid: a neurotoxic from the seeds of Lathyrus sativus. Biochem. 3:432.

Rao, S.L.N., K. Malathi and P.S. Sarma. 1969. Lathyrism. World Rev. Nutr. Diet. 10:214.

Roberts, L.M. 1970. The food legumes--recommendations for expansion and acceleration of research. The Rockefeller Foundation, New York.

Roy, D.N. 1973. Effect of oral administration of β-N-oxalyl-amino-L-alanine (BOAA) with or without Lathyrus sativus trypsin inhibitor (L-SI) in chicks. Environ. Physiol. Chem. 3:192.

Sarma, P.S. and G. Padmanaban. 1969. Lathyrogens. In I.E. Liener (Ed.) Toxic Constituents of Plant Foodstuffs. Academic Press, New York. p. 267.

Schulze, E. 1891. Basic nitrogen-containing compounds from the seeds of Vicia sativa and Pisum sativum. Z. Physiol. Chem. 15:140.

Scudamore, H.H., G.R. Macy, C.F. Consolazio, G.H. Berryman, L.E. Gordon, H.D. Lightbody and H.L. Fevold. 1949. Nitrogen balance on men consuming raw or heated egg white as a supplemental source of dietary protein. J. Nutr. 39:555.

Shurpalekar, S.R., M.R. Chandrasekhara, M. Swaminathan and V. Subrahmanyan. 1961. Chemical composition and nutritive value of soyabean and soybean products. Food Sci. (Mysore). 11:52.

Smith, A.K. 1963. Foreign uses of soybean protein foods. Cereal Sci. Today. 8:196.

Smith, A.K., J.J. Rackis, C.W. Hesseltine, M. Smith, D.J. Robbins and A.N. Booth. 1964. Tempeh: nutritive value in relation to processing. Cereal Chem. 41:173.

Sreenivasan, V., N.R. Moudgal and P.S. Sarma. 1957. Goitrogenic agents in food. I. Goitrogenic actions of ground nut. J. Nutr. 61:87.

Stead, R.H., H.J.H. DeMuelenaere and G.V. Quicke. 1966. Trypsin inhibition, hemagglutination, and intraperitoneal toxicity in extracts of Phaseolus vulgaris and Glycine max. Arch. Biochem. Biophys. 113:703.

Takahashi, T., G. Funatsu and M. Funatsu. 1962. Biochemical studies on castor bean hemagglutinin. I. Separation and purification. J. Biochem. (Tokyo). 51:288.

Travis, J. and R.C. Roberts. 1969. Human trypsin. Isolation and physical-chemical characterization. Biochemistry. 8:2884.

Turner, R.H. and I.E. Liener. The effect of the selective removal of hemagglutinins on the nutritive value of soybeans. J. Agr. Food Chem. 23:484 (1975).

Van Etten, C.H. 1969. Goitrogens. In I.E. Liener (Ed.) Toxic Constituents of Plant Foodstuffs. Academic Press, New York. p. 103.

Van Wyk, J.J., M.B. Arnold, J. Wynn and F. Pepper. 1959. The effects of a soybean product on thyroid function in humans. Pediatrics. 24:752.

Waldschmidt-Leitz, E. and L. Keller. 1970. Seed proteins. XXII. Toxin and agglutinin from *Ricinus*: purification and composition. Hoppe-Seyler's Z. Physiol. Chem. 351:990.

23

PROBLEMS IN THE DIGESTIBILITY OF DRY BEANS

Alfred C. Olson, Robert Becker, Jackson C. Miers,
Michael R. Gumbmann, and Joseph R. Wagner

Western Regional Research Laboratory
Agricultural Research Service
U. S. Department of Agriculture
Berkeley, California

Dry beans may cause gastrointestinal distress when eaten by humans. A reduction in flatulence would make beans more acceptable as a source of nutritious inexpensive plant protein. We are trying to reduce flatulence by finding out what causes it. This paper presents data which show at least two classes of material in dry beans may cause flatulence. They are the sugars raffinose and stachyose and sugar-free bean residue. A stimulating effect of these components fed together was also demonstrated.

INTRODUCTION

Dry beans contain from 20 to 25% protein on the average and are a very important source of protein to large numbers of the world's peoples (see H. K. Burr, this volume). However, in addition to being deficient in the essential amino acid methionine and containing certain toxic substances, dry beans also produce gastrointestinal distress which may include diarrhea and flatulence when eaten by humans. The first two problems can be solved by supplementing a bean diet with methionine or methionine-rich protein and

by cooking since the toxic substances are heat labile. The
flatulence problem is more difficult to define and identify and
so far has not been solved. Increased consumption generated in
part by interest in using beans as a good source of inexpensive
protein in processed foods for new markets has caused several
research groups to look more closely into what causes flatulence
from dry beans and how it might be removed or reduced.

Blair et al. (1947) were among the first authors to quantitate
the production of flatus in man and to show that soybeans increased
gas production and its carbon dioxide content. At the present time
it is generally recognized that bacterial fermentation of food
residues remaining after digestion and assimilation of available
nutrients is the source of intestinal gases causing gastrointestinal
distress. The identity of all the substances fermented, however, is
not complete. Steggerda (1968) suggested that the α-galactosides,
raffinose and stachyose, were principle sources of gastrointestinal
gases from soybeans ingested by either man or dog. The involvement
of this family of sugars in the flatulence problem has been reviewed
by Cristofaro et al. (1974) and Rackis (1975). These carbohydrates
are not digested because mammalian intestinal mucosa lacks α-galactosidase activity and the α-galactosides themselves are not absorbed
into the blood. Bacteria in the lower intestinal tract then metabolize them to form methane, hydrogen, and carbon dioxide and to lower
the pH.

The techniques used for studying flatulence are discussed by
Cristofaro et al. (1974) and Rackis (1975). The methods include
studies with intestinal microflora, animals (principally rats and
dogs), and humans. The complexity of the methods and the variability
of results have left the conclusions of many experiments in this
field in conflict and open to differing interpretation. Results in
this paper are based on a routine bioassay developed by Gumbmann and
Williams (1971). The method uses a life-support system in which a
rat is fed a test diet, and any hydrogen evolved from bacterial fermentation in the intestine is quantitatively trapped for a period of

approximately 16 hours and determined by gas chromatography. In this system the amount of hydrogen evolved by rats increases with increasing consumption of cooked beans.

The α-galactoside content of California Small White beans (CSW) can be reduced by endogenous α-galactosidase by incubating the beans at 45-65°C at pH 5.2 for 24-48 hours (Becker et al., 1974). The decrease in α-galactosides observed in these experiments correlates with an observable decrease in rat hydrogen production by the Gumbmann procedure. Becker et al. (1974) concluded, however, that other unidentified bean components were also contributing to rat hydrogen production.

This paper presents data which extend the involvement of pure α-galactosides in rat hydrogen production and includes evidence of a stimulating effect of stachyose combined with cooked bean solids which have been extracted with 70% ethanol to remove this sugar. Bean fractions that have been freed of α-galactosides by extraction have also been shown to contribute to hydrogen production in the rat.

EXPERIMENTAL

Autolysis Experiments

California Small White (CSW), mung, and soy beans were obtained from local suppliers. Other beans from a collection of named cultivars and advanced breeding lines were obtained from Dr. D. W. Burke, USDA, Irrigated Agriculture Research and Extension Center, Prosser, Washington. Sugar analyses and autolysis experiments were based on work described by Becker et al. (1974). Five-gram portions of beans ground through 20 mesh were shaken with 50 ml of 0.10 M sodium acetate buffer pH 5.2 for 2 hours at 25°. Ten ml of the slurries were removed, centrifuged, and aliquots of the supernatants lyophilized for analysis of endogenous α-galactosides. The remaining slurries were incubated at 45° with shaking for 48 hours, optimum conditions for autolysis. Aliquots were removed at 24 and 48 hours for analysis of remaining α-galactosides. Sugars were determined on dried aliquots of these supernatants by gas liquid chromatography of their trimethylsilyl derivatives as described by Becker et al. (1974).

Effect of Stachyose on Hydrogen Production by Rats

Whole cooked beans were prepared by soaking CSW beans in 4 times their weight of distilled water for 16 hours at 25°. They were cooked in the same water for one hour with stirring, lyophilized, and ground to pass a 10-mesh screen. An oligosaccharide-free bean residue was prepared from cooked whole bean powder by first defatting with hexane. The air dried defatted meal was then extracted 3 times with 70% ethanol (v/v) for 30 minutes at 70-75°. The mixture was filtered hot through cheesecloth; the filtrate was concentrated in vacuo and both the concentrated filtrate and residue were lyophilized. The 70% alcohol extractable material corresponded to 17.6% and the residue to 80% of the original dry bean solids. An aqueous extract of a portion of the residue was found to be free of sucrose, raffinose, and stachyose by the gas liquid chromatography procedures. Stachyose was obtained form Sigma Chemical Company and its purity verified by the same procedures.

The life-support system of Gumbmann and Williams (1971) was used to determine hydrogen produced over a 16-hour period by rats fed test diets. Feedings consisted of 10-g diet per rat. Test substances were incorporated into a purified basal diet at the expense of the basal diet. Each sample was fed 10-14 times, and differences among means were evaluated by Duncan's multiple range test.

Bean Fractionation Experiments

Uncooked beans ground through 20 mesh were extracted 3 times with 70% ethanol (1:8, w/v) at room temperature. The combined extracts were concentrated under vacuum and both the concentrated extract and the residue were lyophilized. A portion of the residue was extracted 3 times with 0.6 M sodium chloride (1:8, w/v). The combined sodium chloride extracts and the residue suspended in water

were dialyzed against distilled water until the dialysate was free
of chloride ion and then lyophilized. An acid extract of the 70%
ethanol extracted bean residue was also prepared from a slurry of
the residue in water (1:8, w/v) and acidified to pH 2.0 with concentrated hydrochloric acid. The extraction was repeated once with
water acidified to pH 2.0 and once with water with no pH adjustment.
The combined acid extract and the residue resuspended in water were
neutralized to pH 6 with 12 N sodium hydroxide and lyophilized.
Since they were not dialyzed the extract and residue from this extraction contained small amounts of sodium chloride. Kjeldahl
nitrogen values were obtained on beans and bean fractions. In this
series all beans and bean fractions were cooked one hour in distilled
water prior to testing for rat hydrogen production.

RESULTS AND DISCUSSION

Autolysis Experiments

Humans cannot effectively absorb raffinose, stachyose, or
verbascose directly into the blood stream and do not possess the
α-galactosidase necessary to break these sugars down into galactose
and sucrose which are ultimately absorbed and nutritionally utilized
(Taeufel et al., 1965, 1967). As a result these sugars pass into
the lumen of the intestine where they are microbiologically metabo-
lized. One way the contribution of α-galactosides to the problem
of flatulence might be solved would be to enzymatically degrade the
sugars before ingestion with either an exogenous or endogenous source
of α-galactosidase. Enzymatic processes using exogenous microbial
sources of α-galactosidases to hydrolyze α-galactosides have been
developed by several groups (Sugimoto and Van Buren, 1970; Rohm and
Haas Company, 1972; Delente et al., 1974; etc.), but so far they
have not been entirely successful either in hydrolysis efficiency,
final product acceptability, cost, and/or effectiveness in reducing
flatulence. Reynolds (1974) developed an immobilized α-galactosidase
continuous flow reactor which could be applied to water extracts of
beans containing the α-galactosides.

Another approach to removing α-galactosides before ingestion is to use bean α-galactosidase. On germination the sugars disappear in 3-4 days and several processes have been described utilizing this fact (Okumura and Wilkinson, 1968; Kim et al., 1973). A partial separation and characterization of α-galactosidase from dormant, sprouted, and high temperature incubated beans has been completed by Kon and Wagner (1975). A somewhat different approach optimizes the conditions for the endogenous α-galactosidase to hydrolyze α-galacto-sides in CSW bean (Kon et al., 1973; Becker et al., 1974; Wagner et al., 1975a). The data in Table 1 extend these reports to some other bean varieties. The method used to determine endogenous raffinose and stachyose gives results consistent with other reported values for these sugars in dry beans. There is some slight variation in samples from different lots of beans as noted in the first three entries for CSW beans, but the sugar content of all of these beans falls within a fairly narrow range. All the beans examined to date have demonstrated α-galactosidase activity under autolysis conditions to all three substrates, raffinose, stachyose, and verbascose (the latter only found in mung beans in the beans examined). That the disappearance is the result of enzymatic degradation is confirmed by the concomitant increase in galactose and sucrose with the dis-appearance of raffinose and stachyose during autolysis and by the failure of the α-galactosides to disappear during incubation of previously boiled preparations (Becker et al., 1974).

Residual amounts of raffinose and stachyose were found in practically every case after 48 hours autolysis. This is not due to enzyme inactivation since addition of raffinose after 120 hours of autolysis followed by continued autolysis resulted in essentially the same rate of disappearance of raffinose as originally observed (Becker et al., 1974). The soy sample exhibited the most rapid and complete α-galactosidase activity with raffinose content dropping in 48 hours to zero and stachyose to 0.2% from the initial 3.8% found in the beans. This may indicate a significant difference in this enzyme activity between *Phaseolus vulgaris* and *Glycine max.* which

TABLE 1

Autolysis of α-Galactosides in Some Dry Beans

Common name	Code	Scientific name	Raffinose			Stachyose		
			0 hr	24 hr	48 hr	0 hr	24 hr	48 hr
			% dry basis					
California Small White	1968 crop	*Phaseolus vulgaris*	0.3	0.1	0.1	3.1	1.3	0.7
California Small White	1972 crop	*Phaseolus vulgaris*	0.3	0.1	0.1	3.2	1.2	0.7
California Small White	1973 crop	*Phaseolus vulgaris*	0.4	0.2	0.1	3.4	1.4	0.7
Sanilac	UN-1	*Phaseolus vulgaris*	0.4	0.1	0.1	2.6	1.1	0.6
Great Northern	UN-33	*Phaseolus vulgaris*	0.3	0.2	0.1	2.3	1.3	0.8
Black Turtle Soup	UN-44	*Phaseolus vulgaris*	0.3	0.2	0.06	2.4	1.1	0.5
Red Mexican	UN-53	*Phaseolus vulgaris*	0.4	0.3	a	3.3	2.0	a
Sutter Pink	UN-134	*Phaseolus vulgaris*	0.2	0.1	a	3.2	1.3	a
Royal Red Kidney		*Phaseolus vulgaris*	0.2	0.1	0.1	3.1	1.3	1.1
Jacobs Cattle		*Phaseolus vulgaris*	0.2	0.2	0.1	3.5	1.9	1.7
Soy, Yellow Lee		*Glycine max.*	0.5	0.2	0.0	3.8	1.9	0.2
Mung[b]		*Phaseolus aureus*	0.3	0.1	0.05	2.1	1.0	0.9

[a] Not determined.

[b] Verbascose in mung beans initially 2.1%, 24 hours autolysis 1.5%, 48 hours autolysis 0.8%.

could account for differences in the extent of disappearance of
these sugars when these different beans are subjected to various
processing conditions. It may be easier to get rid of α-galactosides
in *Glycine max*. than in *Phaseolus vulgaris* varieties using the bean's
own enzyme. With CSW beans the autolytic reduction in raffinose and
stachyose was found to correlate with a reduction in hydrogen produced by rats (Becker et al., 1974). However, hydrogen production
never dropped below 40-50% of that for non-autolyzed beans. While
this may be due in part to the α-galactosides remaining, the magnitude of the activity remaining suggests other factors are responsible.
It is recognized that other enzymatic changes are occurring during
these autolysis experiments, including the hydrolysis of phytic acid
to inositol and inorganic phosphate (Becker et al., 1974; Schwimmer,
this volume). Phytic acid is not readily digested by humans and is
an excellent metal binder. There is no evidence that it is involved
in the flatulence problem, but because of its potential physiological
activity it could play some role in combination with other as yet
unknown factors, e.g., intestinal microbial activity.

Effect of Stachyose on Hydrogen Production by Rats

When stachyose is added to the basal diet in the range 3-6% in
the hydrogen assay the rats produce hydrogen proportional to the
amount of stachyose fed (Table 2). In the same test series 20, 40,
and 60% CSW beans added to the diet produced 3.9 ± 0.8, 6.6 ± 0.8,
and 15.2 ± 1.1 ml of hydrogen, respectively. Since these amounts of
beans would only amount to approximately 0.6, 1.2, and 1.8% stachyose
in the rat diets (assuming a 3.2% value for stachyose in CSW beans
and neglecting the contribution of 0.4% raffinose), it must be concluded that other factors in the beans are also contributing to rat
hydrogen production. Bean residue prepared by defatting and extracting cooked beans with aqueous ethanol produces about half the
rat hydrogen the cooked whole beans produce at the 40% level (3.7
versus 6.6 ml). However, when stachyose and this bean residue are
fed together, the resulting rat hydrogen produced is not the sum of

PROBLEMS IN THE DIGESTIBILITY OF DRY BEANS

TABLE 2

Rat Hydrogen Production from Stachyose and the
Stimulating Effect of an Oligosaccharide-free Bean Residue

% Stachyose	ml H_2 ± S.E.[a]		Calculated hydrogen production[b]	Stimulating effect
	0% Bean residue	40% Bean residue		
0	0.6 ± 0.1	3.7 ± 0.6	--	--
3.3	4.1 ± 1.1	16.5 ± 1.5	7.8	2.1
6.7	10.2 ± 2.3	25.8 ± 2.1	13.9	1.9

[a]Mean hydrogen production from feeding 10-g diet, repeated 11
or 12 times. Diet composed of designated percentages of stachyose
and bean residue with the remainder casein basal diet.

[b]Sum of (40% bean residue, 0% stachyose) and (stachyose with
0% bean residue).

the contributions of the individual test substances but twice the
sum (Table 2), showing a decided stimulating effect of these
materials to elicit hydrogen production by rats. Essentially the
same results were observed when raffinose was used in a similar set
of experiments although without bean residue stachyose produced more
hydrogen than did raffinose (Wagner et al., 1975b).

Bean Fractionation Experiments

From the foregoing it is clear that the α-galactosides in dry
beans contribute to rat hydrogen production and that there are other
factors particularly in oligosaccharide-free bean residue that also
contribute. Many attempts have been made to separate flatulence
factor(s) out of dry beans and identify them. Since it is not known
exactly what is being looked for, many questions arise as to how to
carry out such a fractionation. For example, cooked material represents what is causing the problem but may be difficult to separate
into components (e.g., consider what has happened to starch and
protein in cooking). Separating uncooked bean material into relatively identifiable components may be easier but if a flatulence

factor(s) is formed during cooking of the whole bean then it will
not easily be found in this way. Keeping these ideas in mind we
have tried fractionation schemes beginning with both cooked (e.g.,
use of extracted cooked bean residue in the rat hydrogen stimulation
experiments described previously) and uncooked beans. In this series
we elected to fractionate uncooked beans, cook the fractions, and
test them for rat hydrogen production. Ground CSW beans were first
extracted with 70% ethanol. This removed all the simple sugars
including the α-galactosides as well as other low molecular substances soluble in this solvent. The fraction contained about 8%
of the nitrogen of the bean which was considered to be principally
non-protein nitrogen. The residue from this extraction was extracted
in two different ways to remove a protein-rich fraction. The first
way used 0.6 N sodium chloride and the second used a pH 2.0 acid
extraction. Both methods removed about 40% of the bean's original
protein (20% of the bean dry weight) into fractions that were 69%
and 48% protein, respectively, based on Kjeldahl nitrogen analysis.
The residues from these extractions contained 60% of the bean's
original protein.

Hydrogen is produced by rats at a significantly higher level
from all of these cooked bean fractions than from the no bean control as shown by the data in Table 3. The fractions were fed at the
level at which they are present in 50% of whole beans. The two
separate confirming alcohol extractions (entries 3 and 6 in Table 3)
contained all the raffinose and stachyose in the beans which were
then being fed at about 1.8% of the diet. From the data in Table 2
for pure stachyose alone this comes close to accounting for all of
the rat hydrogen that might be expected from this sugar-rich fraction.
Both extracted protein fractions (entries 4 and 7) produced hydrogen
just significantly above the base of 1.0 ml while both residues
(entries 5 and 8) produced considerably more hydrogen. The residue
from the acid extraction produced significantly more hydrogen than
that from the salt extraction.

The sum of the hydrogen produced by the several fractions
corrected for hydrogen from the basal diet is roughly 50 and 80% of

TABLE 3

Rat Hydrogen Production from Bean Fractions

Bean fraction in diet	% fed in diet[a]	ml H_2 ± S.E.[b]
1. Zero (100% basal diet, no beans or bean fractions)	--	1.0 ± 0.1 [g]
2. Whole beans (not fractionated)	50	11.8 ± 1.1 [c]
3. 70% alcohol extract (sugars)	6.64	3.3 ± 0.5 [e]
4. Aqueous NaCl extract (protein-rich fraction)	5.92	1.7 ± 0.2 [f]
5. Residue from #4	33.22	3.7 ± 0.5 [e]
6. 70% alcohol extract (sugars)	6.20	3.3 ± 0.5 [e]
7. Aqueous acid extract (protein-rich fraction)	8.35	2.0 ± 0.2 [f]
8. Residue from #7	37.01	6.3 ± 0.8 [d]

[a]Based on 10-g diets repeated 14 or 15 times; diets composed of 50% beans or the amount of the particular fraction in 50% beans with the remainder casein basal diet.

[b]Means without a common superscript letter are significantly different, $P < 0.05$, N = 14 or 15.

that for whole beans (for the whole beans extracted with sodium chloride and with acid). Failure of the rats to produce the expected amount of hydrogen may be the result of feeding the components separately.

Although the fractionation schemes were different, it is worth noting that extracted cooked bean residue (Table 2) and extracted and then cooked bean residue (Table 3) all produced hydrogen significantly above the basal values and that all the residues were free of the α-galactosides, raffinose and stachyose.

CONCLUSIONS

Our work as well as that of previous investigators shows that dry beans contain α-galactosides and an α-galactosidase that can be utilized to hydrolyze them to galactose and sucrose. From previous work it is also clear that these α-galactosides are involved in flatulence caused by the consumption of legume seeds. They also produce hydrogen when ingested by the rat as does α-galactoside-free bean residue and protein-rich fractions. A stimulating effect, which may be a synergistic effect, can also be demonstrated when the rats are fed stachyose and an α-galactoside-free bean residue. More experiments of this kind are clearly called for in order to try to determine exactly which factors are contributing to flatulence and whether they are acting synergistically. It would of course be necessary to confirm the results in humans. An understanding of the problem of flatulence, even if only partial, could aid the breeder, grower, and processor in efforts to ameliorate the problem and ultimately benefit the consumer of dry beans and lead to wider use and utilization of an inexpensive source of plant protein.

NOTE

Reference to a company and/or product named by the Department of Agriculture is only for purposes of information and does not imply approval or recommendation of the product to the exclusion of others which may also be suitable.

REFERENCES

Becker, R., A.C. Olson, Doris P. Frederick, S. Kon, M.R. Gumbmann and J.R. Wagner. 1974. Conditions for the autolysis of alpha-galactosides and phytic acid in California Small White beans. J. Food Sci. 39:766.

Blair, H.A., R.J. Dern and P.L. Bates. 1947. The measurement of volume of gas in the digestive tract. Amer. J. Physiol. 149:688.

Cristofaro, E., F. Mottu and J.J. Wuhrmann. 1974. Involvement of the raffinose family of oligosaccharides in flatulence. In H. Sipple and K. McNutt (Eds.) Sugars in Nutrition. Academic Press, New York. Chapter 20, p. 313.

Delente, J., J.H. Johnson, M.J. Kuo, R.J. O'Connor and L.E. Weeks. 1974. Production of a new thermostable neutral α-galactosidase from a strain of *Bacillus stearothermophilus*. Biotechnol. Bioeng. 16:1227.

PROBLEMS IN THE DIGESTIBILITY OF DRY BEANS

Duncan, D.B. 1955. Multiple range and multiple F tests. Biometrics 11:1.

Gumbmann, M.R. and S.N. Williams. 1971. The quantitative collection and determination of hydrogen gas from the rat and factors affecting its production. Proc. Soc. Exp. Biol. and Med. 137: 4:1171.

Kim, W.J., C.J.B. Smit and T.O.M. Nakayama. 1973. The removal of oligosaccharides from soybeans. Food Sci. & Technol. 6(6):201.

Kon, S., A.C. Olson, D.P. Frederick, S.B. Eggling and J.R. Wagner. 1973. Effect of different treatment on phytate and soluble sugars in California Small White beans (Phaseolus vulgaris). J. Food Sci. 38:215.

Kon, S. and J.R. Wagner. 1975. Partial separation and characterization of α-galactosidase from Phaseolus vulgaris. J. Food Sci. (Submitted for publication).

Okumura, G.K. and J.E. Wilkinson. 1968. Process of producing soy milk from sprouted soybeans. U.S. Patent 3,399,997.

Rackis, J.J. 1975. Oligosaccharides of food legumes: alpha-galactosidase activity and the flatus problem. In Physiological Effects of Carbohydrates. A. Jeanes and J. Hodge, (Eds.) Am. Chem. Society, Washington, D.C.

Reynolds, J.H. 1974. An immobilized α-galactosidase continuous flow reactor. Biotechnol. Bioeng. 16:135.

Rohm and Haas Company. 1972. Process for rendering innocuous flatulence-producing saccharides. U.S. Patent 3,632,346.

Steggerda, F.R. 1968. Gastrointestinal gas following food consumption. Ann. New York Acad. Sci. 150, Art. 1:57.

Sugimoto, H. and G.P. Van Buren. 1970. Removal of oligosaccharides from soy milk by an enzyme from Aspargillus saito. J. Food Sci. 35:655.

Taeufel, K., H. Ruttloff, W. Krause, A. Taeufel and K. Vetter. 1965. Zum intestinalen verhalten von galakto-oligosacchariden beim menschen. Klin. Wochenschr. 43:268.

Taeufel, K., W. Krause, H. Ruttloff and R. Maune. 1967. Zur intestinalen spaltung von oligosacchariden. Z. Gesamte Med. Einschl. Exp. Clin. 144:54.

Wagner, J.R., A.C. Olson, R. Becker and S. Kon. 1975a. Process for increasing digestibility of legume seeds. U.S. Patent 3,876,807.

Wagner, J.R., R. Becker, M.R. Gumbmann and A.C. Olson. 1975b. Hydrogen production in the rat following ingestion of raffinose, stachyose and oligosaccharide free bean residue. J. Nutr. (Submitted for publication).

24

CELIAC DISEASE: MALABSORPTION OF NUTRIENTS INDUCED BY A TOXIC FACTOR IN GLUTEN*

Donald D. Kasarda

Western Regional Research Laboratory
Agricultural Research Service
U.S. Department of Agriculture
Berkeley, California

In certain susceptible individuals, a peptide (or peptides) derived from digestion of gluten proteins of wheat and some related cereal grains produces a specific immune response localized in the tissues of the small intestine. The resulting adverse changes in the intestinal mucosa diminish its ability to absorb nutrients and the resulting malabsorption syndrome is frequently known as celiac disease, but sometimes as celiac sprue or gluten sensitive enteropathy. It has been suggested that celiac individuals lack a particular proteolytic enzyme so that some toxic peptide remains undegraded, thereby triggering the immune response. An abnormal immune response to some normally encountered peptide seems a more likely possibility, however, in view of the association of this condition with a particular histocompatibility antigen (HL-A8) and the failure of researchers to demonstrate a missing enzyme in celiac patients. The toxicity of α-gliadin proteins has been demonstrated in several studies. Should the toxic factor be limited to a relatively few protein components, there seems a good possibility for producing a new type of wheat free of those components.

---

*This is an updated version of an article that appeared in Baker's Digest, 1972, 46(6):25.

INTRODUCTION

For a small number of people, perhaps one in two thousand
(McCrae, 1970), bread and other wheat products are not simply
nourishing foods with a pleasing taste--they are poisons that
destroy the crucial functioning of the epithelial cells covering
the surface of the small intestine. The small intestine is where
important digestive processes occur and where nearly all nutrients
are absorbed; disruption of its function produces widespread
symptoms of disease. Immediate symptoms of celiac disease frequently include diarrhea, cramps, and pale, bulky stools as a consequence of malabsorption of fats in the diet. Eventually, general
malabsorption of nutrients may cause stunting of growth in children
or wasting of the body in adults.

Although the symptoms of celiac disease were clearly recorded
in the nineteenth century, it was only about 25 years ago that
wheat was determined responsible and the toxic factor associated
with the gliadin fraction (see discussion of Goldstein and Heiner,
1970, and of Douglas, 1974). From that time on, a seemingly inor-
dinate amount of research by physicians, physiologists, and chemists
has been devoted to the discovery of the molecular nature of the
toxic factor and the determination of the mechanism by which it
produces its effects on the mucosal tissue of the small intestine.
The extensive research in this area derives its justification,
however, not only from the possibility that celiac disease might be
controlled by a means other than exclusion of wheat from the diet
but also from the likelihood that understanding of this condition
would provide clues to presently puzzling aspects of the digestive
process and the functioning of the immune system.

THE DIGESTIVE PROCESS

When we chew our food, digestion begins with the breakdown of
starch by the α-amylase present in saliva, and this enzyme continues
to act on the food mass as it passes on through the gastro-intestinal tract to the stomach (Figure 1) where the salivary amylase

566

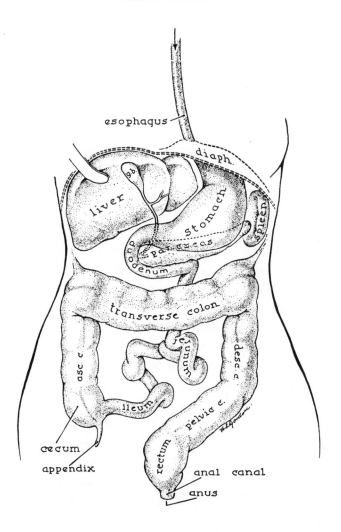

FIG. 1. Diagram of the parts of the digestive tract. (*From* Ham, A. W. 1965. Histology. J. B. Lippincott Co., Philadelphia.)

is eventually inactivated by the low pH. In the stomach, digestion is carried further by hydrochloric acid and pepsin--the hydrochloric acid partially unfolding proteins to make them more susceptible to attack by the pepsin and providing a suitable medium for the action of this acid protease. Next, the partially digested food enters the duodenal portion of the small intestine (Figure 1) where enzymes contributed by both the pancreas and epithelial cells of the small intestine complete digestion. At the same time, the products of digestion are absorbed both passively by diffusion and actively by transport across the membrane of the epithelial absorptive cells as the products of digestion pass through the small intestine. The pancreas supplies the precursors of trypsin, chymotrypsin, carboxypeptidases, and elastase, which, upon activation, continue the digestion of proteins and polypeptides. Pancreatic amylase completes the breakdown of starch to disaccharides, and pancreatic lipase hydrolyzes triglycerides to fatty acids and monoglycerides. Coincident with the introduction of the pancreatic secretions into the duodenum, bile acids from the liver and gallbladder are mixed with the stomach contents in the duodenum to emulsify fats and other nonpolar molecules. This emulsification also promotes the action of lipase in the breakdown of fats. The bile acids subsequently form micelles that transport fatty acids, monoglycerides, and nonpolar molecules, such as cholesterol and fat-soluble vitamins, to the surface of the epithelium.

A considerable number of enzymes are known to be associated with the epithelium of the small intestine and, quite certainly, more will be discovered. These enzymes include peptidases that break down polypeptides to their constituent amino acids, lipases for hydrolyzing fats, and disaccharidases for breaking down maltose, sucrose, and lactose to monosaccharides. Almost all nutrients-- amino acids, monosaccharides, fatty acids, monoglycerides, vitamins, etc.--are absorbed in the small intestine. Even the bile acids are eventually absorbed during their passage through the small intestine to be recirculated by way of the liver and the gall bladder for subsequent use.

The large intestine (colon-Figure 1) serves largely to extract water and electrolytes from the remains of the digested food and to provide an opportunity for bacteria to continue breakdown of those materials, such as cellulose, that are intractable to human enzymes, thereby reducing bulk. A small amount of nutrient absorption does occur from the colon, however, and some important nutrients may even be contributed by the bacterial action.

EPITHELIUM OF THE SMALL INTESTINE

The surface of the small intestine contains a number of features that maximize surface area, including folds and finger-like projections called villi (Figures 2 and 3). In between villi, the surface has many openings called crypts (Figure 2) that extend below the surface. The entire surface of the intestine is covered by a single layer of epithelial cells that extends from the bases of the crypts all the way to the tips of the villi. New cells are formed at the base of the crypts and migrate up the walls of the crypts to the surface, perhaps in response to the pressures from cell division occurring in the crypts. From the surface, the epithelial cells continue their migration up the walls of the villi to the tips where they eventually break off into the interior passage

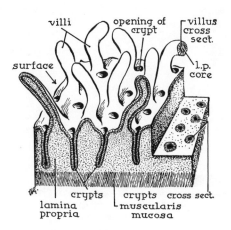

FIG. 2. Three-dimensional drawing of the lining of the small intestine. (*From* Ham, A. W. 1965. Histology. J. B. Lippincott Co., Philadelphia.)

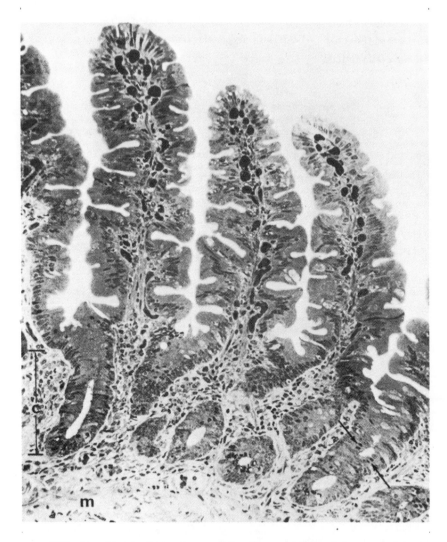

FIG. 3. Light photomicrograph of a section of human jejunum that has been stained with toluidine blue. Villi with lengths of about 1 mm are shown. The depths of the crypts are denoted by the arrows at C.   m represents the muscularis mucosa, the thin layer of smooth muscle that separates the mucosa from the submucosa below. The other arrows indicate dividing cells. (*From*   Rubin, W. 1971. Am. J. Clin. Nutr. 24:45.)

(lumen) of the intestine. Thus the entire population of cells is
continually renewed, with a renewal time of three to seven days
(see discussion of Rubin, 1971). During the migration from base of
crypt to tip of villus, the cells undergo a maturation process
whereby they increase their enzymatic activities and absorptive ca-
pabilities (Falchuk et al., 1974b).

Differentiation of the immature cells formed in the crypts
results in several types of cells with different functions, but the
concern here shall be with the absorptive cells that cover the
villi. The role of these cells in the digestive process is an area
of active research; what has been learned, however, reveals a complex array of interrelated reactions concerned with transport,
breakdown, and absorption of nutrients. Sections of normal absorptive cells are shown in Figure 4. The normal villous absorptive
cell is tall and columnar; the cell surface exposed to the lumen is
covered by many small projections called microvilli (Figure 5). The
microvilli are usually less than a micron long and have a diameter
of about 0.1 micron. They serve to extend the cell surface, and
enzymes organized at their surfaces catalyze many reactions that
occur at this surface (Crane, 1969). Many of the enzymes associated
with the absorptive cells--disaccharidases, alkaline phosphatase,
ATPase, aminopeptidase, dipeptidases--and receptor and carrier systems are associated with the plasma membrane covering the microvilli
(Rubin, 1971). The microvilli are covered with a fuzzy coat that
seems to be an extension of the cell membrane surface. Its function
is not well understood although it may be responsible for the
apparent adsorption of the pancreatic enzymes to the mucosal surface
(Crane, 1969).

The organization of enzymes in the epithelial cell membranes
or beneath them is not understood in detail, but it seems likely that
molecules are transported in a "hand-to-hand" fashion from enzyme
to enzyme and through the membrane (Crane, 1969). For example, a
disaccharide molecule such as maltose might be bound to the active
site of a maltase enzyme ordered on the membrane surface. Splitting

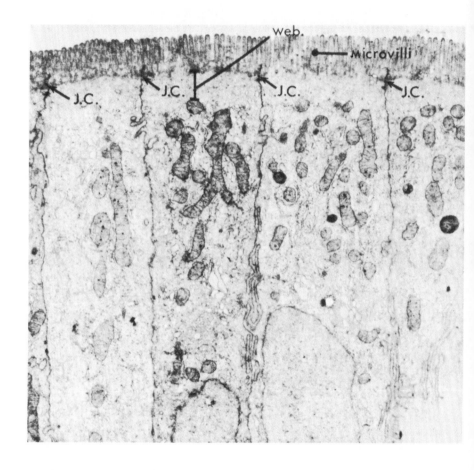

FIG. 4. Low power electron micrograph of section of rat intestine showing several contiguous cells. The arrows labeled J. C. point to junctional complexes, where the membranes of contiguous cells are fused. The terminal web (labeled) is a fibrillar material that probably serves as a supporting and anchoring structure. Microvilli cover the absorptive surface of the cells. (*From* Ham, A. W. 1965. Histology. J. B. Lippincott Co., Philadelphia.)

of the disaccharide to form two units of glucose results in these monosaccharide molecules diffusing only a short distance to be bound immediately by carrier molecules capable of transporting the glucose formed across the membrane. The obviously important

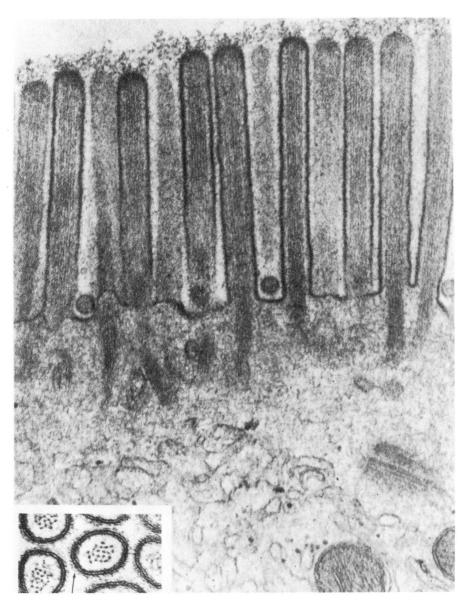

FIG. 5. Electron micrograph of microvilli on the surface of an epithelial cell from a human intestine. The inset shows a section through the microvilli cut at a 90° angle to the first section. The arrow points to the glycocalyx--thin filaments that extend from the surface of the microvilli into the lumen. (*From* Rubin, W. 1971. Am. J. Clin. Nutr. 24:45.)

functions of the surface membrane depend in a critical way on reactions that take place at other sites in the cell. Active transport requires energy that is derived from metabolic processes that occur elsewhere; disaccharidases and other proteins are probably synthesized elsewhere in the cell. These and other epithelial cell processes are so interdependent that breakdown at any point may prevent the epithelial cell from functioning.

CELIAC DISEASE

In the past, the name celiac disease usually has been applied when a particular set of symptoms developed in children, but it seems generally agreed that the similar set of symptoms in adults represents the same condition. Celiac disease is also known as gluten-sensitive enteropathy, celiac sprue, non-tropical sprue, and adult celiac disease. The most frequently reported symptoms include diarrhea, pale bulky stools, abdominal cramps, flatulence, and weight loss or a failure to grow. Malabsorption of fats (steatorrhea) is usually noted, but almost all nutrients such as sugars, amino acids, and vitamins are poorly absorbed; minerals are poorly absorbed as well. Any of the symptoms that accompany vitamin or mineral deficiencies may be observed, for example, diffuse bone pain and a susceptibility to fractures resulting from the malabsorption of calcium and vitamin D. Obviously, the retardation of growth or weight loss of celiac patients is directly related to the failure of the small intestine to absorb nutrients adequately.

A depression of many enzymes associated with the epithelial cells of the small intestine has been noted in celiac disease (Berg et al., 1970; Douglas et al., 1970; Jos et al., 1967). The low levels of the disaccharidase enzymes permit disaccharides to move along and through the small intestine without breakdown to monosacharrides and subsequent absorption. Upon reaching the colon, these disaccharides contribute an osmotic pressure to the system such as to retard or even reverse the usual flow of water from the intestinal lumen through the epithelial cells to the blood and lymph systems so that the fecal matter remains watery, causing diarrhea. At the same time, bacterial fermentation of these sugars and other unabsorbed nutrients results in gas production with accompanying cramps and flatulence.

Examination of tiny samples of epithelial tissue obtained from celiac patients by intestinal biopsy (which involves insertion of a capsule attached to fine tubing into the intestine by way of the esophagus) showed striking changes from the normal (Rubin et al., 1962, Weinstein et al., 1970). The villi were no longer visible and the surface had acquired a flat appearance with a mosaic pattern. Plasma cells had infiltrated the lamina propria (Figure 2) indicating that an immunological response was taking place. These changes were noted most frequently and with most severity in the duodenum and the jejunum (Figure 1) of the small intestine; involvement of the ileum was much less frequent. The histological changes observed in the epithelial tissue of the jejunum are usually considered the definitive test for celiac disease when clinical symptoms are present, and when such changes are observed in the duodenum or jejunum in the absence of clinical symptoms, a mild form of the disease may be present with insufficient surface area of the small intestine affected for obvious symptoms to be manifest. Similar changes have been observed, however, in other diseases (Weinstein et al., 1970).

Role of Wheat

In 1950 and shortly thereafter, Dicke and others (see discussion of Frazer, 1956) showed that wheat ingestion was responsible for the symptoms of celiac disease in the great majority of cases. Removal of wheat from the diet produced immediate improvement in many cases--sometimes in days--and a more gradual improvement over a period of weeks to months in most others (Benson et al., 1964). Return of the duodenal and jejunal mucosa to a normal appearance

was somewhat slower than the disappearance of the general symptoms
of intestinal distress and the improvement in the absorptive capacity of the intestine, but over a period of months during which
the patients were kept on a gluten-free diet, the villous structure
approached the normal state. When recovered patients return to
a normal diet that includes wheat, they sometimes do not show any
of the obvious symptoms of celiac disease, but they may develop
steatorrhea, and usually develop the typical lesions of the intestinal mucosa as evidenced by biopsy and histological examination
of the tissue (Benson et al., 1964; Visakorpi and Savilahti, 1970).
McNicholl et al. (1974) have reported, however, that reversion of
the mucosa to the flat state may take several years to occur in
some patients.

Rye also produces the symptoms of celiac disease and must be
avoided by celiac patients. Many investigators think that barley
and oats also contain the toxic factor (Frazer, 1956; Visakorpi
and Savilahti, 1970; Rubin et al., 1962). In this respect, it is
interesting to note that Ewart (1966b) found rye closely related
to wheat, barley less closely related, and oats and maize not
related at all on the basis of common antigens to an antigliadin
serum and Rossipal (1974) found cross reaction of the antibodies
to α-gliadin with at least one component in rye, barley, and oats.
Dissanayake et al. (1974) concluded, however, that oats are harmless to celiac individuals. Corn and rice products have usually
been considered non-toxic to celiac patients (Dicke et al., 1953)
although a clearly allergic response of a conventional type to
these grains is known. In the latter case, symptoms might include
respiratory distress, headache, joint pains, or hives. Unfortunately, neither corn nor rice flour produces a bread with the
unusually good texture and flavor of wheat bread.

Fractionation of Wheat

Dicke and coworkers found that wheat flour, but not wheat
starch, produced symptoms of celiac disease in susceptible individuals. Van de Kamer et al. (1953) reported that a water extract

was less toxic than the residue, that gliadin (the protein fraction soluble in 70% ethanol) was toxic when fed to patients in amounts as small as 3 g per day, and that glutenin (the insoluble residue after extraction of gluten with 70% ethanol) was much less toxic than gliadin. Complete hydrolysis of gliadin rendered it harmless as did partial hydrolysis with 1 M HCl for 45 min. at 100°C (Van de Kamer and Weijers, 1955). The principal effect of the latter treatment should be to convert glutamine side chains to glutamic acid side chains through loss of ammonia, which points to a possible role of glutamine in the toxicity of gliadin (Van de Kamer and Weijers, 1955) although such treatment could result in the hydrolysis of some susceptible peptide bonds as well. About one of every three amino acid residues in gliadin is glutamine (Kasarda et al., 1971). Glutamine itself seems to produce no effect when fed to celiac patients (Van de Kamer and Weijers, 1955; Weijers et al., 1957), however, and I am unaware of any attempts to administer peptides of glutamine to celiac patients. Presumably, some sequence of amino acids is responsible for the toxic effect of certain peptides derived from gluten proteins and although this sequence could consist of a series of glutamine residues only, it is also possible that glutamine combined with other amino acids makes up the toxic sequence. And since the partial hydrolysis of Van de Kamer and Weijers (1955) could conceivably break some susceptible peptide bonds, it may be that glutamine is not a constituent residue of the toxic sequence at all.

Frazer (1962) reported that digestion of gliadin with the pancreatic proteases pepsin and trypsin did not destroy the toxicity. He also reported that passage of a peptic-tryptic digest through a dialysis membrane (ultrafiltration) resulted in a fraction that was toxic to celiac patients, which indicated that the toxic peptide must be relatively small since the membrane would retain large peptides with molecular weights greater than about 12,000 Daltons. Krainick and Mohn (1959) concluded from their experiments that the toxic peptides obtained from an ultrafiltrate

have an average molecular weight of 874 and consist chiefly of
glutamine and proline residues. Other investigators (Cornell,
1974; Cornell and Townley, 1973) found that digestion of gliadin
with pepsin, trypsin, and pancreatin yielded peptides with molecular weights up to 3,000 Daltons that were still toxic; chromatography of this digest on sulfoethyl-Sephadex yielded a fraction
(designated fraction nine) in which most of the activity was concentrated. A similar fraction was obtained from glutenin (Cornell,
1974). Jos et al. (1974) note, however, that digestion with pepsin, trypsin, and chymotrypsin destroyed the toxicity of gliadin
as measured by the effect on cultures of biopsied intestinal tissue
when each step of the enzymatic digestion was carried out for 16
hrs. This suggests that the toxic peptides may represent partial
digestion products of gliadin.

It may be that both intact gliadin molecules and certain small
peptides that result from enzymatic digestion of gliadin are toxic
to celiac patients since instillation of gliadin by means of a
tube directly into the jejunum of a celiac patient produced immediate histological changes in the intestinal mucosa characteristic
of those seen in untreated celiac patients (Hekkens et al., 1970).
Falchuk et al. (1974b) also noted toxic effects on tissue cultures
from celiac patients for intact α-gliadin protein as well as for
a peptic-tryptic digest of gliadin. It is conceivable that some
enzymatic breakdown of the native protein could have occurred
during the course of these experiments although this seems unlikely
in the experiments of Falchuk et al. (1974b).

Bronstein et al. (1966) and Kowlessar et al. (1970) studied
toxic peptides in the ultrafiltrate of a peptic-tryptic-Cotazym
digest of gliadin. They found that the ultrafiltrate contained at
least 14 different free amino acids, but noted that glutamine and
proline were not among them--these amino acids remained bound. The
peptides in the digest were separated into an "acidic group" of
peptides that was not retained on a cation exchange resin in the
H^+ form and a group of peptides that was removed from the resin

with 3 M NH$_4$OH. The acidic group of peptides contained N-pyrroli-
done carboxylyl end groups that presumably resulted from the cyclization of N-terminal glutamine residues under the slightly
alkaline conditions employed for tryptic digestion (Bronstein et
al., 1966). These acidic peptides, which contained large amounts
of glutamine and proline, were shown to have toxic effects.
Accordingly, these workers suggested that N-terminal pyrrolidone
carboxylyl peptides may be the toxic factor in enzymatic digests
of gliadin. Kowlessar et al. (1970) reported that further fractionation of the acidic peptides on an anion exchange column
yielded a fraction containing glycopeptides and another fraction,
free of carbohydrate but with an extremely high glutamine content.
Van de Kamer et al. (1970) have also discussed the possible importance of peptides containing pyrrolidone carboxylic acid groups.
Woodley (1972) found, however, no impairment in the ability of
the intestinal mucosa of untreated celiac patients to split the
terminal pyrrolidone carboxylyl residue from peptides and other
workers (Cornell, 1974; Jos et al., 1974) have found no, or low,
toxicity for peptide fractions containing such end groups.

Most of the attempts to define the toxic peptide of gliadin
have involved fractionation of the whole gliadin. The relatively
large amounts of protein required for testing with patients have
made this necessary. Whole gliadin, however, contains at least 40
components (Wrigley and Shephard, 1973). These components can
differ substantially in their amino acid compositions (Booth and
Ewart, 1970) with consequent complication of the problem of
sorting out all the various peptides that result from enzymatic
degradation of whole gliadin. In addition, the question arises
as to whether all the gliadin components, or just some of the
components, contain the sequences of amino acids responsible for
the toxic effect. Kendall et al. (1972) and Schneider et al. (1974)
reported that only one of twelve gliadin fractions separated by
ion exchange was toxic to celiac patients on the basis of the xy-
lose absorption test. Hekkens et al. (1970) sought to simplify

the situation with regard to the complexity of the mixture of
gliadin proteins by separating α-gliadin from the mixture and testing its effect on celiac patients. One of the methods they chose
was that of Bernardin et al. (1967) whose aggregation method yields
large amounts of a relatively pure gliadin fraction. The α-gliadin
prepared in this way still contains several closely similar components (Platt and Kasarda, 1971), but represents a considerably
more homogeneous protein fraction than does whole gliadin and one
that has been extensively characterized (Kasarda et al., 1971;
Kasarda et al., 1974). When 7.5 g of α-gliadin were instilled over
a period of eight hours into the jejunum of a patient in remission,
there were changes in the epithelial tissue characteristic of
celiac disease after eight hours (Hekkens et al., 1970).

Enzymatic Aspects

The mechanism by which the toxic factor from wheat exerts its
effect on the epithelium of the small intestine is still unknown.
Early observations (Frazer, 1962; Alvey et al., 1957) indicated
that digestion of gluten or gliadin with pepsin and trypsin did
not destroy the toxicity of these wheat fractions, but Frazer
(1956) reported that an enzyme extract prepared from pig intestinal
mucous membrane was capable of destroying the toxicity. He suggested that an enzyme associated with the epithelial cells of the
small intestine of normal persons and capable of digesting peptides
of gluten that contain glutamine was missing or deficient in those
persons with celiac disease. Since then, many workers have tried
to find such a missing enzyme. The sensitivity of celiac patients
to gliadin proteins suggests that the enzyme would be a peptidase
capable of splitting a sequence of amino acids that occurs only in
these proteins.

The gastric and pancreatic enzymes of celiac patients seem to
be normal (Messer et al., 1961) although depression of enzyme activity associated with the epithelial tissue of the small intestine
has been observed. Berg et al. (1970) reported that enzyme

activities of epithelial tissue for dipeptide substrates containing proline were reduced to about 50% of the normal level, whereas the reduction of activity was about 30% for splitting of the following substrates: glycyl-leucine, glycyl-valine, alanyl-glutamic acid, and glutamyl-valine. Disaccharidase activities were reduced to about 10-20% of the controls for sucrase, maltase, lactase, isomaltase, and trehalase. They concluded that the diminished enzyme activities were a secondary effect resulting from primary damage to the epithelial tissue, but did not exclude the possibility that a lack in celiac patients of some as yet undiscovered peptidase is responsible for the disease.

Enzyme activities are generally found to be higher in treated celiac patients on a gluten-free diet than in untreated patients (Berg et al., 1970) although lactase and the dipeptidase responsible for splitting glutamyl-proline dipeptides remained low even in treated patients. Lactase is one of the first enzymes affected when wheat is introduced to the diet of a treated celiac patient (Bayless et al., 1970), and returns to normal slowly after removal of wheat from the diet; these changes in lactase levels may be responsible for the milk intolerance that frequently accompanies celiac disease. Jos et al. (1967) consider that lactose in the diet prevents restoration of the villi in patients on a wheat-free diet. Nevertheless, they consider lactose intolerance transient; when the epithelial tissue returns to normal, the intolerance disappears.

Low levels of the enzyme gamma-glutamyl transpeptidase were found in celiac patients on a gluten-free diet and with the disease in remission (Cohen et al,, 1970). This enzyme is capable of breaking the gamma-carboxyl-amide linkage, and Cohen et al. (1970) claimed that such linkages do occur in gliadin and its fractions. Pyrrolidone carboxylyl peptidase (PCA-peptidase), an enzyme that cleaves N-terminal pyrrolidone carboxylate groups formed by cyclization of N-terminal glutamine residues of peptides, has been considered as possibly being the missing enzyme in celiac individuals (Kowlessar, 1970). The results of Woodley (1972), however, indicate that normal levels of this enzyme are present in celiac patients.

Phelan et al. (1974) have claimed that the toxicity of gliadin peptides resides in glycosidic residues bound to the amino acid side chains and that gliadin can be detoxified by treatment with carbohydrases. However, Hekkens et al. (1974) reported that a toxic fragment obtained by tryptic digestion of α-gliadin contained not more than one half glucose residue per mole of peptide (M.W. 18,000). This result would seem to indicate that the glucose found represents an impurity rather than being chemically bound.

Strumeyer (1972) has speculated that an α-amylase inhibitor found in the whole gliadin fraction of wheat may be responsible for celiac disease by blocking the action of pancreatic α-amylase, which may be present only in low levels in susceptible individuals. This hypothesis seems unlikely in consideration of the toxic effects observed for α-gliadin and gliadin peptides included in the culture medium of organ-cultured biopsies from celiac patients (Falchuk et al., 1974b). Auricchio et al. (1974) fed α-amylase inhibitors from wheat to a celiac patient and found no effect on starch and fat absorption. They suggest that α-gliadin toxicity is not related to inhibitory activity toward α-amylase.

Regardless of the mechanism by which the toxic factor from wheat exerts its effects, the most important immediate effect seems to be a destruction of mature absorptive cells on the upper surfaces of the villi. In consequence, an increase in the rate of cell division begins in the crypts with more rapid migration of these cells up from the base of the crypts to take the place of those damaged cells sloughed from the surface into the intestinal lumen (Trier and Browning, 1970; Clark and Senior, 1969). Trier and Browning (1970) consider this cell proliferation responsible for the increase in crypt thickness, which, along with the loss of cells from the villous tips, contribute the flat appearance of the epithelial surface characteristic of celiac disease.

CELIAC DISEASE

Immunochemical Aspects

Involvement of the immune system in celiac disease is unquestionable as evidenced by the infiltration of lymphocytes and plasma cells into the lamina propria as one of the first observable events resulting from wheat ingestion by celiac patients in remission (Shiner, 1974; Shmerling and Shiner, 1970), the improvement that occurs in celiac patients following treatment with corticosteroids even when wheat is included in their diets (Wall et al., 1970), and the presence of precipitating antibodies to wheat antigens in the blood serum (Heiner et al., 1962; Rossipal, 1971, 1974), in intestinal secretions (Katz et al., 1968), and in biopsied intestinal tissue (Falchuk et al., 1971). It seems likely that the immune response is responsible for the destruction of the mature epithelial cells, but it is not clear whether this immune response is the result of an abnormal immune system reacting to a peptide formed by the normal digestive process or whether the response is a normal one to an antigenic peptide that is undegraded as a consequence of an enzyme defect in individuals with celiac disease.

The finding by Falchuk et al. (1972) and Stokes et al. (1972) that certain cell surface proteins (HL-A8 histocompatibility antigens) are found with unusually high frequencies in celiac patients (about 80%) as compared to normal individuals (about 20% with HL-A8) suggests that individuals with celiac disease may indeed have an abnormality of the immune system. Strober (1974) has suggested that gluten proteins, or peptides derived from them, may bind to the epithelial cells with the HL-A8 histocompatibility antigen providing at least part of the binding site. This binding could then trigger an immunogenic response that results in cell destruction. Loeb et al. (1971) showed that gluten challenge triggered production of immunoglobulins within the gastrointestinal mucosa in celiac disease and that these immunoglobulins were of the *IgA* and *IgM* classes. This conclusion has been supported by Savilahti (1974). Falchuk et al. (1971) showed that a major part of the immunoglobulin increase was composed of anti-gliadin antibodies. These antibodies could be responsible for cell destruction as suggested by Booth (1970) and Strober (1974).

Heiner et al. (1962) reported that celiac patients have a high frequency of precipitins to a particular gliadin protein fraction. In later work, Beckwith and Heiner (1966) showed this protein fraction to be identical with α-gliadin (because of the wheat variety used, equivalent to the A-gliadin of Platt et al., 1974). It has often been considered that these circulating antibodies represent a secondary effect in celiac disease and result from increased permeability of the mucosa to proteins and peptides. However, Katz et al. (1968) found antibodies to a peptic-tryptic digest of gluten in the intestinal secretions and stool of celiac patients. They point out that the immune system of the small bowel mucosa is independent of the system responsible for circulating antibodies (Crabbé and Heremans, 1966; Shiner, 1974) and that the circulating antibodies may have their origin in the increased production of antibodies by this intestinal system. Scott et al. (1974) noted that individuals with the HL-A8 histocompatibility antigen tended to have higher serum antibodies to a tryptic digest of gliadin than those without this antigen. This was true whether or not they had celiac disease although the highest antibody levels were found for celiac patients. They conclude that the HL-A8 histocompatibility antigen is either linked to an immune response gene for gliadin or that HL-A8 on the surface of small intestinal epithelial cells acts as a receptor for binding of gliadin.

Falchuk et al. (1974b) developed an *in vitro* model of gluten sensitive enteropathy (celiac disease) based on the tissue culture of intestinal biopsy specimens first described by Browning and Trier (1969). Falchuk et al. (1974b) showed that the activity of alkaline phosphatase in the cultured tissue increased over a 48 hr period for tissue from normal individuals or celiac individuals. This increase was presumably due to maturation of epithelial cells in the culture. When intact α-gliadin or a peptic-tryptic digest of gliadin was included in the culture medium, however, there was

a significant inhibition of the development of alkaline phosphatase
activity for tissue taken from a celiac patient with active disease.
The gliadin had no effect on tissue from patients with the disease
in remission (on a gluten-free diet) indicating that gliadin is
not directly toxic to the epithelial tissue; an endogenous effector mechanism must first be activated by gluten challenge.   In
later work, Falchuk et al., 1974a, showed that when tissue from samples
active and inactive celiac patients were cultured in the same
medium, gliadin affected both cultures--indicating that the endogenous effector was a diffusible substance.   This substance was
not identified, but might be anti-gliadin antibody.

Polygenic Nature

Although the incidence of celiac disease in Western Europe
seems to be roughly 1 in 2,000, there are regional differences--
most notably in the West of Ireland where Mylotte et al. (1973)
have estimated that the incidence may be as high as 1 in 300.   The
disease seems to be genetically determined, but the inheritance
does not follow simple Mendelian laws.   McCarthy et al. (1974)
concluded that the incidence would fit either a polygenic inheritance with a high heritability or dominant inheritance with a low
rate of manifestation in heterozygotes.   McCrae (1970) had concluded earlier that expression of celiac disease is controlled by
more than one gene.   He suggested that susceptibility to celiac
disease may vary continuously throughout the population depending
upon the number of contributing genetic factors expressed in any
individual.

The appearance of celiac disease symptoms is apparently
dependent on environmental factors as well as genetic factors.
Many celiac patients return to a normal diet after excluding
wheat without immediate return of obvious symptoms of the disease
(Visakorpi and Savilahti, 1970; McNicholl et al., 1974) although
biopsies taken during this period may show the flat mucosa characteristic of celiac disease.   After periods ranging from weeks to

years, relapse usually occurs. It is conceivable that emotional or physical stress serves as a triggering factor in such relapses. The finding that one of a pair of identical twins developed celiac disease (Walker-Smith, 1973) lends supports the possibility that factors other than genetic are involved in the appearance of symptoms.

McNeish et al. (1974) note that there seems to be a racial difference in susceptibility to celiac disease. They attempted to relate incidence throughout the world to the incidence of the HL-A8 histocompatibility antigen in a given population, the time at which wheat is first introduced in the diet of infants, and the amount of wheat in the diet.

Dohan (1969) has noted that celiac disease and schizophrenia appear to occur in the same individual somewhat more frequently than could be expected from chance alone. He suggested that both diseases may have genes in common.

DISCUSSION

For those who suffer from celiac disease, removal of wheat from the diet presents a difficult problem--partly because of the importance of bread and other baked goods in our culture, and partly because of the pervasiveness of wheat as an ingredient in so many foods that are not immediately associated with wheat, ranging from soups to candies. This problem is compounded by the need to exclude rye and barley from the diet as well as wheat. Labeling can be confusing. Baked products sold in health food stores as wheat-free have been found to contain wheat (Lietze et al., 1967). A major manufacturer of baby food listed malt flour as an ingredient in rice cereal. Relatively few housewives would be sophisticated enough to recognize the possible relation of this ingredient to wheat or barley when they are trying to exclude these cereals from their baby's diet. It would be best to exclude additives derived from wheat, rye, or barley from rice cereals.

CELIAC DISEASE

Because the onset of celiac disease might be related to the age of an infant when wheat (or related grains) is first introduced to the diet (McNeish et al., 1974; Mylotte et al., 1973) the possibility of recommending a delay in the introduction of wheat products to the diet until the age of about 9 months has been considered (Asquith, 1974). The situation is not clear, however, and the relationship of early wheat feeding to celiac disease is speculative.

Since there is a possibility that only a fraction of the gliadin proteins in wheat may be responsible for producing the toxic effects in celiac disease (Kendall et al., 1972), it may be possible to develop a wheat variety free of these particular protein components by genetic means. The many components (40 or more) of the gliadin mixture appear to be related to one another through partial common amino acid sequences as indicated by peptide mapping techniques (Bietz et al., 1970; Ewart, 1966a). In the event that the toxic amino acid sequence turns out to be widely distributed among the gliadin proteins, it will be impossible to produce a non-toxic wheat.

The toxicity in celiac disease of the α-gliadin proteins from wheat seems established (Hekkens et al., 1970, 1974; Falchuk et al., 1974b; Kendall et al., 1972; Ezeoke et al., 1974). Breakdown of this protein into peptides, combined with tests for toxicity of the sort developed by Strober's group (Falchuk et al., 1974b) which require relatively small sample sizes (milligram amounts), should lead to definition of the smallest toxic peptide and its amino acid sequence in the near future.

REFERENCES

Alvey, C., C. M. Anderson, and M. Freeman. 1957. Wheat gluten and coeliac disease. Arch. Dis. Childhood (London). 32:434.

Asquith, P. 1974. Discussion of paper by McNeish et al. *In* Coeliac Disease, W. Th. J. M. Hekkens and A. S. Peña (Editors), Proc. 2nd Int. Symp. Stenfert Kroese, Leiden. p. 337.

Auricchio, S., B. De Viria, L. Carta De Angelis, and V. Silano. 1974. Alpha-amylase protein inhibitors in coeliac disease. Lancet. I:98.

Bayless, T. M., S. E. Rubin, T. M. Topping, J. H. Yardley, and T. R. Hendrix. 1970. Morphologic and functional effects of gluten feeding on jejunal mucosa in celiac disease. *In* Coeliac Disease, C. C. Booth and R. H. Dowling (Editors). Proc. Int. Symp. Churchill Livingstone, Edinburgh, p. 76.

Beckwith, A. C., and D. C. Heiner. 1966. An immunological study of wheat gluten proteins and derivatives. Arch. Biochem. Biophys. 117:239.

Benson, G. D., O. D. Kowlessar, and M. H. Sleisenger. 1964. Adult celiac disease with emphasis upon response to the gluten-free diet. Medicine 43:1.

Berg, N. O., A. Dahlqvist, T. Lindberg, and A. Nordén. 1970. Intestinal dipeptidases and disaccharidases in celiac disease in adults. Gastroenterology. 59:575.

Bernardin, J. E., D. D. Kasarda, and D. K. Mecham. 1967. Preparation and characterization of α-gliadin. J. Biol. Chem. 242:445.

Bietz, J. A., F. R. Huebner, and J. A. Rothfus. 1970. Chromatographic comparisons of individual gliadin proteins. Cereal Chem. 47:393.

Booth, C. C. 1970. The enterocyte in coeliac disease. Br. Med. J. 4:14.

Booth, M. R., and J. A. D. Ewart. 1970. Relationship between wheat proteins. J. Sci. Food Agr. 21:187.

Bronstein, H. D., L. J. Haeffner, and O. D. Kowlessar. 1966. Enzymatic digestion of gliadin: The effect of the resultant peptides in adult celiac disease. Clin. Chim. Acta 14:141.

Browning, T. H. and J. S. Trier. 1969. Organ culture of mucosal biopsies of human small intestine. J. Clin. Invest. 48:1423.

Clark, M. L. and J. R. Senior. 1969. Small gut mucosal activities of pyrimidine precursor enzymes in celiac disease. Gastroenterology 56:887.

Cohen, M. I., H. McNamara, D. Blumenfeld, and I. M. Arias. 1970. The relationship between glutamyl transpeptidase and the syndrome of celiac-sprue. *In* Coeliac Disease, C. C. Booth and R. H. Dowling (Editors). Proc. Int. Symp. Churchill Livingstone, Edinburgh, p. 91.

Cornell, H. J. 1974. Gliadin degradation and fractionation. *In* Coeliac Disease, W. Th. J. M. Hekkens and A. S. Peña (Editors), Proc. 2nd Int. Symp. Stenfert Kroese, Leiden, p. 74.

Cornell, H. J. and R. R. W. Townley. 1973. Investigation of possible intestinal peptidase deficiency in coeliac disease. Clin. Chim. Acta 43:113.

Crabbé, P. A., and J. F. Heremans. 1966. The distribution of immunoglobulin-containing cells along the human gastrointestinal tract. Gastroenterology 51:305.

Crane, R. K. 1969. A perspective of digestive-absorptive function. Am. J. Clin. Nutr. 22:242.

Dissanayake, A. S., S. C. Truelove, and R. Whitehead. 1974. Lack of harmful effect of oats on small-intestinal mucosa in coeliac disease. Brit. Med. J. 4:189.

Dohan, F. C. 1969. Schizophrenia: Possible relationship to cereal grains and celiac disease. *In* Schizophrenia: Current Concepts and Research. D. V. Sankar (Editor). P. J. D. Publications, Ltd., Hicksville, New York, p. 539.

Douglas, A. P. 1974. Long term prognosis and relation to diets. *In* Coeliac Disease. W. Th. J. M. Hekkens and A. S. Peña (Editors). Proc. 2nd Int. Symp. Stenfert Kroese, Leiden, p. 399.

Douglas, A. P., T. J. Peters, A. V. Hoffbrand, and C. C. Booth. 1970. Studies of intestinal peptidases with special reference to coeliac disease. *In* Coeliac Disease. C. C. Booth and R. H. Dowling (Editors). Proc. Int. Symp. Churchill Livingstone, Edinburgh, p. 115.

Ewart, J. A. D. 1966a. Fingerprinting of glutenin and gliadin. J. Sci. Food Agr. 17:30.

Ewart, J. A. D. 1966b. Cereal proteins: Immunological studies. J. Sci. Food Agr. 17:279.

Ezeoke, A., N. Ferguson, O. Fakhri, W. Th. J. M. Hekkens, and J. R. Hobbs. 1974. Antibodies in the sera of coeliac patients which can coopt K-cells to attack gluten-labelled targets. *In* Coeliac Disease. W. Th. J. M. Hekkens and A. S. Peña (Editors). Proc. 2nd Int. Symp. Stenfert Kroese, Leiden, p. 176.

Falchuk, Z. M., R. L. Gebhard, and W. Strober. 1974a. The pathogenesis of gluten-sensitive enteropathy (celiac sprue): Organ culture studies. *In* Coeliac Disease. W. Th. J. M. Hekkens and A. S. Peña (Editors). Proc. 2nd Int. Symp. Stenfert Kroese, Leiden, p. 107.

Falchuk, Z. M., R. L. Gebhard, C. Sessoms, and W. Strober. 1974b. An *in vitro* model of gluten-sensitive enteropathy: Effect of gliadin on intestinal epithelial cells of patients with gluten-sensitive enteropathy in organ culture. J. Clin. Invest. 53:487.

Falchuk, Z. M., L. Laster, and W. Strober. 1971. Gluten sensitive enteropathy: Intestinal synthesis of anti-gluten antibody *in vitro*. Abstract. Clin. Res. 19:390.

Falchuk, Z. M., G. N. Rogentine, and W. Strober. 1972. Predominance of histocompatability antigen HL-A8 in patients with gluten-sensitive enteropathy. J. Clin. Invest. 51:160.

Frazer, A. C. 1956. Discussion on some problems of steatorrhea and reduced stature. Proc. Roy. Soc. Med. 49:1009.

Frazer, A. C. 1962. On the significance of mucosal damage. *In* Intestinal Biopsy. G. E. W. Wolstenholme and M. P. Cameron (Editors). Ciba Foundation Study Group No. 14. Little, Brown and Co., Boston, p. 54.

Goldstein, G. B., and D. C. Heiner. 1970. Clinical and immunological perspectives in food sensitivity. J. Allergy 46:270.

Heiner, D. C., M. E. Lahey, J. F. Wilson, J. W. Gerrard, H. Shwachman, and K. T. Khaw. 1962. Precipitins to antigens of wheat and cow's milk in celiac disease. J. Pediatrics 61:813.

Hekkens, W. Th. J. M., A. J. Ch. Haex, and R. G. J. Willighagen. 1970. Some aspects of gliadin fractionation and testing by a histochemical method. *In* Coeliac Disease. C. C. Booth and R. H. Dowling (Editors). Proc. Int. Symp. Churchill Livingstone, Edinburgh, p. 11.

Hekkens, W. Th. J. M., C. J. Van den Aarsen, J. P. Gilliams, Ph. Lems-Van Kan, and G. Bouma-Frölich. 1974. α-Gliadin structure and degradation. *In* Coeliac Disease. W. Th. J. M. Hekkens and A. S. Peña (Editors). Proc. 2nd Int. Symp. Stenfert Kroese, Leiden, p. 39.

Jos, J., J. Frézal, J. Rey, and M. Lamy. 1967. Étude histochimique de la muqueuse duodéno-jéjunale dans la maladie coeliaque. Pediat. Res. 1:27.

Jos, J., G. Lenoir, G. de Ritis, and J. Rey. 1974. *In vitro* culturing of biopsies from children. *In* Coeliac Disease. W. Th. J. M. Hekkens and A. S. Peña (Editors). Proc. 2nd Int. Symp. Stenfert Kroese, Leiden, p. 91.

Kasarda, D. D., D. A. da Roza, and J. I. Ohms. 1974. N-terminal sequence of α_2-gliadin. Biochim. Biophys. Acta 351:290.

Kasarda, D. D., C. C. Nimmo, and G. O. Kohler. 1971. Proteins and the amino acid composition of wheat fractions. *In* Wheat: Chemistry and Technology. Y. Pomerantz (Editor). American Assn. Cereal Chemists, St. Paul, Minnesota, p. 227.

Katz, J., F. S. Kantor, and T. Herskovic. 1968. Intestinal antibodies to wheat fractions in celiac disease. Ann. Int. Med. 69:1149.

Kendall, M. J., R. Schneider, P. S. Cox, and C. F. Hawkins. 1972. Gluten subfractions in coeliac disease. Lancet. II:1065.

Kowlessar, O. D., R. E. Warren, and H. D. Bronstein. 1970. Celiac Disease: Enzyme defect or immune mechanism? *In* Progress in Gastroenterology. Vol. II. G. B. J. Glass (Editor). Grune and Stratton, New York, p. 409.

Krainick, H. G., and G. Mohn. 1959. Weitere Untersuchungen über den schädlichen Weizenmehle-effekt bei der Cöliakie. 2. Die Wirkung der enzymatischen Abbauprodukte des Gliadin. Helv. Paediat. Acta 14:124.

Lietze, A., A. H. Rowe, A. Rowe, Jr., and C. E. Sinclair. 1967. Unlisted wheat in hypoallergenic bread and other bakery products. Ann. Allergy 25:175.

Loeb, P. M., W. Strober, Z. M. Falchuk, and L. Laster. 1971. Incorporation of L-leucine-^{14}C into immunoglobulins by jejunal biopsies of patients with celiac sprue and other gastrointestinal diseases. J. Clin. Invest. 50:559.

McCarthy, C. F., M. Mylotte, F. Stevens, B. Egan-Mitchell, P. F. Fottrell, and B. McNicholl. 1974. Family studies on coeliac disease in Ireland. *In* Coeliac Disease. W. Th. J. M. Hekkens and A. S. Peña (Editors). Proc. 2nd Int. Symp. Stenfert Kroese, Leiden, p. 311.

McCrae, W. M. 1970. The inheritance of coeliac disease. *In* Coeliac Disease. C. C. Booth and R. H. Dowling (Editors). Proc. Int. Symp. Churchill Livingstone, Edinburgh, p. 55.

McNeish, A. S., C. J. Rolles, R. Nelson, T. O. Kyaw-Myint, P. Mackintosh, and A. F. Williams. 1974. Factors affecting the differing racial incidence of coeliac disease. *In* Coeliac Disease. W. Th. J. M. Hekkens and A. S. Peña (Editors). Proc. 2nd Int. Symp. Stenfert Kroese, Leiden, p. 330.

McNicholl, B., B. Egan-Mitchell, and P. F. Fottrell. 1974. Varying gluten susceptibility in coeliac disease. *In* Coeliac Disease. W. Th. J. M. Hekkens and A. S. Peña (Editors). Proc. 2nd Int. Symp. Stenfert Kroese, Leiden, p. 413.

Messer, M., C. M. Anderson, and R. R. W. Townley. 1961. Peptidase activity of biopsies of the duodenal mucosa of children with and without coeliac disease. Clin. Chim. Acta 6:768.

Mylotte, M., B. Egan-Mitchell, C. F. McCarthy, and B. McNicholl. 1973. Incidence of coeliac disease in the West of Ireland. Br. Med. J. 1:703.

Phelan, J. J., C. F. McCarthy, F. M. Stevens, B. McNicholl, and P. F. Fottrell. 1974. The nature of gliadin toxicity in coeliac disease: A new concept. *In* Coeliac Disease. W. Th. J. M. Hekkens and A. S. Peña (Editors). Proc. 2nd Int. Symp. Stenfert Kroese, Leiden, p. 60.

Platt, S. G., and D. D. Kasarda. 1971. Separation and characterization of α-gliadin fractions. Biochim. Biophys. Acta 243: 407.

Platt, S. G., D. D. Kasarda, and C. O. Qualset. 1974. Varietal relationships of the α-gliadin proteins in wheat. J. Sci. Food Agr. 25:1555.

Rossipal, E. 1971. Nachweis von präcipitierenden Antikörpern gegen wässrige Mehlextrakte bei Cöliakie. Z. Kinderheilk. 110:188.

Rossipal, E. 1974. Antigenic properties of gliadin proteins. *In* Coeliac Disease. W. Th. J. M. Hekkens and A. S. Peña (Editors). Proc. 2nd Int. Symp. Stenfert Kroese, Leiden, p. 76.

Rubin, C. E., L. L. Brandborg, A. Flick, W. C. MacDonald, R. A. Parkins, C. M. Parmentier, P. Phelps, S. Sribhibhadh, and J. S. Trier. 1962. Biopsy studies on the pathogenesis of coeliac sprue. *In* Intestinal Biopsy. G. E. W. Wolstenholme and M. P. Cameron (Editors). Ciba Foundation Study Group No. 14. Little, Brown and Co., Boston, p. 67.

Rubin, W. 1971. The epithelial "membrane" of the small intestine. Am. J. Clin. Nutr. 24:45.

Savilahti, E. 1974. Immunofluorescence in coeliac disease. *In* Coeliac Disease. W. Th. J. M. Hekkens and A. S. Peña (Editors). Proc. 2nd Int. Symp. Stenfert Kroese, Leiden, p. 163.

Schneider, R., M. J. Kendall, and C. F. Hawkins. 1974. Gliadin subfractionation. *In* Coeliac Disease. W. Th. J. M. Hekkens and A. S. Peña (Editors). Proc. 2nd Int. Symp. Stenfert Kroese, Leiden, p. 72.

Scott, B. B., S. M. Rajah, M. L. Swinburne, and M. S. Losowsky. 1974. HL-A8 and the immune response to gluten. Lancet. II: 374.

Shiner, M. 1974. Cell distribution in the jejunal mucosa in coeliac disease. *In* Coeliac Disease. W. Th. J. M. Hekkens and A. S. Peña (Editors). Proc. 2nd Int. Symp. Stenfert Kroese, Leiden, p. 121.

Shmerling, D. H., and M. Shiner. 1970. The response of the intestinal mucosa to the intraduodenal instillation of gluten in patients with coeliac disease during remission. *In* Coeliac Disease. C. C. Booth and R. H. Dowling (Editors). Proc. Int. Symp. Churchill Livingstone, Edinburgh, p. 64.

Stokes, P. L., P. Asquith, G. K. T. Holmes, P. Mackintosh, and W. T. Cooke. 1972. Histocompatibility antigens associated with adult coeliac disease. Lancet. II:162.

Strober, W. 1974. HL-A in relation to coeliac disease. *In*

Coeliac Disease. W. Th. J. M. Hekkens and A. S. Peña (Editors). Proc. 2nd Int. Symp. Stenfert Kroese, Leiden, p. 203.

Strumeyer, D. H. 1972. Protein amylase inhibitors in the gliadin fraction of wheat and rye flour: Possible factors in celiac disease. Nutr. Reports Int. 5:45.

Trier, J. S., and T. H. Browning. 1970. Epithelial cell renewal in cultured duodenal biopsies in celiac sprue. New Eng. J. Med. 283:1245.

Van de Kamer, J. H., and H. A. Weijers. 1955. Coeliac Disease. V. Some experiments on the cause of the harmful effect of wheat gliadin. Acta Paediat. 44:465.

Van de Kamer, J. H., H. A. Weijers, and W. K. Dicke. 1953. Coeliac Disease. IV. An investigation into the injurious constituents of wheat in connection with their action on patients with coeliac disease. Acta Paediat. 42:223.

Van de Kamer, J. H., H. A. Weijers, and E. A. K. Wauters. 1970. Some biochemical aspects of coeliac disease: Past, present, and future. *In* Coeliac Disease. C. C. Booth and R. H. Dowling (Editors). Proc. Int. Symp. Churchill Livingstone, Edinburgh, p. 106.

Visakorpi, J. K., and E. Savilahti. 1970. A clinical and morphological study of the permanence of gluten tolerance. *In* Coeliac Disease. C. C. Booth and R. H. Dowling (Editors). Proc. Int. Symp. Churchill Livingstone, Edinburgh, p. 224.

Wall, A. J., A. P. Douglas, C. C. Booth, and A. G. E. Pearse. 1970. Response of the jejunal mucosa in adult coeliac disease to oral prednisolone. Gut. 11:7.

Walker-Smith, J. A. 1973. Discordance for childhood coeliac disease in monozygotic twins. Gut. 14:374.

Weijers, H. A., J. H. Van de Kamer, and W. K. Dicke. 1957. Celiac disease. Advanc. Pediat. 9:277.

Weinstein, W. M., S. S. Shimoda, J. R. Brow, and C. E. Rubin. 1970. What is celiac sprue? *In* Coeliac Disease. C. C. Booth and R. H. Dowling (Editors). Proc. Int. Symp. Churchill Livingstone, Edinburgh, p. 232.

Woodley, J. F. 1972. Pyrrolidonecarboxylyl peptidase activity in normal intestinal biopsies and those from coeliac patients. Clin. Chim. Acta 42:211.

Wrigley, C. W., and K. W. Shepherd. 1973. Electrofocusing of grain proteins from wheat genotypes. Annals N.Y. Acad. Sci. 209:154.

BIOLOGIC EFFECTS OF
N^ε-(DL-2-AMINO-2-CARBOXYETHYL)-L-LYSINE, LYSINOALANINE

J. Carroll Woodard, Dennis D. Short,
Marvin R. Alvarez, and Jon Reyniers

Department of Pathology
College of Medicine
University of Florida
Gainesville, Florida

INTRODUCTION

Soybean meal, when properly processed, is considered an excellent source of amino acids for human needs. The globulin proteins isolated from soybean meal are used extensively in infant
formulas and in adult nutrition as meat extenders. For many years,
alkali treatment of soyprotein has been used by some cultural
groups to make a food known as "tofu," the washed soybean curd
formed by alkaline protein coagulation from a liquid dispersion of
meal (Standal, 1963, 1967). Alkali treatment is being increasingly
investigated by food technologists as a protein-processing method.
Within the past few years, food manufacturers have developed a process for forming fibers from isolated soyprotein and for incorporating these fibers into meat-like analogues which are finding consumer
acceptance as low-cholesterol meat substitutes. The steps involved
in fiber formation involve alkali treatment by dispersal of the soyprotein isolate in sodium hydroxide at pH 12 (Thulin and Kuramoto,
1967).

Although there have been increased investigations on processing methods and uses of alkali-treated proteins, there have not been paralleled research efforts to determine the nutritional effects of alkali treatment. De Groot and Slump (1969) investigated the effects of alkali treatment on food proteins under varying conditions of pH, temperature, and time. Their study showed that the exposure of several high-protein products to aqueous alkali resulted in the formation of the amino acid lysinoalanine. When the alkali treatment was made more severe, the protein's lysinoalanine content increased; and large increases were attended by decreased net protein utilization and protein digestibility.

A number of investigators have observed that alkali treatment of different proteins may cause chemical changes which lead to formation of new amino acids such as lanthionine (Horn et al., 1941), ornithinoalanine (Ziegler et al., 1967), and lysinoalanine (Patchornik and Sokolovsky, 1964; Bohak, 1964). Studies in our laboratory indicate that one of these, lysinoalanine, has a nephrotoxic effect in rats. Although this amino acid has not been reported in soyprotein textured foods, large quantities have been demonstrated in an animal confectionery product used as a commercial foaming agent (De Groot and Slump, 1969).

The biologic effects of this amino acid should be investigated to determine its potential effects on human and animal health. The purpose of this paper is to describe renal alterations that occurred in rats fed semi-purified diets containing either an alkali-treated protein (alpha protein) or organically synthesized lysinoalanine.

ALKALI-TREATED SOYPROTEINS

It was originally demonstrated that weanling rats fed semi-purified diets containing 20% of alpha protein developed unique renal lesions characterized by cytomegalic changes in the straight portion of the proximal tubule (Woodard and Alvarez, 1967). Alpha protein is an industrial soyprotein which has been modified by alkali treatment to develop maximum adhesive properties.

Subsequently, it was shown that the toxicity of the alpha protein
was related to alkaline modification, and such treatment also induced the formation of lysinoalanine (Woodard and Short, 1973).
Investigations of the renal morphologic changes induced by alkali-
treated soyproteins have been carried out over a period of several
years. Even though similar diets and strains of animals have been
used, the morphologic lesions observed during the earlier investi-
gative periods were found to be more severe than those observed
during the past year. Limited attempts to determine the reason for
the variation of expression have shown that the differences are not
related to the dietary level of protein, mineral composition, or
level of methionine. Since the majority of our morphologic investigations were carried out prior to finding that renal lesions were
caused by lysinoalanine, the dietary content of lysinoalanine was
not determined in the earlier experiments. Lysinoalanine analysis
of three separate batches of alpha protein varied between 0.4 and
0.7 percent (w/w).

Methods

The specific details of the methods used in the various experiments have been described elsewhere (Woodard and Alvarez, 1967;
Woodard and Short, 1973; Woodard, 1969; Reyniers et al., 1974).
The composition of the various animal diets is shown in Table 1
because typographical errors appear in one of the original reports
(Woodard and Short, 1973). Animals were fed semi-purified diets
containing either an edible soyprotein (Promine D), or alkali-
treated soyprotein (alpha protein). The 20 percent soyprotein diets
were similar in each experiment except the mineral composition was
changed; and in one study of the nuclear cytochemical alterations,
the level of protein was increased from 20 to 30 percent (Reyniers
et al., 1974). During each experimental period, animals were fed
alpha protein from a single batch; and the data which is presented
was collected from animals which demonstrated lesions of renal
tubular cytomegalia. Investigations were carried out on weanling

TABLE 1

Composition of Diets

Item	Portion of diet, %	
	I	II
Sucrose	54.5	44.5
Soyprotein[a]	20.0	30.0
Minerals[b]	5.0	5.0
Cottonseed oil[c]	10.0	10.0
DL-methionine	0.3	0.3
Choline bitartrate	0.2	0.2
Vitamins[d]	10.0	10.0

[a]Promine D or Alpha Protein, Central Soya Co., Chicago. (0.1% methionine).

[b]i. Hegstead Salts, Nutritional Biochemical Corporation, Cleveland, Ohio. Hegsted, M. et al. : Choline in the nutrition of chicks. J. Biol. Chem. 1941. 138:459.

ii. Mineral mixture was added to the diet in sucrose carrier and contained the following, (g/100 g mixture): dibasic calcium phosphate, 43.33; calcium carbonate, 7.59; sodium chloride, 3.81; potassium chloride, 6.43; potassium sulfate, 3.63; magnesium oxide, 1.99; ferric citrate, 0.30; zinc carbonate, 0.043; magnesium carbonate, 0.22; cupric carbonate, 0.018; potassium iodide, 0.0004; mineral mixture was prepared by the method of Bernhart and Tomarelli; a salt mixture supplying the National Research Council estimates of the mineral requirements of the rat. J. Nutr. 1966. 89:495.

iii. Mineral mixture was added to diet in sucrose carrier and contained the following, (g/100 g mixture): dibasic calcium phosphate, 43.33; calcium carbonate, 7.59; magnesium chloride, 19.0; potassium citrate, 8.28; potassium chloride, 7.88; sodium chloride, 3.28; potassium sulfate, 0.84; ferric citrate, 0.64; potassium iodine, 0.016; manganeous sulfate, 0.38; aluminum potassium sulfate, 0.0032; zinc chloride, 0.05; cupric sulfate, 0.04.

[c]Wesson Oil, Wesson Oil Sales Company, Fullerton, California.

[d]Vitamins were added to the diet in sucrose carrier and contained the following, (mg/100 g diet): thiamine $\cdot$ HCl, 1.6; pyridoxide $\cdot$ HCl, 1.6; riboflavin, 1.6; D-calcium pantothenate, 4.0; nicotinic acid amide, 5.0; folic acid, 0.5; inositol (meso), 10.0; DL-α-tochopheryl acetate, 1.0; menadione, 1.0; vitamin B_{12}, 0.0005 (IU/100 g diet); vitamin A palmitate, 2,500; vitamin D_2, 600.

albino rats of the Sprague-Dawley strain. During the various experiments, single animals or pairs were housed in raised, screen-wire cages in air-conditioned animal quarters; food and water were supplied ad libitum. Some animals were maintained on the dietary regimens as long as nine months. Other animals were killed at weekly intervals for the first three weeks, and every other week thereafter until the fourteenth week of experimental feeding. Kidney tissue was placed in fixative and processed by standard methods for light and electron microscopic examination. Autoradio-graphic and colchicine injection techniques were used to study DNA synthesis and to compare the number of cells within the synthetic and mitotic phases of the cell cycle (Woodard, 1969). Quantitative measurements of nuclear DNA, total protein, total histones, protein-bound sulfhydryl groups, chromatin thermal denaturation, acridine-orange dye binding by DNA, and bromphenol blue binding by arginine and lysine residues of histones were made on nuclei isolated from treated- or control-rat kidneys (Woodard, 1969; Reyniers et al., 1974). In addition, an attempt was made to determine if there was any alteration in the renal function of cytomegalic tubular cells. Four animals from both the treated and control groups were anesthe-tized after the eighth experimental week and given hypertonic mannitol solution. After their canulated ureters were occluded, intravenous injections of 5.4 mg C^{14}-labeled inulin (sp. act. 1 x 10^{-4} mC/mg) and 1.0 mg tritium-labeled para aminohippurate (sp. act. 2 x 10^{-3} mC/mg) were given, and stop-flow urine analysis of each radioactive substance was determined.

Results

After two weeks on the diet, an increased number of polyploid cells in alpha protein-fed animals were detected by quantitative techniques, and at the end of the third week, marked photometric differences were obtained. At the end of the fourth week of exper-imental feeding, animals receiving the alkali-treated protein had microscopic evidence of cytomegalia which could be detected by

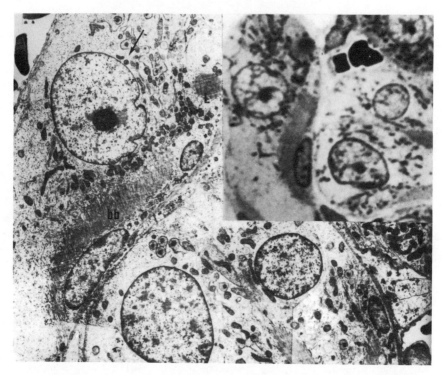

FIG. 1. Electron micrograph montage and light micrograph
(inset) of cytomegalic cells of pars recta from animal fed alpha
protein diet. Areas shown at higher magnification in Figures 5
and 6 are marked (↑). Correspondence of the light and electron
micrographs between the cytoplasmic organelles, brush border (bb),
and lipid inclusion (L) can be noted. Inset, X 920.

observing occasional large nuclei with increased amounts of

Feulgen-positive nuclear material. There was only a slight in-

crease in the maximal nuclear size between the fourth and fourteenth

experimental week; however, there was an obvious increase in the

number of karyomegalic nuclei and polyploid cells which reached a

maximum during the eighth to tenth week. At nine months, nuclei

could be detected having a much larger nuclear volume than that

demonstrated at fourteen weeks.

Electron microscopic studies showed that the cytomegalic

changes induced by alpha protein feeding were limited to the pars

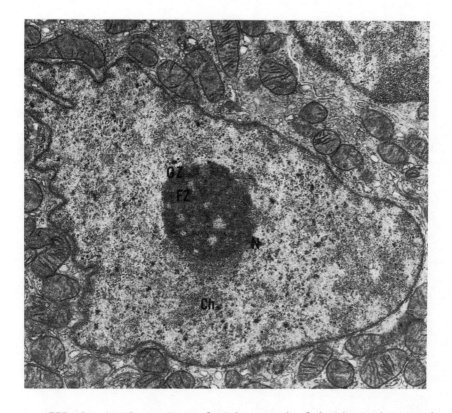

FIG. 2. As the nucleus of alpha protein-fed animals increased in size, the nuclear envelope became ruffled or scalloped. The nucleolus (N) shows DNA-containing fibrillar zones (FZ) and RNA-rich granular zones (GZ). Clumps of chromatin (heterochromatin) can also be observed (Ch), X 8,855.

recta of the renal ·tubule and were characterized by increases in both the nuclear and cytoplasmic portions of the cell (Figure 1). When the nucleus began to enlarge, the nuclear envelope frequently became ruffled or scalloped (Figure 2). With continued enlargement, cytoplasmic invaginations into the nucleus formed intranuclear inclusions containing lysosomes, endoplasmic reticulum, and lipid (Figures 3 and 4). Although the megalic cells often had multiple or enlarged nucleoli, no differences in the morphologic characteristics of the nuclear chromatin or cytoplasmic organelles

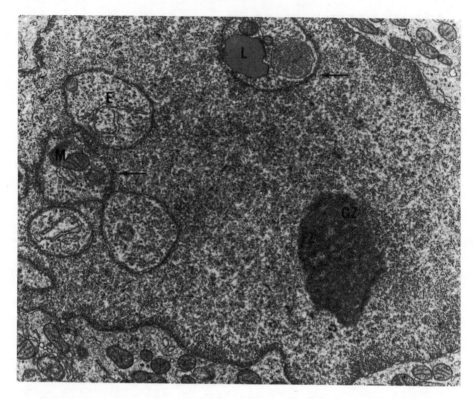

FIG. 3. Irregularity of the nuclear envelope led to invagina-
tion and to development of intranuclear inclusions (↑) which contain
mitochondria (M), endoplasmic reticulum (E), and lipid (L). The
fibrillar (FZ) and granular nucleolar zones (GZ) can be seen,
X 8,788.

were observed between enlarged cells and cells of normal size
(Figures 5 and 6).

Quantitative measurements of nuclear DNA, protein-bound sulfhydryl groups, and total histones in isolated cytomegalic nuclei
indicated that the majority, but not all, had increased quantities
of DNA and chromosomal proteins (Figures 7 and 8). Increased
nuclear size was accompanied by a proportional increase in the
amount of total nuclear protein (Figure 9). In some animals, there
were a large number of cytomegalic nuclei that had values intermediate between the 2C and 4C amounts of DNA, and nuclei

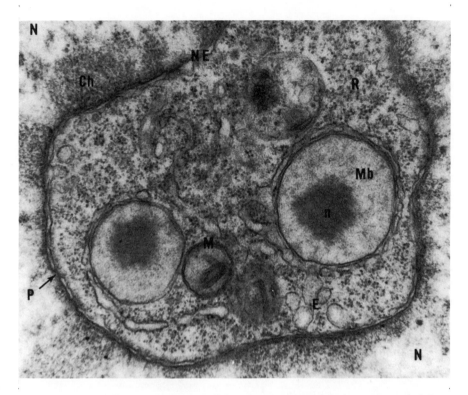

FIG. 4. The inclusion within the nucleus (N) is surrounded by a system of two membranes [nuclear envelope (NE)] which is interrupted by pores (P). Chromatin (Ch) is clumped around the outside, and the inclusion contains normal cytoplasmic constituents : ribosomes (R), mitochondria (M), smooth endoplasmic reticulum (E), and microbodies (Mb) with homogeneous matrix enclosing nucleoid (n), X 38,996.

representing the 6C and 8C DNA levels were observed. Intermediate DNA values could represent interphase nuclei that were in the process of doubling their DNA content.

During the second and third experimental weeks, the synthesis of DNA and number of mitoses were increased within the inner cortical stripe of the kidney of the alpha protein-fed animals. This is the zone where cytomegalic cells later developed. After cytomegalia was manifested, a number of cells with enlarged nuclei were found synthesizing DNA; and the size of the nuclei continued to increase

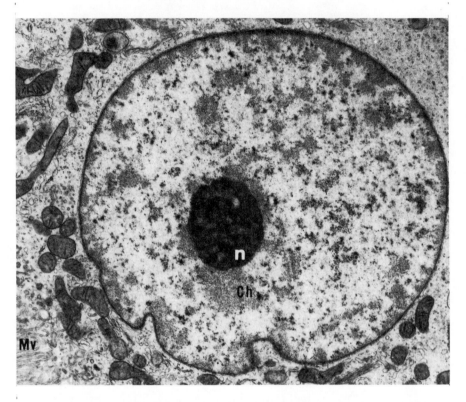

FIG. 5. Karyomegalic nucleus of renal tubular cell shown in
Figure 1. Chromatin (Ch) is clumped around the large nucleolus (N).
Microvilli (Mv), X 6,255.

after cessation of DNA synthesis. Microfluorometric measurements
of acridine orange bound by the chromatin complex of the nuclei revealed approximately a 2.5 fold increase in the dye-binding capacity
of megalocytes over cells of normal size (Figure 10). There were
also significant differences in the chromatin thermal stability
(Figure 11), and there was an altered ratio of histone residues of
arginine and lysine between megalic and normal-sized nuclei
(Table 2).

In order to determine if there was a functional impairment in
the cells of the proximal renal tubule to secrete para aminohippurate, stop-flow urine analysis was performed. There was no

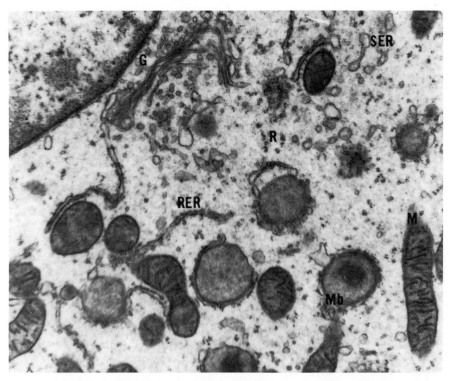

FIG. 6. The cytomegalic cell (Figure 1) contains normal cytoplasmic constituents including golgi complex (G), mitochondria (M), microbodies (Mb), rough endoplasmic reticulum (RER), ribosomes (R), and smooth endoplasmic reticulum (SER), X 13,282.

statistical difference in the values from treated and control groups (Figure 12).

SYNTHESIZED LYSINOALANINE

Methods

Lysinoalanine was synthesized by a modification of the method of Okuda and Zahn (1965). The amino acid gave a single peak on a Durrum amino acid analyzer and contained a single spot by thin-layer chromatography. The detailed synthetic methods and results of feeding experiments will be reported in detail elsewhere.

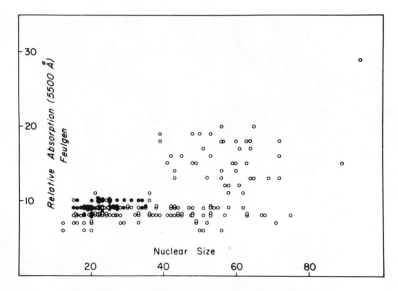

FIG. 7. Kidney cell DNA values obtained from treated (open circles) and control (closed circles) animals. Cells of normal size (less than 40) have diploid amounts of DNA. Some large nuclei contain diploid amounts of DNA; whereas, others are tetraploid. One octaploid nucleus is observed, as well as many others with values intermediate between the diploid and tetraploid level.

Female, weanling, 45-55 g albino rats of the Sprague-Dawley strain were divided into groups of three animals, and each group was fed a semi-purified diet containing 0, 0.025, 0.05, 0.1, and 0.3 percent lysinoalanine. Animals were killed after they had been on the diets for four weeks, and kidney tissues were processed by standard methods for light microscopic examination.

In addition, two animals were given daily intraperitoneal injections of 30 mg of lysinoalanine (dissolved in 1 ml of water with the aid of a sonicator). Two control animals were given daily intraperitoneal injections of 30 mg of L-lysine monohydrochloride. Other groups were given 30 mg of lysinoalanine or 30 mg L-lysine monohydrochloride daily by stomach tube. All animals were killed the day after the seventh treatment, and the kidney tissues processed for light microscopic examination.

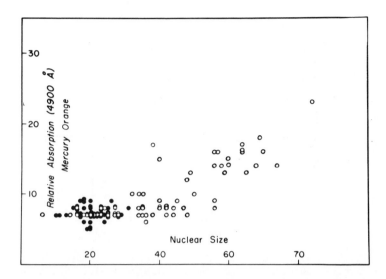

FIG. 8. Values for nuclear protein-bound sulfhydryl groups (chromosomal protein) obtained from treated (open circles) and control (closed circles) animals. The distribution pattern in karyomegalic nuclei coincides with the values obtained for DNA (Figure 7), and cells with values intermediate between diploid and tetraploid values can be noted. Similar results were obtained when stainable histones were determined.

Results

Kidney lesions were observed in all animals fed the lysinoalanine diets, and the lesions were more severe with the higher dose levels. A marked karyomegalic reaction was observed in both the inner and outer cortical zones of animals receiving the 0.3 percent level (Figure 13). Many of the tubular cells within the pars recta lacked their normal brush border, some cells had pyknotic nuclei, and intraluminal protein casts were present. Tubular dilitation and regeneration were also observed.

The lesions were not as severe in animals receiving the 0.1 percent lysinoalanine diets. The histopathologic reaction was more or less limited to the inner cortical zone. Tubules in this region were dilated, and many giant nuclei were present. There appeared to be loss of some tubular epithelial cells, and the remaining cells

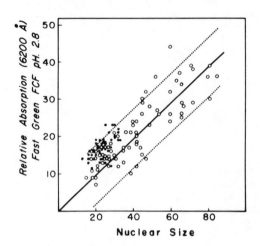

FIG. 9. Values for total nuclear protein obtained from treated (open circles) and control (closed circles) animals. The total nuclear-protein content increased in a linear fashion and was proportional to the degree of nuclear enlargement. This is in contrast to the results obtained for DNA (Figure 7) or chromosomal protein (Figure 8).

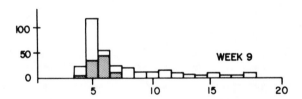

FIG. 10. Frequency distribution of acridine orange binding by kidney nuclei of rats fed control (stippled bars) or alpha protein diets (open bars) for 9 weeks. Approximately 15 percent of the nuclei from alpha protein animals show increased dye-binding capacity, and the maximal dye binding is increased approximately 2.5 fold.

lacked their normal eosinophilic staining properties. The kidneys of animals receiving either 0.05 or 0.025 percent lysinoalanine did not differ markedly from the 0.1 percent group. Many cells in the inner cortical zone had giant nuclei, but there was not as much evidence of tubular destruction (Figure 14).

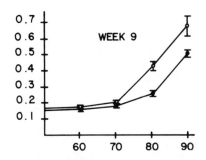

FIG. 11. Chromatin thermal stability in megalic (open circles) and normal (closed circles) nuclei isolated from animal fed alpha protein diet for 9 weeks. Abscissa: temperature, in °C; ord. 590/530 nm fluorescence emission ratio (metachromatic ratio) in arbitrary units. Mean values for normal nuclei from the alpha protein animal were similar to those from animals fed the control diet. The differences in mean metachromatic ratio of megalic and normal nuclei at 90° are significant at the 5 percent level of probability. This implies that karyomegalic transformation involves a decreased thermal stability of the chromatin as well as a relative increase in the availability of DNA phosphates.

TABLE 2

Bromphenol-blue Dye Binding by Lysine and Arginine
Residues in Kidney Cell Nuclear Histones of Rats
Fed Alpha Protein or Control Diets for 9 Weeks

Binding	Nuclei from control animals	Nuclei from alpha protein animals	
		Normal size	Megalic
Binding by lysine and arginine residues (total histones)	10.5±0.125	10.5±0.204	18.1±0.255[a]
Binding by lysine residues	5.5±0.095	5.3±0.105	10.4±0.224
Binding by arginine residues	5.0	5.1	7.6
Lysine/arginine	1.1	1.1	1.4[b]

[a]Mean dye binding by both lysine and arginine was higher in megalic nuclei than normal-sized nuclei, a reflection of their increased chromatin content.

[b]The increase in lysine staining of megalic nuclei is proportionally greater (significant at the 5 percent level) than that of arginine, an indication that karyomegalia is accompanied by an altered availability of lysine residues in histones in relation to the amount of stainable lysine.

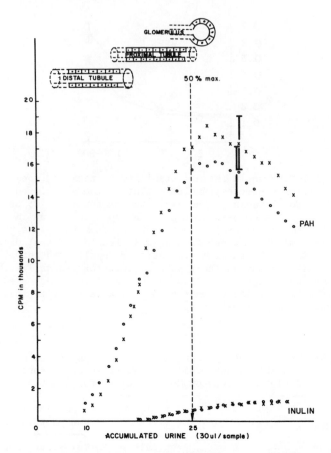

FIG. 12. Stop-flow urine analysis of para aminohippurate secretion in alpha protein (0) and control (X) animals. Each point represents the mean of four animals, and the data range is indicated. Fifty percent of the maximum inulin secretion marks the appearance of new glomerular filtrate. No significant differences in the two treatments could be detected.

Renal lesions were observed when 30 mg of lysinoalanine were given orally or intraperitoneally for seven days, but no reaction was observed in animals given the lysine. Lesions were limited almost exclusively to the inner cortical zone, and dilitation of the proximal tubules, necrosis of epithelial cells, and karyomegalia were observed in this region (Figure 15).

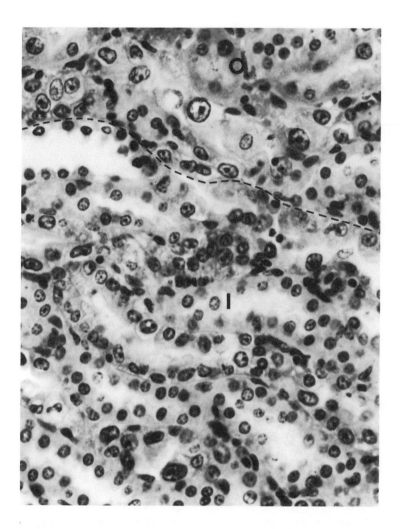

FIG. 13. Junction of the inner (I) and outer (O) renal cortical zones (dotted line) of animal receiving the 0.3% lysinoalanine
diet for four weeks. Karyomegalia can be observed in proximal
tubules from both the inner and outer cortical regions. Notice
nuclear enlargement in the inner cortex is not as marked as those
fed lower doses of lysinoalanine (Figure 14), and the cells of the
pars recta no longer contain their normal brush border. Hematoxylin
and eosin, X 116.

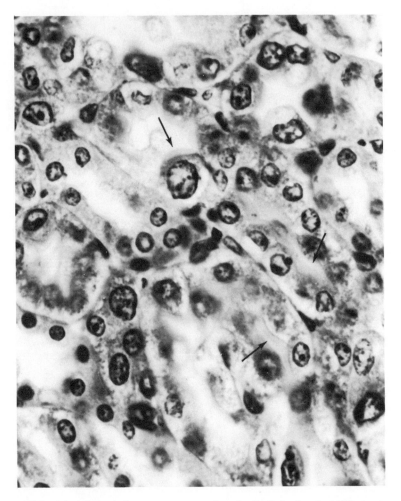

FIG. 14.   Renal inner cortex of animal fed the 0.025% lysinoalanine diet for four weeks.   Karyomegalia and the tubular brush
border (↑) are evident.   Destruction of renal tubular cells in the
inner cortex was not as marked in animals given lower doses of
lysinoalanine.   Hematoxylin and eosin, X 450.

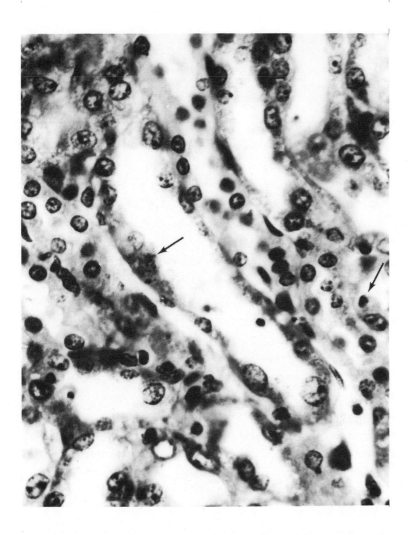

FIG. 15. Renal inner cortex from rat receiving intraperitoneal injections of lysinoalanine for one week. There is tubular dilitation and necrosis (↑) of epithelial cells of the pars recta. There has been loss of the normal brush border, and karyomegalic alterations are already present. Hematoxylin and eosin, X 450.

DISCUSSION

It can now be conclusively stated that the cytomegalic lesions in rats fed alpha protein or alkali-treated edible soyprotein (Woodard and Short, 1973) are the result of the lysinoalanine formed during alkaline modification. It appears that semi-purified diets are more toxic when the free amino acid is used than when the amino acid forms an integral part of the protein molecule. Since both oral and intraperitoneal injections of lysinoalanine produced a similar effect, it is the absorbed amino acid that is the nephrotoxic agent. Differences in protein digestibility might explain the variability observed in the production of renal lesions with alkali-treated proteins of high lysinoalanine content. De Groot and Slump (1969) reported that treatment of isolated soyprotein at pH 12.2 and room temperature for 60 or 10 minutes resulted in 0.2 and 0.03 g lysinoalanine/16 g protein nitrogen. If this protein constituted 20% of the diet, the ingested lysinoalanine would be in the same concentration range as that used in the low-level nephrotoxic experimental diets (0.025% free amino acid).

The mode of action of this renal toxin is speculative. Its selectivity for the pars recta is reminiscent of the action of low levels of mercuric bichloride or transient anoxia. Unlike mercuric bichloride, however, high levels (0.3%) of lysinoalanine destroy the inner cortical zone before the cells of the outer cortex are affected. In addition, lysinoalanine causes karyomegalia which is not observed with mercuric bichloride or anoxia. The nuclear reaction probably proceeds independently of the necrotic changes which were observed in the high dose groups. The data on the physiochemical properties of chromatin of hyperdiploid nuclei are consistent with the view that megalocytes represent "activated" renal tubular cells, and these cells probably have an altered functional state (Reyniers et al., 1974).

Although the renal proximal tubule is divided into three distinct morphologic regions, little is known concerning differences in their physiologic functions. The cells of the pars recta are capable of endocytosis of macromolecules, and they are active in both the secretion of para aminohippurate and in the transport of amino acids (McDowell, 1974). The basic amino acids are thought to be resorbed in this portion of the nephron by a single transport mechanism (Meister, 1973). Reduction in the excretion of para aminohippurate could not be demonstrated in animals whose kidneys had megalia nuclei but no morphologic evidence of cell necrosis. This probably results because the excretion of para aminohippurate by the proximal tubule is not limited to the pars recta. The nephron units vary considerably in length, and a given sample of urine is not derived from exactly the same nephron segment. Since the functions of the renal tubular cells of the pars recta have not been adequately defined, it may be difficult to access physiologic alterations in lysinoalanine-induced karyomegalic cells.

This work has significance because it illustrates the difficulties involved in determining the quality of a protein. Many questions remain unanswered as to whether lysinoalanine is of practical importance in human or animal health. Many substances (e.g., lead, dimethylgold, pyrrolizidine alkaloids) which induce renal karyomegalia have been shown to be tumorogenic. There is no evidence that lysinoalanine has this potential; however, the possibility that lysinoalanine may be carcinogenic must be ruled out by animal experimentation.

A model has been established by which renal lesions can be induced by the parenteral administration of relatively small quantities of lysinoalanine. Lesions are analogous to those seen in rats fed alkali-treated proteins for much longer periods of time. Such a model should prove useful in further evaluations of the biologic significance of this unusual amino acid.

REFERENCES

Bohak, Z. 1964. N^{ε}-(DL-2-amino-2-carboxyethyl)-L-lysine, a new amino acid formed on alkaline treatment of proteins. J. Biol. Chem. 239:2878.

De Groot, A.P. and P. Slump. 1969. Effects of severe alkali treatment of proteins on amino acid composition and nutritive value. J. Nutr. 98:45.

Horn, M.J., D.B. Jones and S.J. Ringel. 1941. Isolation of a new sulfur-containing amino acid (lanthionine) from sodium carbonate-treated wool. J. Biol. Chem. 138:141.

McDowell, Elizabeth M. 1974. Unbuffered osmium staining in pars recta of the proximal tubule from rat kidney studied by thin and semi-thin section cytochemistry. Histochemistry. 39:335.

Meister, Alton. 1973. On the enzymology of amino acid transport. Science. 180:33.

Okuda, Toru and Helmut Zahn. 1965. Synthese von N^{ε}-(2-Amino-2-caboxy-äthyl)-L-lysin, einer neuen Aminosäure aus alkalibehandelter Wolle. Chem. Ber. 98:1164.

Patchornik, A. and M. Sokolovsky. 1964. Chemical interactions between lysine and dehydroalanine in modified bovine pancreatic ribonuclease. J. Amer. Chem. Soc. 86:1860.

Reyniers, Jon P., James C. Woodard and Marvin R. Alvarez. 1974. Nuclear cytochemical alterations in α-protein-induced nephrocytomegalia. Lab. Investigation. 30:582.

Standal, B.R. 1963. Nutritional value of proteins of oriental soybean foods. J. Nutr. 81:279.

Standal, B.R. 1967. Amino acids in oriental soybean foods. J. Amer. Dietetics Association. 50:397.

Thulin, W.W. and S. Kuramoto. 1967. Bontrae, a new meat-like ingredient for convenience foods. Food Technol. 21:168.

Woodard, James C. 1969. On the pathogenesis of alpha protein-induced nephrocytomegalia. Lab. Investigation. 20:9.

Woodard, James C. and Marvin R. Alvarez. 1967. Renal lesions in rats fed diets containing alpha protein. Arch. Path. 84:153.

Woodard, James C. and Dennis D. Short. 1973. Toxicity of alkali-treated soyprotein in rats. J. Nutr. 103:569.

Ziegler, K., I. Melchert and C. Lurken. 1967. N^{ε}-(2-amino-2-carboxyethyl)-ornithine, a new amino acid from alkali-treated proteins. Nature. 214:404.

Editor's Note

I wish to comment on the preceding paper by Woodard et al. concerning lysinoalanine. Rate studies show that SH groups react about three to thirteen hundred times faster than NH_2 groups with reactive vinyl compounds (Friedman, 1973; Friedman et al., 1965; Cavins and Friedman, 1968; Snow et al., 1975 a, b). For this reason, adding thiol compounds such as cysteine and reduced glutathione during alkali treatment of soy (or other) protein could trap residues of dehydroalanine or methyldehydroalanine (reactive vinyl compounds) formed by alkali as transient products. Lysinoalanine formation would be minimized by this competitive reaction; lanthionine and methyllanthionine residues would be produced instead. This expectation appears to have been realized (Finley et al., 1975).

Two additional points are noteworthy. First, the above reasoning implies that dehydroalanine may react with enzymatic or other essential sulfhydryl groups in vivo. Such reactions have been postulated by Gross for dehydroalanine- and methyldehydroalanine-containing peptide antibiotics (Gross 1971; 1974). Pharmacological consequences of such reactions are worth exploring. It is similarly possible that lysinoalanine exerts its pharmacological effect on kidneys by undergoing a reverse-Michael reaction in situ to form dehydroalanine as the reactive agent. Second, metal ions, especially transition metal ions, also show strong, varied affinity for thiols and amines (Friedman, 1974). Metal ions may therefore also effectively compete with dehydroalanine for SH or NH_2 groups, both in vivo and in vitro, and thus affect the relative reactivity of sulfhydryl and amino groups. These possibilities deserve careful study.

References

Cavins, J.F. and M. Friedman. 1968. Specific modification of protein sulfhydryl groups with α,β-unsaturated compounds. J. Biol. Chem. 243:3357.

EDITOR'S NOTE

REFERENCES

Cavins, J.F. and M. Friedman. 1968. Specific modification of
protein sulfhydryl groups with α,β-unsaturated compounds.
J. Biol. Chem. 243:3357.

Finley, J.W., J.T. Snow, and M. Friedman. 1975. Inhibiting the
formation of lysinoalanine. USDA Patent Case No 6115.

Friedman, M., Editor. 1974. Protein-Metal Interactions.
Plenum, New York, N.Y. Chapters 2, 15, 24. See also
Chapter 2 of the following reference.

Friedman, M. 1973. The Chemistry and Biochemistry of the Sulfhydryl
Group in Amino Acids, Peptides, and Proteins. Pergamon Press,
Oxford, England and Elmsford, New York. Chapter 4.

Friedman, M., J.F. Cavins, and J.S. Wall. 1965. Relative nucleophilic reactivities of amino groups and mercaptide ions
with α,β-unsaturated compounds. J. Am. Chem. Soc. 87:3572.

Gross, E. 1971. Structure and function of peptides with α,β-unsatu-
rated amino acids. Intra-Science Chem. Repts. 5:405.

Gross, E. 1974. α,β-Unsaturated amino acids in peptides and proteins:
formation, chemistry and biological role. Abstracts, 168th
Meeting of the American Chemical Society, Atlantic City,
New Jersey. p. AGFD 13.

Snow, J.T., J.W. Finley, and M. Friedman. 1975a. A kinetic study
of the hydrolysis of N-acetyldehydroalanine and N-acetyldehydroalanine methyl ester. Int. J. Peptide Protein Res.
(In press).

Snow, J.T., J.W. Finley, and M. Friedman. 1975b. Relative reactivi-
ties of sulfhydryl groups with N-acetyldehydroalanine and
N-acetyl dehydroalanine methyl ester. Int. J. Peptide Protein
Res. (In press).

618

PROTEIN:ENERGY RATIOS--
GUIDELINES IN THE ASSESSMENT OF PROTEIN NUTRITIONAL QUALITY

G. H. Beaton

Department of Nutrition and Food Science
Faculty of Medicine
University of Toronto
Toronto, Canada

Protein:energy ratios are useful, albeit limited, criteria of
the nutritional quality of the diets of individuals or groups of
individuals. Many of the interpretative criteria published in the
literature at present have been erroneously calculated for their
intended purpose. Appropriate criteria have been derived through a
probability approach taking into account the variabilities of requirements for energy and for protein, the correlation between them,
and, for population groups, the variability of the observed protein:
energy ratio in self-selected diets. Empirically the derived ratios
appear to be relatively independent of growth rate, age, and sex
(except perhaps in the cases of young infants and pregnant or
lactating women where appropriate criteria could not be derived with
existing data). The "safe" or "desirable" protein:energy ratios
were found to be dependent upon protein quality, habitual level of
voluntary activity, and, in population groups, variability of the
protein:energy ratio of self-selected diets. A number of limitations to the application and interpretation of these criteria have
been outlined and potential uses have been identified. While the
orientation of this paper and the calculations therein have been

toward the assessment of human diets, certain of the principles are applicable to animal feeds. The principles and approaches outlined in this paper may also be applicable to the assessment of the quality of diets with reference to other nutrients.

In the present paper, the estimates of energy and protein requirements published by an FAO/WHO committee have been used as the basis of calculation. While these estimates, and hence the derived protein:energy ratios may be altered as additional data become available, the underlying principles governing the derivation and interpretation of "safe" or "desirable" protein:energy ratios should remain unaltered.

INTRODUCTION

The calculation of the protein:energy ratio (protein energy as percent of total energy) has found wide use as one of the descriptors of quality of foods and diets. However, it is an imperfectly understood concept and the criteria for the interpretation of observed ratios have often been miscalculated, perhaps leading to seriously erroneous interpretations.

Properly used, the protein:energy ratio is a valid and useful measurement. Conceptually, it is a measure of the ability of a given food, feed, or diet to meet protein requirements when consumed in sufficient quantity to meet the energy needs of the host. Thus, a basic assumption in the establishment of interpretative criteria is that food intake is regulated in accord with energy requirement among free-living individuals given free access to food. There is much evidence that over long periods this assumption is valid provided that the diet is nutritionally adequate and is free of noxious materials or undesirable flavors that inhibit appetite.

The interpretative criterion then must consider both the protein requirement and the energy requirement (determinant of energy intake) of the host. It is well known that both of these are subject to individual variation. Human dietary standards commonly cite a level of protein intake that is sufficiently high to meet the needs of almost all individuals, thereby exceeding the actual needs of most individuals. This level of intake may be described as the "recommended," "desirable," or "safe" level of intake; it is a level which, for the individual, carries very little risk of inadequate intake (Beaton, 1972). In contrast, although energy requirements also exhibit individual variability, dietary standards commonly cite only the average requirement figure; in the case of energy, both inadequate and excess intakes are thought of as carrying a risk to the individual.

The use of the numbers in a dietary standard for the calculation of an interpretative criterion for protein:energy ratios therefore presents a problem. This may be illustrated from the requirement estimates reported by an FAO/WHO committee (1973). For adult man average protein requirement was estimated to be 0.44 g egg or milk protein/kg body weight; average energy requirement was estimated to be 46 kcal/kg body weight. The coefficient of variation of protein requirement was reported as 15% and the "safe level of intake" was set at 0.57 g egg or milk protein/kg body weight. The FAO/WHO group did not stipulate a coefficient of variation for energy, but Beaton and Swiss (1974) found a value of about 15% from a search of the literature. Using these figures and assuming a value of 4 kcal/g as the energy equivalent of protein, four different protein:energy ratios may be calculated as shown in Table 1.

The first two of the ratios in Table 1 are of the types that are usually cited in the literature. While the third and fourth examples represent types of calculations that have not been used in the literature, they are cited for the sake of completeness. They are just as logical as the first two examples.

This, then, portrays the basic quandary. What ratio should be calculated as the criterion for the assessment of diets? A subsidiary, but equally important, question relates to the use of the criterion for the observed diet of an individual or the average diet of a group of individuals. Since not all individuals in the population

TABLE 1

Some Simple Protein:Energy Ratios for Adult Men[a,b]

Protein requirement	Energy requirement	Derived ratio (protein[c] as % energy)
Average	Average	3.8
Average + 2 S. D.[d]	Average	5.0
Average	Average + 2 S. D.	2.6
Average + 2 S. D.	Average + 2 S. D.	3.7

[a]None of these ratios are correct criteria for the interpretation of observed dietary ratios (see Tables 2 and 3).

[b]Based on FAO/WHO requirement figures (1973).

[c]Egg or milk protein.

[d]Mean requirement + 2 S.D. would meet or exceed the requirements of 97.5% of individuals. By convention, this is the level that is customarily published in human dietary standards.

will consume identical diets, a moment's reflection will reveal that it would be illogical to adopt the same criterion to judge the adequacy of an individual diet and the average diet of a number of individuals.

Beaton and Swiss (1974) have examined these problems and have offered interpretative guidelines. Their approach has been severely criticized by Sukhatme (1974, 1975) and by Payne (1975). These criticisms have been answered by Corey and Beaton (1975) who again assert the validity of the statistical approaches while recognizing some qualifications that should be applied to the interpretation of protein:energy ratios. The mathematical basis of the calculations will not be discussed here (see A.R. Schulz, Part 1, this volume). Rather, emphasis will be placed upon the underlying concepts and interpretation of protein:energy ratios of human diets.

CRITERIA FOR THE ASSESSMENT OF INDIVIDUAL DIETS

Theoretical Basis

The protein:energy ratio of a diet would be judged inadequate if it is probable that when the diet is consumed at a level that satiated the energy requirement of the host, his protein requirement remains unmet. Beaton and Swiss (1974) approached the definition of the criterion on a probability basis employing the bivariate distribution of protein and energy requirements (Lörstad, 1971). As in the case of "recommended," "desirable," or "safe" levels of nutrient intakes, it was decided to adopt a criterion that would ensure that protein requirements were met or exceeded for 97.5% of individuals when their personal energy requirements were met. In this approach, the variability of energy requirement and of protein requirement were considered as well as the correlation between them. "Safe" or "desirable" ratios were calculated for several age groups using requirement estimates published by the FAO/WHO group (1973).

In his criticism of Beaton and Swiss (1974), Payne (1975) pointed out that while they had restricted their calculations to persons with "moderate" or "average" levels of voluntary activity, not all population groups exhibited activity levels this high. If activity were reduced, energy requirements would fall and the necessary protein:energy ratio would rise. He pointed out that in areas where food was not readily available, children might compensate through a reduction of voluntary activity without interference with growth rate. While this may or may not be a desirable situation from the standpoint of behavioral and social development, it appears to be a practical situation in some areas of the world (Rutishauser and Whitehead, 1972). Shortage of food is not the only reason for low voluntary activity levels. In North America, energy requirements appear to be appreciably lower than that of the moderately active man described by the FAO/WHO group (1973) presumably because of the customary life style.

Table 2 presents criteria for "safe" or "desirable" protein:energy ratios based upon the requirement estimates published by

623

TABLE 2

Criteria for the Interpretation
of the Protein:Energy Ratio of Individual Diets

Age/sex group	Activity level	"Desirable" or "safe" protein:energy ratio (protein[a] as % energy)
Children, 2-3 years	Average[b]	5.3
	"Maintenance"[c]	6.7
Children, 6-8 years	Average	5.1
Male adolescents	Average	5.1
Male adults	Moderate	5.4
	Light	6.1
	U.S. figures for energy requirement[d]	6.4

[a]As egg or milk protein.

[b]As described by FAO/WHO group (1973) unless otherwise noted.

[c]As estimated by Payne (1975); this is about 80% of the level suggested in the FAO/WHO report (1973).

[d]Food and Nutrition Board (1974).

FAO/WHO (Beaton and Swiss, 1974; Corey and Beaton, 1975). Also shown are ratios appropriate to individuals with lower levels of voluntary activity as suggested by Payne (1975). The similarity of predictions based upon moderate activity in adults and average activity in children is readily apparent. Empirically, the ratio seems to be relatively independent of age or growth rate. This may not be true for young infants or for pregnant or lactating women. Present data are inadequate to estimate correlation between protein and energy requirements in these groups and hence to calculate "safe" protein:energy ratios (a high correlation would reduce the required ratio).

In contrast, it is readily apparent that the ratio is highly dependent upon the expected level of voluntary activity. While 5.1-5.4% of the energy as milk or egg protein appears to be sufficient for moderately active individuals, the required level rises to 6.4-6.7% with low levels of voluntary activity.

All of these values are expressed in terms of egg or milk protein. In practice freely-chosen diets customarily contain a mixture of protein sources with biological value below that of egg or milk protein. Two approaches are possible. The values in Table 2 may be adjusted upward in accord with the deviation in utilizability of protein in the observed diets (see Table 3 for example). Conversely, the observed dietary protein intake may be adjusted downward to the equivalent of egg or milk protein on the basis of its relative biological utilizability. This approach is analogous to the calculation of net dietary protein as percent of calories (NDP Cals %) put forward by Platt and Miller (1958) and by Miller and Payne (1961a, b, c). While the particular interpretative guidelines used by these authors have been criticized (Njaa, 1962), the concept of NDP Cals % is quite useful.

Practical Limitations

Regardless of the approach to the adjustment for protein quality, practical difficulties in the determination of the expected protein utilizability of mixed diets are sufficiently great that it may be preferable to make general assumptions about the probable quality of diets of different types. For example, the FAO/WHO group (1973) suggested that, in general, diets rich in animal foods may have a quality of about 80% relative to that of egg or milk protein. In regions where the staple diet is of mixed plant sources with only a small amount of animal source foods, the relative quality may be about 70%. In some areas, particularly those where the predominant food is cassava or corn and virtually no animal sources are present, the relative value may be about 60%.

Hegsted (1972) has emphasized the need to observe dietary intakes for a sufficiently long period that an estimate of usual or habitual intake is obtained. The protein:energy ratio of an individual's diet would be expected to vary somewhat from day to day.

625

The effect of this variation must be minimized by extension of the observation period. The criteria described in Table 2 are applicable to the usual diet of the individual (e.g., the average ratio over a week of observation). The criteria are not applicable to one day intake data or to data for household units in which the relative distribution among the individual members remains unknown.

While the derivation of the "desirable" or "safe" protein:energy ratio takes into account the correlation between protein and energy requirements, it ignores interactions that may occur as energy intakes and protein intakes are varied above and below the requirement level. Rather, the present model assumes that energy requirements are met. Calloway (1975) has demonstrated that over a limited range of marginal intakes, there are inverse relationships between energy intake and protein requirement. The effect of ignoring this interaction (which could raise or lower the requisite ratio depending upon the levels under consideration) cannot be estimated at present. Severe restrictions of energy intake with associated weight loss are likely to induce a net catabolism of protein, relatively unaffected by dietary protein, except in the special situation of the obese subject with an endogenous source of energy. In this situation, appropriate manipulation of the diet can lead to the maintenance of nitrogen balance in spite of a severely restricted energy intake (Flatt and Blackburn, 1974). Obviously, the protein:energy ratio is meaningless in the first situation in which catabolism predominates and inappropriate in the special situation of the obese subject where diet provides only a part of the energy.

In spite of these limitations, the protein:energy ratio, as calculated in Table 2, has empirical value in the assessment of an individual's diet.

Practical Application

The fundamental application of the protein:energy ratio is in the assessment of the quality of the diet of the individual. It is a criterion that is intended to answer the question "If the subject

consumes this diet in accord with his/her energy requirements, is it
expected that his/her protein requirements will be met?". In this
regard it differs from direct comparison of observed intake of protein to a dietary standard.

If observed protein intake is below the recommended level, it
may be because the diet has too low a protein concentration or because
not enough of the diet is consumed. The protein:energy ratio offers
an approach to distinguishing which reason is correct.

It seems probable that a major practical application of the ratio
for individual diets will be in the establishment of quality standards.
If applied to an individual food, it must be recognized that no account
is being taken of how that food is consumed. The "safe" or "desirable"
protein:energy ratio is intended for application to the total diet as
consumed. Nevertheless, as the North American market moves toward an
increasing use of "meal replacements" and similar products constituting
a major part of the day's food intake, the present ratios may find increasing applicability. The ratios may also find use as a guideline
in the assignment of minimal specifications for institutional meals or
analogous situations. Here a very careful distinction must be made
between standards applicable to a meal to be consumed by a large number
of persons and to the average composition of differing meals consumed
by groups of individuals. The criteria must be different as is discussed in the next section.

CRITERIA FOR THE ASSESSMENT OF NATIONAL OR REGIONAL AVERAGE DIETS

Theoretical Basis

The above discussion has focused upon the definition of
"safe" or "desirable" protein:energy ratios for individual diets.
However, in the literature it has been a common practice to use such
ratios in assessing the quality of national or regional average or
typical diets. Such an approach presents a conceptual problem beyond
those described above. Application of the criteria presented in Table
2 would be valid only if it could be assumed that all of the individuals

consumed exactly the same diet. This is not the situation in populations consuming self-selected diets. In point of fact the observed
protein:energy ratio shows variability among the individuals. This
variability must be taken into account in establishing interpretative
criteria applicable to the average diet. As the coefficient of variation of the protein:energy ratio increases, the required mean level
would be expected to increase if the same level of protection is to
be afforded the individuals in the population.

Beaton and Swiss (1974) calculated interpretative criteria for
national or regional diets as shown in Table 3. Again, the levels
shown are intended to cover the needs of 97.5% of the individuals in
the population. The table demonstrates the effect of an increase in
the coefficient of variation of the ratio in observed intakes. In
practice, there must be available an estimate of the magnitude of
this coefficient. Desirably, this should be derived from the population under consideration; in practice, it may be derived from a
sample of that population or may be based upon data derived from
seemingly similar populations.

In North American population groups, the coefficient of variation seems to be about 15% (Beaton and Swiss, 1974). Whitehead
(personal communication) reported a coefficient of variation of 24%
for 31 Ugandan children. He also noted that the distribution of
observed ratios was skewed (mean 9.5% of energy as protein, median
9.2%), suggesting the need for logarithmic or other appropriate conversion of the data, particularly in situations where the general
diets are relatively low in the quantity and/or quality of protein
and some individuals have access to sources of food with higher
quantity/quality of protein.

Table 3 also portrays the effect of change in the biological
utilizability of dietary protein. As noted earlier, another approach
would be the calculation of a variant of the NDP Cals %. This table
does not take into account the possible existence of low voluntary
activity levels. As was illustrated in Table 2, "safe" or "desirable"
protein:energy ratios would have to increase if voluntary activity of
the population under study was low.

TABLE 3

Predicted "Desirable" or "Safe"
Protein:Calorie Ratios for National or Regional Average Diets

Observed coefficient of variation of dietary protein concentration (% of mean)	Children 2-3 years	Children 6-8 years	Male adolescents	Male adults
	(% of energy as protein)			
A. *Egg or milk protein*				
10	5.4	5.3	5.3	5.8
15	5.9	5.7	5.8	6.3
20	6.6	6.4	6.4	7.1
25	7.7	7.5	7.5	8.2
B. *Protein with utilization 80% that of egg or milk protein*[a]				
10	6.8	6.6	6.6	7.2
15	7.4	7.1	7.2	7.9
20	8.3	8.0	8.1	8.8
25	9.6	9.3	9.4	10.2
C. *Protein with utilization 70% that of egg or milk protein*				
10	7.7	7.5	7.6	8.3
15	8.4	8.2	8.2	9.0
20	9.4	9.1	9.2	10.1
25	10.9	10.6	10.7	11.7
D. *Protein with utilization 60% that of egg or milk protein*				
10	9.0	8.8	8.8	9.7
15	9.8	9.5	9.6	10.5
20	11.0	10.7	10.7	11.8
25	12.8	12.4	12.5	13.6

[a]The relative utilization of mixed dietary protein is expressed as $\frac{\text{NPU diet}}{\text{NPU egg or milk}}$ x 100 or on the basis of the amino acid score (FAO/WHO, 1973). The quality correction may overestimate the needs of adults.

Practical Limitations

The protein:energy ratio criteria described in Table 3 represent a generalized approach applicable to groups or populations. Table 2 is the special case involving a single person. The limitations noted in connection with Table 2 also apply here.

However, a major practical limitation is the need for data on the variability of the protein:energy ratios among the usual diets of the population group. Reference has already been made to Hegsted's caution (1972). Unless the effect of day-by-day variation within the individual's diet is minimized by extension of the observation period, there can be a serious overestimation of the coefficient of variation (Sukhatme, 1975). As noted above, there may be need to transform the data if there is evidence of skewing; the criteria presented in Table 3 are based on the assumption of a normal of Gaussian distribution of observed protein:energy ratios.

It is also to be recognized that although Table 3 refers to data for populations, and although the "safe" protein:energy ratios are empirically similar across a series of age groups, the coefficient of variation of the observed ratios should be computed for particular age/sex groups rather than a total population. It is quite conceivable that the variabilities will be found to be different with different age/sex groups; if groups are combined, the coefficient of variation will be increased and assessment of the quality of the diet will be less precise.

Practical Application

The criteria of "safe" protein:energy ratios set down in Table 3 are applicable to a judgment of the quality of average diets available in particular areas, regions, or socio-economic strata. These criteria do not contribute to the assessment of nutritional status of the individual. However, they may find application in interpreting the etiology of existing problems or looking toward alternative approaches to the rectification of problems.

The criteria were originally developed in an attempt to provide another approach to the resolution of a continuing controversy in the literature. In Third World countries in which protein-energy malnutrition appears to be prevalent, is the nature of the food supply (protein concentration in the diets) a major limiting factor or is the level of consumption of the diet more limiting?

Unfortunately, while interpretative criteria have been developed, available data about food supplies, and particularly about the coefficient of variation of the protein:energy ratio in the various regions, are limiting. Nevertheless, if one compares the criteria set forth in Table 3 with the average protein:energy ratios observed in surveys by the Interdepartmental Committee on Nutrition for National Defense (ICNND) (Table 4), certain general postulates may be reached; these are subject to further examination with more refined data.

1) In most areas of the world, the concentration of protein in national/regional diets is above critical levels.

2) In these regions, protein-energy malnutrition is more likely to be the result of factors that limit the intake of food (e.g., food accessibility, recurrent infections with associated anorexia and/or cultural practices in the treatment of disease, caloric density of the diet, etc.).

3) In a few areas, the concentration of protein in usual diets is below critical levels and probably represents a primary limiting factor.

4) In many areas, the concentration of protein, taking into account its biological value, is sufficiently close to the criterion of an adequate diet that any action that would add energy sources not providing additional protein, and thereby "diluting" the existing protein concentration, must be viewed with concern.

5) Population groups, or subgroups with unusually low levels of voluntary activity have need of a higher concentration of dietary protein and may be particularly at risk in regions where the usual diet is marginal in comparison to the criterion set forth in Table 3.

TABLE 4

Apparent Average Protein Concentrations
Observed in Dietary Surveys Conducted by the
Interdepartmental Committee on Nutrition for National Defense

Area and group	Average protein concentration (% kcal)
Latin America	
Bolivia,[a] families	12.2
Chile, families	12.6
Colombia, families	10.2
Ecuador,[a] families	13.0
Northeast Brazil[a]	
Families	14.0
Pregnant women	16.5
Infants under 2 years	11.9
Uruguay[a]	
Families	14.0
Children, 3-4 years	21.1
Children, 1-2 years	21.1
Caribbean	
Trinidad, families	13.2
St. Lucia, families	12.8
St. Kitts, families	17.1
Nevis, families	17.3
Anguilla, families	13.6
Alaska, males, all ages	29.3
Middle East	
Ethiopia, families	12.4
Jordan,[b] families	12.6
Lebanon,[b] families	12.6
Far East	
Burma, families	9.1
East Pakistan, families	
Rural	10.2
Urban	11.2
Malaya	
Families	11.2
Children	10.7
Thailand, families	10.7
Vietnam, families	
Vietnamese[a]	10.4
Highlanders	10.4

[a]Two or more regions studied; concentrations generally comparable.

[b]Refugees and non-refugees studied; concentrations generally comparable.

PROTEIN:ENERGY RATIOS

The criteria of "safe" or "desirable" protein:energy ratios for population groups can find use in the initial assessment of the quality of regional or national diets. In this sense they constitute an adjunct in the identification of high risk diets and high risk populations or population groups. However, as Payne (1975) has emphasized, in planning programs or actions for the amelioration of nutritional problems, it is necessary to look at the high risk people and their particular social and biological situation. It is not enough to plan on the basis of calculated deficits in national or regional diets.

REFERENCES

Beaton, G.H. 1972. The use of nutritional requirements and allowances. *In* P.L. White (Ed.) Proceedings of the Western Hemisphere Nutrition Congress III. Mount Kisko, New York. Futura, p. 356.

Beaton, G.H. and L. Swiss. 1974. Evaluation of the nutritional quality of food supplies: prediction of "desirable" or "safe" protein: calorie ratios. Amer. J. Clin. Nutr. 27:485.

Calloway, D.H. 1975. Nitrogen balance of men with marginal intakes of protein and energy. J. Nutr. 105:914.

Corey, P. and G.H. Beaton. 1975. Letter to the editor. Amer. J. Clin. Nutr. (In press).

FAO/WHO. 1973. Energy and protein requirements. WHO Report Series No. 522, Geneva; FAO Nutrition Meetings Report Series No. 52, Rome.

Flatt, J.P. and G.L. Blackburn. 1974. The metabolic fuel regulatory system: implications for protein-sparing therapies during caloric deprivation and disease. Amer. J. Clin. Nutr. 27:175.

Food and Nutrition Board. 1974. Recommended dietary allowances (80 revised edition). National Academy of Sciences, Washington.

Hegsted, D.M. 1972. Problems in the use and interpretation of the recommended dietary allowances. Ecol. Food Nutr. 1:255.

Lörstad, M.H. 1971. Recommended intake and its relation to nutrient deficiency. FAO Nutrition Newsletter 9, No. 1:18.

Miller, D.S. and P.R. Payne. 1961a. Problems in the prediction of protein values of diets: caloric restriction. J. Nutr. 75:225.

Miller, D.S. and P.R. Payne. 1961b. Problems in the prediction of protein values of diets: the influence of protein concentration. Brit. J. Nutr. 15:11.

Miller, D.S. and P.R. Payne. 1961c. Problems in the prediction of protein values of diets: the use of food composition tables. J. Nutr. 74:413.

Njaa, L.R. 1962. A note on the method of Miller and Payne for prediction of protein value. Brit. J. Nutr. 16:185.

Payne, P.R. 1975. Safe protein:calorie ratios in diets. The relative importance of protein and energy intake as causal factors in malnutrition. Amer. J. Clin. Nutr. 28:281.

Platt, B.S. and D.S. Miller. 1958. The quantity and quality of protein for human nutrition. Proc. Nutr. Soc. 7:106.

Rutishauser, I.H.E. and R.G. Whitehead. 1972. Energy intake and expenditure in 1-3 year old Ugandan children living in a rural environment. Brit. J. Nutr. 28:145.

Sukhatme, P.V. 1974. The protein problem: its size and nature. J. Roy. Statist. Soc. 137:166.

Sukhatme, P.V. 1975. Letter to the editor. Amer. J. Clin. Nutr. 28:568.

APPENDIX

SELECTED ABBREVIATIONS

(This list complements a similar list on page 597, Part 1.)

AACC	American Association of Cereal Chemists
AOAC	Association of Official Agricultural Chemists
A:TE RATIO	ratio of specific essential amino acids to the sum of essential amino acids
CP	crude protein
CMC	carboxymethyl cellulose
CSIRO	Commonwealth Scientific and Industrial Research Organization
CSM	corn-soy-milk
CSW	California small white beans
CV %	percent coefficient of variation
DCP	digestibility of crude protein
DSM	dried skim milk
EAAI	essential amino acid index
EAF LYSINE	ε-amino free lysine
E:T RATIO	ratio of essential to total amino acids
FAO/WHO	Food and Agriculture Organization and World Health Organization of the United Nations
FER	feed efficiency ratio
GPV	gross protein value
HPHPQ	high protein and high protein quality
IBP	isolated beef protein
LBP	lima bean protein
LCP	liquid cyclone process
LPC	leaf protein concentrate
MEAA	modified essential amino acid index
MHA	methionine hydroxy analogue
NDP	net dietary protein
NFE	nitrogen-free extract
NPUC	net protein utilization count
NRC/NAS	National Research Council of the National Academy of Sciences
NSP	nonstorage protein
PAG/UN	Protein Advisory Group of the United Nations
PC	protein concentrate
PKU	phenylketonuria
PPO	polyphenol oxidase
PUFA	polyunsaturated fatty acid

635

SELECTED ABBREVIATIONS

RDA	recommended daily allowance
SBOM	soybean oil meal
SBH	soybean hemagglutinin
SCP	single cell protein
SP	storage protein
SSL	sodium-2-stearoyl-2-lactylate
TAAV	total amino acid value
TCB	trypsin carboxypeptidase-B
TDN	total digestible nutrients
TIU	trypsin inhibitor units
UN	utilizable nitrogen
VFA	volatile fatty acid
WSB	wheat-soy blend
WPC	whey protein concentrate

AUTHOR INDEX

Holzer, Z. 470
Honavar, P.M. 531, 532, 533, 547
Hontz, L. 518
Hoover, W.H. 259, 304
Hopkins, D.T. 361, 363, 373, 548
Horigome, T. 344, 352, 511, 516
Horn, M.J. 596, 616
Horney, F.D. 254, 298
Hoseney, R.C. 76
Houston, D.F. 103, 104, 105, 115, 116
Hove, E.L. 329, 338, 353, 354
Howe, E.E. 24, 73
Howe, J.M. 466
Howard, A. 545
Hrdlicka, J. 512, 516
Hron, R.J. Sr. 373
Huber, J.T. 258, 303
Huber, T.L. 246, 291
Hudson, J.F. 349, 352
Hudson, L.W. 233, 252, 265, 295, 296
Hudson, W.R. 352
Huebner, F.R. 588
Hughes, B.P. 17, 73, 476, 483, 484, 486
Hughes, J.G. 243, 252, 280, 297
Hullah, W.A. 213, 247
Hulse, J.H. 11, 12
Hume, I.D. 215, 216, 252, 262, 297
Hungate, R.E. 213, 214, 215, 216, 222, 228, 252, 262, 297
Hunnell, J.W. 116
Hunscher, H.A. 468
Hutchison, J.C.D. 479, 486
Hutton, J.B. 279, 297
Hutton, J.T. 464, 468
Hydowitz, J.D. 536, 547

Idler, D.R. 517
Ikekawa, T. 317
Imondi, A.R. 501, 516
Indirama, K. 486
Ingalls, J.R. 243, 256, 257, 281, 301, 302
Inglett, G.E. 72, 78
Ingversen, J. 9, 12, 29, 73
Iriarte, R.J.R. 479, 486

Irvine, G.N. 48, 64, 77
Isaacs, J. 266, 297
Ivanko, S. 23, 74
Ivy, C.A. 548
Iwasaki, T. 116

Jacko, V.P. 47, 74
Jacobs, H.L. 469
Jacobsen, D.H. 439, 468
Jacobson, D.R. 268, 296
Jaffe, W.G. 201, 209, 533, 534, 535, 545, 547
Jambunathan, R. 12
Janicek, G. 512, 516
Jansen, G.R. 73
Janson, J.C. 506, 517
Jasasingke, J.B. 248
Jaschik, S. 486
Jaswal, A.F. 482, 483, 486
Jayasinghe, J.B. 236, 252
Jeffery, R.S. 256
Jekat, F. 461, 480, 481, 486
Jenkins, G. 44, 74
Jensen, L.S. 545, 547
Jeswani, L.M. 542, 547
Johnson, B.C. 184, 339
Johnson, D.E. 276, 289, 290, 296, 297
Johnson, J.H. 562
Johnson, R.M. 376, 388, 391
Johnson, V.A. 18, 59, 64, 74
Johnston, P.H. 395, 415
Jones, D.B. 479, 486, 616
Jones, G.M. 263, 297
Jones, H.W. 185
Jones, J.D. 518
Jones, M. 54, 59, 74
Jorgenson, N.A. 256, 298, 301
Jos, J. 574, 578, 579, 581, 590
Josefsson, E. 496, 516
Joseph, A.A. 479, 486
Joyce, J.P. 255, 281, 282, 283, 300
Judge, M.D. 174, 183
Judson, G.J. 279, 297
Juliano, B.O. 17, 74, 102, 105, 116, 117
Julien, J.P. 466

Labuza, T.P. 389, 390
Lachance, P.A. 501, 502, 508,
  517, 518
Lahey, M.E. 590
Laing, E.M. 11, 12
Laird, W.M. 351
Lal, B.M. 547
Lambou, M.G. 185
Lamy, M. 590
Landman, W.A. 183, 185
Landry, J. 4, 9, 10, 12
Lane, G.T. 242, 248
Lane, M.D. 340
Langer, P.N. 225, 252
Langlands, J.P. 241, 243, 252
Larmond, E. 143, 159
Larsen, A.E. 99
Larson, B.L. 469
Laster, L. 590, 591
Lau, H.C.K. 133
Laver, B.H. 209
Lazar, M.E. 339, 497, 517
Lazarchik, V.M. 49, 73
Lea, C.H. 390
Lems-Van Kan, Ph. 590
Leng, E.R. 73
Leng, R.A. 279, 297
Lenoir, J. 590
Leopold, A. 491, 517
Leroy, F. 233, 253
Lettner, F. 440, 468
Leverton, R.M. 128, 133
Levin, E. 185
Levy, A. 545
Lewis, D. 214, 222, 246, 252,
  253
Lewis, R.W. 185
Lewis, T.R. 222, 253
Lexander, K. 345, 353
Liener, I.E. 128, 133, 493,
  517, 523, 525, 526, 527, 530,
  531, 547, 548, 550
Lietze, A. 586, 591
Lightbody, H.D. 549
Lima, I.H. 349, 353
Lindberg, T. 588
Lindner, K. 472, 486
Lindquist, L.O. 448, 468
Lindsay, D.B. 246, 279, 297
Linklater, P. 491, 519
Linn, J.N. 300

Linson, E.V. 506, 517
Linton, J.H. 257, 287, 297, 302
Linzell, J.L. 268, 269, 297, 298
Lis, H. 530, 548
Little, C.O. 220, 249, 250, 251,
  252, 262, 265, 276, 297, 298
Little, R.R. 102, 117
Liu, T.Y. 165, 184
Livingston, A.L. 320, 339
Lo, Y.Y. 507, 517
Lobay, W. 75
Loeb, P.M. 583, 591
Lofgreen, G.P. 215, 218, 253
Lohrey, E. 338, 346, 353, 354
Lombard, J.H. 324, 339
Lönnerdal, B. 454, 468, 506, 517
Loosli, J.K. 215, 253
Lorentsson, R. 467
Lörstad, M.H. 623, 633
Losowsky, M.S. 592
Loughheed, T.C. 257, 297, 302
Loveen, M.K. 390
Lowry, O.H. 395, 415
Lugay, J.C. 74
Luh, B.S. 159
Luke, H.H. 75
Lum, K.C.J. 506, 517
Lund, D.B. 497, 517
Lundborg, T. 353
Lundin, R.E. 518
Lurken, C. 616
Luther, R.M. 298
Lutwak, L. 470
Lykes, A.H. 17, 74
Lyman, C.M. 48, 74, 372
Lyman, R.L. 546
Lynn, L. 116
Lyon, C.K. 294
Lyster, L.R.J. 446, 468

McAllan, A.B. 216, 257
McAtee, J.W. 279, 298
McBeath, D.K. 30, 74
McBride, J.R. 506, 517
McCarthy, C.F. 585, 591
McCarthy, R.D. 255, 295
Maccioni, A. 431
McCollum, E.V. 477, 486
McDaniel, M.E. 38, 75

AUTHOR INDEX

Robbins, G.S. 21, 22, 23, 31,
  33, 37, 39, 49, 50, 51, 52,
  54, 56, 58, 61, 64, 71, 73,
  76, 77
Roberts, E.A.H. 344, 353
Roberts, L.H. 174, 184
Roberts, L.M. 523, 549
Roberts, R.C. 529, 550
Robinson, I.M. 215, 248
Rockland, L.B. 136, 148, 158,
  160
Rodier, W.I. 464, 469
Rodriguiz, R. 12
Roessler, E.R. 143, 158
Roffler, R.E. 214, 217, 255,
  266, 301
Rogentine, G.N. 590
Roilfe, E.J. 390
Roitman, E. 487
Rolles, C.J. 591
Rolz, C. 514
Root, W. 188, 191, 196
Rose, D. 447, 469
Rose, M.S. 480, 487
Rose, W.C. 167, 184
Rosenbrough, N.J. 415
Rossipal, E. 576, 583, 592
Rothfus, J.A. 588
Roubal, W.T. 512, 519
Rouelle, H.M. 345, 353
Rowe, A. Jr. 591
Rowe, A.H. 591
Roy, D.N. 541, 549
Roy, J.H.B. 441, 469
Royan, G.F. 514
Rubin, C.E. 593
Rubin, S.E. 588, 592
Rubin, W. 570, 571, 573, 575,
  576, 592
Rucker, R.B. 159
Rutger, J.N. 131, 134
Rutishauser, I.H.E. 623, 634
Ruttloff, H. 563

St. Angelo, A.J. 512, 520
Saint-Rat, L. 502, 519
Salam, A. 339
Salsburg, R.L. 224, 255, 281,
  301

Sanne, S. 99
Santos, F.O. 201, 209
Saperstein, S. 470
Sarma, P.S. 540, 545, 549
Satter, D.N. 376, 390
Satter, L.D. 214, 217, 248, 255,
  258, 262, 292, 301
Satterlee, L.D. 172, 185
Saunders, R.M. 323, 339, 508, 519
Savage, J.E. 539, 540, 549
Savilahti, E. 583, 592, 593
Saville, D.G. 243, 256, 304
Saxena, H.C. 545
Schalen, V. 353
Schelling, G.T. 219, 220, 226,
  246, 249, 250, 256, 276, 278,
  289, 301
Schelstraete, M. 106, 107, 111,
  112, 117
Schiftan, H. 479, 487
Schiller, K. 96, 97, 100
Schinckel, P.G. 219, 255, 276,
  278, 300
Schisler, L.C. 307, 317
Schlehuber, A.M. 78
Schmidt, J.W. 74
Schmidt, S.P. 239, 242, 256,
  281, 285, 286, 301
Schmitz, A.A. 196
Schneider, R. 579, 591, 594
Schreiber, K. 472, 473, 487
Schroeder, M.E. 306, 317
Schulz, A.R. 622
Schulze, E. 543, 549
Schuphan, W. 129, 134, 473, 477,
  487
Schuster, H. 308, 312, 317
Schwab, C.G. 218, 221, 256, 268,
  269, 273, 301
Schwachman, H. 590
Schweiger, R.G. 174, 185
Schwerdtfeger, E. 474, 487
Schwimmer, S. 477, 487, 496,
  500, 513, 516, 519, 558
Scott, B.B. 584, 592
Scott, G.C. 256, 301, 303
Scott, H.M. 387, 389, 390, 391
Scott, T.W. 212, 256
Scrimshaw, N.S. 78, 500, 519
Scudamore, H.H. 529, 549
Sechler, D. 75

651

SUBJECT INDEX